Management Principles for Health Professionals

Fifth Edition

Joan Gratto Liebler, MA, MPA, RHIA
Professor Emeritus, Health Information Management
Temple University
Philadelphia, Pennsylvania

Charles R. McConnell, MBA, CM
Consultant
Human Resource and
Health Care Management
Ontario, New York

JONES AND BARTLETT PUBLISHERS
Sudbury, Massachusetts
BOSTON   TORONTO   LONDON   SINGAPORE

World Headquarters

Jones and Bartlett Publishers
40 Tall Pine Drive
Sudbury, MA 01776
978-443-5000
info@jbpub.com
www.jbpub.com

Jones and Bartlett Publishers
Canada
6339 Ormindale Way
Mississauga, Ontario L5V 1J2
CANADA

Jones and Bartlett Publishers
International
Barb House, Barb Mews
London W6 7PA
UK

Jones and Bartlett's books and products are available through most bookstores and online booksellers. To contact Jones and Bartlett Publishers directly, call 800-832-0034, fax 978-443-8000, or visit our website, www.jbpub.com.

Substantial discounts on bulk quantities of Jones and Bartlett's publications are available to corporations, professional associations, and other qualified organizations. For details and specific discount information, contact the special sales department at Jones and Bartlett via the above contact information or send an email to specialsales@jbpub.com.

Production Credits
Chief Executive Officer: Clayton Jones
Chief Operating Officer: Don W. Jones, Jr.
President, Higher Education and Production Publishing: Robert W. Holland, Jr.
V.P., Design and Production: Anne Spencer
V.P., Manufacturing and Inventory Control: Therese Connell
V.P., Sales and Marketing: William J. Kane
Publisher: Michael Brown
Associate Editor: Katey Birtcher
Associate Production Editor: Jennifer Ryan
Marketing Manager: Sophie Fleck
Composition: Publishers' Design and Production Services, Inc.
Cover Design: Anne Spencer
Cover Image: © VisualField/ShutterStock, Inc.
Printing and Binding: Malloy, Inc.
Cover Printing: Malloy, Inc.

Library of Congress Cataloging-in-Publication Data

Liebler, Joan Gratto.
   Management principles for health professionals / Joan Gratto Liebler,
Charles R. McConnell.— 5th ed.
      p. ; cm.
Includes bibliographical references and index.
   ISBN 978-0-7637-4617-9 (alk. paper)
   1. Health services administration. 2. Management. I. McConnell, Charles, R. II. Title.
[DNLM: 1. Health Services Administration. 2. Health Facilities—organization & administration.
3. Health Personnel—organization & administration.
WX 150 L716m 2008]
   RA393.L53 2008
   362.1'068—dc22

                                                                    2007010551
                                                                    6048

Printed in the United States of America
12 11 10 09 08   10 9 8 7 6 5 4 3 2

Contents

Preface

This book is intended for health care professionals who engage in the classic functions of a manager—planning, organizing, decision making, staffing, leading or directing, communicating, and motivating—yet have not had extensive management training. Health care practitioners may exercise these functions on a continuing basis in their roles as department directors or unit supervisors, or they may participate in only a few of these traditional functions such as training and development of unit staff. In any case, knowledge of management theory is an essential element in professional training, as no single function is ever addressed independently of all others. In this book, emphasis is placed on definitions of terms, clarification of concepts, and, in some cases, highly detailed explanations of processes and concepts. All examples presented are drawn from the health care setting.

Every author must decide what material to include and what level of detail to provide. The philosopher and pundit Samuel Johnson observed, "A man will turn over half a library to make one book." We have been guided by experience gained in the classroom and in many training and development workshops for health care practitioners. Three basic objectives determined the final selection and development of material:

1. Acquaint the health care practitioner with management concepts essential to the understanding of the organizational environment within which the functions of the manager are performed. Some material challenges assumptions about such concepts as power, authority, influence, and leadership. Some of the discussions focus on relatively new concepts such as appreciative inquiry approaches to motivation and conflict management and Six Sigma applications for quality control. Practitioners must keep abreast of developing trends in management, guarding against "being the last to know."

2. Provide a base for further study of management concepts. Therefore, the classic literature in the field is cited, major theorists are noted, and terms are defined, especially where there is a divergence of opinion in management literature. We all stand on the shoulders of the management "giants" who paved the way in the field; a return to original sources is encouraged.

3. Provide sufficient detail in selected areas to enable the practitioner to apply the concepts in day-to-day situations. Several tools of planning and control, such as budget preparation and justification, training design, and labor union contracts are explained in detail.

We have attempted to provide enough information to make it possible for the reader to use these tools with ease at their basic level. It is the authors' hope that the readers themselves, as they grow in their professional practice and management roles, will, in turn, contribute to the literature and practice of health care management. We are grateful to our many colleagues who have journeyed with us over many years and who have shared ideas with us.

Joan Gratto Liebler
Charles R. McConnell

About the Authors

Joan Gratto Liebler is Professor Emeritus, Health Information Management, at Temple University, Philadelphia, Pennsylvania. She has over 36 years of professional experience in teaching and research in health care settings. In addition to teaching, her work and consulting experience include community health centers, behavioral health settings, schools, industrial clinics, prisons, and long-term care, acute care, and hospice facilities. She has also been an active participant in areawide health-care planning, end-of-life care coalitions, and areawide emergency and disaster planning.

She is also the author of *Medical Records: Policies and Guidelines* and has authored numerous journal articles and contributed chapters relating to health information management.

Ms. Liebler holds the degrees of Master of Arts (concentration in Medical Ethics), St. Charles Borromeo Seminary, Philadelphia, Pennsylvania, and Master of Public Administration, Temple University, Philadelphia, Pennsylvania. She is a credentialed Registered Health Information Administrator.

Charles McConnell is an independent health care management and human resources consultant and freelance writer specializing in business, management, and human resource topics. For 11 years he was active as a management engineering consultant with the Management and Planning Services (MAPS) division of the Hospital Association of New York State (HANYS) and later spent 18 years as a hospital human resources manager. As author, coauthor, and anthology editor he has published 25 books and has contributed nearly 400 articles to various publications. He is in his 26th year as editor of the quarterly professional journal *The Health Care Manager.*

Mr. McConnell received a Masters of Business Administration and a Bachelor of Science degree in Engineering from the State University of New York at Buffalo.

What's New to the Fifth Edition?

Examples have been updated throughout, new examples have been provided in several chapters, and dated material carried over from the earlier editions has in most instances been either eliminated or replaced with more pertinent material.

SPECIFIC CHAPTER UPDATES:

- **Chapter 2—New!** A completely new chapter, concerned largely with the management of change and the manager's role as a change agent. This chapter anchors and complements the balance of the book with significant examples relevant to what's occurring today in health care. Much has been added concerning addressing change with employees, and developments such as the advent of the Health Insurance Portability and Accountability Act (HIPAA) are addressed in detail.
- **Chapter 6—**The chapter entitled "Organizing" (formerly Chapter 5) has been expanded to include enlarged consideration of outsourcing and information on telecommuting and using temporary workers.
- **Chapter 10—New!** This revised and reorganized section combines the former Chapter 6 ("Staffing: Recruiting and Retaining Quality Employees") and the former Chapter 10 ("Adaptation, Motivation, and Conflict Management).
- **Chapter 11—**The chapter entitled "Training and Development: The Backbone of Motivation and Retention" now covers considerable new information about both all-employee and departmental orientation, including comprehensive orientation checklists.
- **Chapter 14—**This revised chapter, "Communication: The Glue that Binds Us Together," features a greatly expanded section on written communication.

CHAPTER 1

The Changing Scene: Organizational Adaptation and Survival

CHAPTER OBJECTIVES

- Describe the health care environment as it has evolved since the middle to late 1960s.
- Examine megatrends in the health care environment.
- Identify the need for organizational survival as a fundamental goal of organizational effort.
- Identify selected management strategies used to enhance organizational survival.
- Identify the phases of the organizational life cycle that reflect major changes and relate these to the functions of the manager.

THE CHANGING HEALTH CARE SCENE

A great deal is said about change. We are constantly adapting to change, probably to a greater extent than we realize. Although we are aware that nothing stays the same for very long, people who enter contemporary health care careers soon discover that change in health care has for some time been more dramatic and more rapid than in most other dimensions of modern life.

The management of health care organizations must, therefore, monitor change to anticipate the points of convergence in trends so as to effectively meet the challenges presented. It is helpful and in fact necessary to be knowledgeable of such continuing trends as:

- regulation of the health care industry
- ongoing managed care mandates
- restructuring of health care organizations through mergers, affiliations, and the virtual enterprise model
- impact of technology
- ongoing social and ethical factors

REGULATION OF THE HEALTH CARE INDUSTRY

When an organization provides goods and services central to the common good of the overall population, state and federal governments place strict regulatory requirements on their practices. In government organization terminology, these oversight organizations are called regulatory agencies or independent commissions or corporations. Familiar examples of this model of extensive industry regulation include the Nuclear Regulatory Commission, the National Transportation Safety Board, the U.S. Postal Service, and the National Railroad Passenger Corporation (Amtrak). Such agencies are created when the government exercises tight control but does not directly render the service or produce the goods. How closely does the regulation of health care fit the classic model of an officially regulated industry, to the point where health care will fall under a centralized federal regulatory body? Compare the characteristics of the formally regulated agency or commission with the net effect of health care regulations. A federal (or state) regulatory agency generally has these features:

- It is an official unit of the federal or state government.
- It is established by lawmakers to closely regulate a specific industry.
- A distinct regulatory agency promulgates a coordinated set of regulations appropriate to the industry.
- It is governed by a board of regulators, appointed by the president (or governor), and not subject to removal except for cause.

Given the amount of detail in laws and regulations at both the state and federal levels, the health care industry is, at the very least, a quasi-regulated industry. There is not yet one overall regulatory body with the classic board of regulators. However, initiatives to overhaul the health care delivery system include such consideration, making this a trend to be monitored and assessed. The extensive literature (especially in the field of public administration) concerning the pros and cons of the centrally regulated industry provides managers with insights into this process. The position papers developed by major health care associations, political parties, and labor unions are another source of information about this debate. The issue is usually tied to the increasing cost of health care.

Concern for health care costs and efforts to control or reduce these costs have been gathering momentum since the 1960s. Costs clearly took a leap upward immediately following the introduction of Medicare and Medicaid in the mid-1960s; however, Medicare and Medicaid are not the sole cause for the cost escalation. Rather, costs have been driven up by a complex combination of forces that include the aforementioned programs and other government undertakings, private not-for-profit and commercial insurers, changes in medical practice and advancements in technology, proliferation of medical specialties, increases in physician fees, advances in pharmaceuticals, overexpansion of the country's hospital system, economic improvements in the lot of health care workers, and the desires and demands of the public. These and other forces have kept health care costs rising at a rate that has outpaced overall inflation two- or three-fold in some years.

As concern for health care costs has spread, so have attempts to control costs without adversely affecting quality or hindering access. The final two decades of the 20th century and the beginning of this century have seen some significant dollar-driven phenomena that are dramatically changing the face of health care delivery, specifically:

- the rise of competition among providers in this industry that was long considered essentially devoid of competition
- changes in the structure of care delivery, such as system shrinkage as hospitals decertify beds or close altogether, an increase in mergers and other affiliations that catalyzed the growth of health care systems, and the proliferation of independent specialty practices
- the growth and expansion of managed care to its present level

In one way or another most modern societal concerns for health care relate directly to cost or, in some instances, to issues of access to health care, which in turn translates directly to concern for cost. Massive change in health care has become a way of life, and dollars are the driver of this change. One of the significant directions taken has been the path of managed care.

THE MANAGED CARE ERA

Driven by Dollars

Technological advances aside, nearly everything that has occurred in recent decades in the organization of health care delivery and payment has been driven by concern for costs. Changes have been inspired primarily by the desire to stem alarming cost increases and in some instances to reduce costs overall. These efforts have been variously focused. Government and insurers have acted upon health care's money supply, essentially forcing providers to operate on less money than they feel they require. Provider organizations have taken steps to adjust expenditures to fall within the income limitations imposed on them—steps that have included closures, downsizing, forming large systems to take advantage of economies of scale, and generally looking for ways to deliver care more economically and efficiently. Evolving in this cost-conscious environment, managed care seemed to offer workable solutions to the problem of providing reasonable access to quality care at an affordable cost.

Managed Care Proliferates

With the advent of managed care, for the first time in the history of American health care, significant restrictions were placed on the use of services. Managed care introduced the concept of the primary care physician as "gatekeeper" to control access to specialists and various other services. Previously, an insured individual could self-refer, going to any specialist at will, and the person's insurance would generally pay for the service. With the gatekeeper in place, however, a subscriber's visits to a specialist are covered only if the subscriber is referred by the primary care physician. Certain ancillary services, such as X-rays or laboratory tests, were ordered by the primary care physician; under managed care the services of medical specialists were also ordered by the primary care physician. Subscribers who went to specialists without benefit of referral suddenly found themselves being billed for the specialists' entire costs.

By placing limitations on what services would be paid for and under what circumstances these services could be accessed, managed care plans reduced health insurance premium costs to employers and subscribers. In return for lower costs, subscribers had to accept limitations on their choice of physicians, having to choose from among those physicians who agreed to participate in a given plan and accept that plan's payments, accepting limitations on the services that could be accessed, and, in most cases, having to pay certain specified deductibles and copayments.

Managed care organizations and elements of government brought pressure to bear on hospitals as well. Hospitals and physicians were encouraged to reduce the length of hospital stays, cut back on the use of ancillary services, and meet more medical needs on an outpatient basis. Review processes were established such that hospitals were penalized financially if their costs were determined to be too high or their inpatient stays too long. Eventually payment became linked to a standard, or target, length of stay so that any given diagnosis was compensated at a specific amount regardless of how long the patient was hospitalized.

As they grew larger, managed care organizations began to deal directly with hospitals, negotiating the use of their services. As various plans contracted with hospitals that would give the best price breaks for the plan's patients, price competition between and among providers became a factor to be reckoned with.

Cost concerns moved even the federal Medicare program into more controlled directions, so that as managed care grew and placed limits on providers for their subscribers, these same providers began to feel the financial pinch stemming from their Medicare patients as well. Medicare has helped its target population a great deal, but runaway cost increases have had their effects here as well. When Medicare began in the mid-1960s its projected 1990 cost was about $10 billion per year, an estimate that fell short of reality several times over. Not too many years ago the actual cost of Medicare surpassed $100 billion per year. It seems that with Medicare, for the first time in American history, a government benefit was separated from any form of financial control, and steps had to be instituted to bring expenditures into line.[1]

Including Medicare and Medicaid, more than 160 million Americans are enrolled in managed care plans, encompassing what may well be the overwhelming majority of people who are suitable for managed care. In-and-out participation of some groups continues, such as the younger elderly and Medicaid patients, but the bulk of people on whom managed care plans could best make their money are already enrolled.[2]

Reaching the Managed Care Limit

Much of the movement into managed care was spurred by employers attempting to contain health care benefit costs. The movement has been rapid. In 1994, half of the covered work force was in managed care plans, but by 1998 this proportion had grown to 85 percent.[3] However, shortly after 1998 the growth curve flattened out and the proportion of the workforce covered under managed care remains at about 85 percent.

Managed care was able to slow the rate of health insurance premium increases throughout most of the 1990s. However, it is evident in the second half of the present decade that the slowdown of premium increases in the 1990s was temporary. In most of the years since 2000, health insurance premiums have increased at an alarming rate, in some instances registering more than 10 percent per year. The cost of health insurance coverage continues to climb, with no end in sight. Some see this as a trend that is likely to continue and believe that this could be the early stages of some considerable difficulties in the organization of medical coverage provided to Americans.[4]

Discontent with managed care continues to be a major campaign issue during election cycles. Politicians are reacting to consumer complaints amid charges that health maintenance organizations and managed care plans in general are putting profits ahead of patients, an argument heard frequently.[5]

There is continuing pressure on Congress from elements of government and the public to place legal controls or constraints on some aspects of managed care operations. Amid the cries for controls we also frequently hear reiterated the long-standing complaint of caregivers about managed are: medical professionals do not want business people—accountants and such—to tell them how to practice medicine.[6]

Labor unions, seeing a greater share of premium costs passed along to their members and retirees, have become active participants in the managed care debate. Some unions have become involved to the extent of cutting their own deals with providers for both active employees and retirees. Organized labor has seemed increasingly accepting of managed care plans in exchange for less cost-sharing and a greater say in the evaluation and selection of those plans, especially for post-retirement medical benefits.[7]

By mid-1998 it appeared that the majority of average middle-class subscribers had reached a negative consensus about managed care, an attitude that could damage the political viability of for-profit managed care and hurt managed care overall. Indeed, it is increasingly clear that managed care may not be financially affordable in the long run. Experts predicted that the first decade of the new century would not see a stable health care system providing adequate care to an overwhelming percentage of citizens.[8] As judged from the vantage point of early 2007, the "experts" were correct.

Some have proposed legally mandated external review processes that allow patients to file malpractice-type suits against plans covered by the Employee Retirement Income Security Act (ERISA) and that force plans to provide out-of-network coverage options. Those opposed to such mandates, mainly managed care plans and their supporters, contend that mandates would sharply increase costs, cause millions to lose coverage, and lead to a government-controlled system.[9]

Concerning denials of service or payment under managed care plans, patients are now finding they have somewhere to go to protest when their plans turn them down.[10] Managed care organizations are becoming increasingly vulnerable to litigation arising out of the actions of parties with whom they have contractual relationships. This is but one manifestation of political efforts to hold managed care entities more accountable than in the past.

While some have argued that the profit motive is needed in managed care to control costs, while competition supposedly keeps quality sharp, a 1998 study of a dozen key measures of quality and productivity submitted by 329 health plans to the National Committee for Quality Assurance found that not-for-profit plans had higher patient satisfaction ratings and did better in offering preventive care than did the for-profit plans. Patient satisfaction ratings were 62 percent for not-for-profits and 54 percent for the for-profits. Also, the not-for-profits tended to spend more—and lose more—than the for-profits.[11]

There is also Medicaid to consider in the overall picture of health care access and cost. In addition, the numbers of those who are completely uninsured continue to increase. The current situation could easily lead to a day when the government provides basic health insurance for everyone. It may not be a particularly appealing level of care, but nevertheless some care would be provided for everyone but supplemented in most instances by private insurance and self-pay.[12]

It is becoming increasingly clear that managed care plans probably will not be able to keep their promises of delivering efficient and cost-effective care. The converging trends in health care delivery are forcing many managed care companies to reevaluate their pricing structures. An aging population, newer and more expensive technology, newer and higher priced prescription drugs, new federal and state mandates, and pressure from health care providers for higher fees will significantly diminish the savings from managed care enjoyed by employers.[13]

CAPITATION: A LOGICAL PROGRESSION?

For many years employers and insurers have prodded hospitals to streamline their operations, cut costs, and form networks with others—all activities that can be interpreted as readying the health care system for capitation.[14] From the vantage point of the year 2007, it appears that the system is still "getting ready" for capitation.

Capitation, under which a provider is paid a specific amount of money to attend to all of the health care needs of a given population—literally, so much "per head," as the term indicates—has long had its strong proponents among insurers and health plans. Capitation was for many years resisted by most providers, however; outside of California and neighboring states discounted charges and per diem fees still dominate most health care markets. The West Coast has been home to 80 percent of all hospital capitation in the country, but it is now predominantly hospitals, not health plans, that are demanding capitation.[15]

PROVIDER GROWTH: MERGERS AND AFFILIATIONS

It should be no secret to even the casual observer that the structure of the nation's health care delivery system changed dramatically over the last few decades of the 20th century and continues to change into the new century.

Restructuring through mergers and affiliations and the trend toward the creation of the virtual enterprise characterize these efforts to adapt and survive. Why do health care organizations seek such restructuring? The reasons are several and include:

- the desire to increase size so as to have greater clout in negotiations with managed care providers who tend to bypass smaller enterprises
- the desire to penetrate new markets to attract additional customers
- the need for improved efficiencies resulting from centralized administrative practices such as financial and health information resource streamlining, or public relations and marketing intensification
- the desire to express an overall value of promoting comprehensive, readily accessible care by shoring up smaller community-based facilities, keeping them from closure

As cost containment pressure grew, providers, primarily hospitals, initially moved into mergers mostly to secure economies of scale and other operating efficiencies and sometimes for reasons as basic as survival. The growth and expansion of managed care plans spurred further incentive to merge among hospitals, which in turn seems to have inspired health plan mergers in return. Each time a significant merger occurs, one side gains more leverage in negotiating contracts. The larger the managed care plan, the greater the clout in negotiating with hospitals and physicians, and vice versa.

Clarification of Terms

The term *merger* is used to describe the blending of two or more corporate entities to create one new organization with one licensure and one provider number for reimbursement purposes. One central board of trustees or directors is created, usually with representation from each of the merged facilities. Debts and assets are consolidated. For example, a university medical center buys a smaller community-based hospital. Ownership and control of the smaller facility is now shifted to the new organization. Sometimes the names of the original facilities are retained as part of public relations and marketing, as when a community group or religious-affiliated group has great loyalty and ties to the organization. Alternatively, a combined name is used, e.g., Mayfair Hospital of the University Medical System.

An affiliation is a formal agreement between or among member facilities to officially coordinate and share one or several activities. Ownership and control of each party remains distinct, but binding agreements, beneficial to all parties, are developed. Shared activities typically include managed care negotiations, group purchasing discounts, staff development and education offerings, and shared management services.

Such restructuring efforts, especially the formal merger, are preceded with mutual due diligence reviews in which operational, financial, and legal issues are assessed. Federal regulations and state licensing regulations must be followed. Details of the impact of the restructuring on operational levels are considered with each manager providing reports, statistics, contractual information, leases (as of equipment), and staffing arrangements, including independent contractors and outsourced work.

Practical considerations constitute major points of focus, such as redesign of forms, merging the master patient index and record system into one new system, merging finance and billing processes, and the specifics of officially discharging and readmitting patients when the legally binding merger has taken place.

Present-day mergers and affiliations can have a pronounced effect on the health professional entering a management position. Consider the example of the laboratory manager who must now oversee a geographically divided department because a two-hospital merger has left this person responsible for a department with two sites that are miles apart. There is far more to consider in managing a split department than in managing a single-site operation; the manager's job is made all the more difficult. Overall, mergers and affiliations are blessing the professional-as-manager with greatly increased responsibility and accountability and a role of increasing complexity.

THE VIRTUAL ENTERPRISE

In the business community, the concept of the virtual enterprise (or corporation) has emerged as a result of available technology. The virtual enterprise is a relatively temporary partnership of independent companies or individuals, composed of suppliers of certain goods, services, or customers. Two or more organizations temporarily join together into a meta-enterprise to take advantage of rapidly changing technology. The meta-enterprise seeks to capitalize on this technology by making it readily available. These virtual services or products (e.g., one-hour eyeglasses, on-line prescription processing, clinical decision support information) rapidly adapt to user needs and demands. A key feature of many virtual enterprises is heavy reliance on outsourcing, with only a small, centralized corporate core staff and physical facility. Information exchange is highly dependent on computer networks. Health care organizations already have some of these characteristics, a trend that is likely to increase.[16] The contemporary health information department reflects some of these trends: outsourcing of dictation-transcription function and home-based coding are common practices.

IMPACT OF TECHNOLOGY

A survey of any health care discipline would readily provide examples of the impact of technology. New treatment modalities emerge; specialty care is taken to the patient (e.g., bedside anesthesia, mobile van with chemotherapy, portable diagnostic equipment). The need for large, dedicated space within one central facility is reduced; staffing patterns change.

Information technology is yet another area with major impact on health care delivery. As organizations merge or affiliate, more freestanding facilities develop, independent practitioners provide service in their own facilities, and patients access e-health information right in their own homes, information sharing becomes all the more vital. Several interrelated concepts are associated with contemporary information technology. These practices incorporate and enhance the more historical methods of the paper record, decentralized indexes and registries, and special studies:

- Data warehousing—centralized depository of data collected from all aspects of the organization (for example, patient demographics, financial/billing transactions, and clinical decision making) gathered into one consistent computerized format. Easy connectivity to national and international databases (e.g., National Library of Medicine) is yet another feature of this process.

- Data mining—analyzing and extracting data to find meaningful facts and trends for "real-time" intervention in clinical decision-making support, studies and oversight review of administrative and clinical practice by designated review groups, budget support, and related data usage. With proper safeguards (e.g., patient confidentiality, data security) data are made more accessible to approved users in the organization.

- Informatic standards and common language—these include standard vocabulary and classification systems—for example, the National Library of Medicine's Unified Medical Language System© (UMLs) and the Institute of Electrical and Electronics Engineers (IEEE). The current Health Insurance Portability and Accountability Act of 1996 (HIPAA) regulations require the adoption of the American National Standards Institute (ANSI) protocols for electronic transactions. These standards cover both format and content for data capture and transmission.

- Development of a national health care information infrastructure—the American Health Information Association supports the development of such an infrastructure to advance capture, access, use, exchange, and storage of quality health care data, along with comprehensive, uniform standards for transmission, content, and terminologies.[17]

Other current technologies having impact on timely data recoding include the handheld personal digital assistant (PDA), portable computer, e-mail communications, and speech recognition technologies. The evolution of improved technology shows no signs of letting up, making this aspect of change one needing constant monitoring.

Technology also impacts social and therefore ethical norms.

SOCIAL AND ETHICAL FACTORS

Given the continuing activity in genetic research, ethical questions intensify. Consideration of social and ethical norms has always been a part of the health care ethos, but from time to time a more urgent debate is required. As noted here, a technological breakthrough occasions such renewed interest. At another time, a new legislative mandate, such as the Patient Self-Determination Act, brings about fresh consideration of enduring concerns. Increased sensitivity to patient or consumer wishes is yet another source of attentiveness to social and ethical issues; for example, the increased use by patients of alternative therapies and interventions has reopened the questions about the proper integration of nontraditional care with the accepted modes. This debate reaches into the question of reimbursement as well; health care plans increasingly consider some alternative/complementary interventions as reimbursable costs.

Ethical considerations such as the foregoing result in the increased use of the ethics review committee, the institutional review board, and similar clinical and administrative review groups.

These trends and the ways that health care organizations respond to them lead to a discussion of organizational strategies for both survival and growth. The groundwork for the theoretical and practical aspects of organizational survival and growth strategies was extensively developed in the 1950s and 1960s. These concepts of bureaucratic imperialism, co-optation, goal expansion, and organizational life cycle continue to have application today in the continuing challenge of responding to change.

INTRODUCING ORGANIZATIONAL SURVIVAL STRATEGIES

Organizational survival and growth are implicit organizational goals requiring the investment of energy and resources. Normally, only higher levels of management need give attention to organizational survival; it may be taken for granted by most employees or members, some of whom may even take actions that threaten survival (for example, a prolonged strike). There may be an unwillingness to admit the legitimacy of survival as a goal because it seems self-serving; however, managers disregard the concept of organizational survival—whether whole corporation or even just department or unit—at their own peril.

So fundamental is the goal of organizational survival that it underpins all other goals. Fostering this goal contributes to the satisfaction of the more explicit goals of the group or organization. Bertram Gross described this implicit goal as "the iron law of survival." The unwritten law of every organization, he said, is that its survival is an absolute prerequisite for its serving any interest whatsoever.[18]

Survival is articulated as a goal in certain phases of organizational development—for example, when competition threatens. The clientele network includes competitors, rivals, enemies, and opponents that must be faced. Certain threats to organizational survival may be identified:

- lack of strong, formal leadership after the early charismatic leadership of the founders
- too-rapid change either within or outside the organization

- shifting client demand, either with the loss of clients or with the increased exercise of control by clients
- competition from stronger organizations
- high turnover rate in the rank and file or the leadership
- failure to recognize and accept organizational survival as a legitimate, although not the sole, organizational purpose

These factors drain from the organization the energy that should be goal directed.

An organization ensures its survival through certain strategies and processes, such as bureaucratic imperialism, co-optation, patterns of adaptation, goal multiplication and expansion, use of organizational roles, conflict limitation, and integration of the individual into the organization. Astute managers recognize such patterns of organizational behavior and assess them realistically. A weak organization or unit cannot pull together the money, resources, and power to serve clients effectively.

BUREAUCRATIC IMPERIALISM

Organizations develop to foster a particular goal, serve a specific client group, or promote the good of a certain group. In effect, an organization stakes out its territory. Thus, a professional association seeks to represent the interests of members who have something in common, such as specific academic training and professional practice. A hospital or home health agency seeks to serve a particular area. A union focuses on the needs of one or several categories of workers. A political party attempts to bring in members who hold a particular political philosophy. A government agency seeks to serve a specific constituency.

The classic definition of bureaucratic imperialism reflects the idea that a bureaucratic organization exerts a kind of pressure to develop a particular client group and then to expand it. It becomes imperialistic in the underlying power struggle and competition that ensues when any other group seeks to deal with the same clients, members, or area of jurisdiction. Matthew Holden, Jr., coined the term *bureaucratic imperialism* and defined it in the context of federal government agencies that must consider such factors as clients to be served, political aspects to be assessed, and benefits to be shared among administrative officials and key political clients. According to Holden's definition of the concept, bureaucratic imperialism is "a matter of interagency conflict in which two or more agencies try to assert permanent control over the same jurisdiction, or in which one agency actually seeks to take over another agency as well as the jurisdiction of that agency."[19] The idea of agency can be expanded to include any organization, the various components of the clientele network can be substituted for the constituency, and the role of manager can replace that of the administrative politician in those organizations that are not in the formal political setting.

Managers in many organizations can recognize the elements of this competitive mode of interaction among organizations. There may even be such competition among departments and units within an organization. In the health care field, competition may be seen in the areas of professional licensure and practice, accrediting processes for the organizations as a whole, the delineation of clients to be served, and similar areas.

Professional licensure has the effect of annexing specific "territory" as the proper domain of a given professional group, but other groups may seek to carry out the same, or at least similar, activities. For example, there is the question of the role of chiropractors in traditional health care settings. Is the use of radiological techniques the exclusive jurisdiction of physicians and trained radiological technicians or should the law be changed to permit chiropractors greater use of these techniques? Psychiatrists question the expanding role of others who have entered the field of behavioral health. As each health care profession develops, the question of jurisdiction emerges.

The accrediting process in health care reflects similar struggles for jurisdiction. Which shall be the definitive accreditation process for mental health facilities—that approved by the American Psychiatric Association or that approved by the Joint Commission on the Accreditation of Healthcare Organizations (Joint Commission)? Should all these processes be set aside, leaving only state governments to exercise such control through the licensure of institutions?

Other examples may be drawn from the health care setting. There has been the jurisdictional dispute over blood banking between the American Red Cross and the American Association of Blood Banks, as well as the competition of health maintenance organizations (HMOs) with the more traditional Blue Cross and Blue Shield plans and commercial medical insurance companies. The area of health care planning also reflects this territorial question; several agencies, including both government and private agencies, require hospitals and other health care institutions to submit to several sets of planning mandates.

Although the charitable nature of health care has been emphasized traditionally, the elements of competition and underlying conflict must be recognized. With shifts in patient populations and changes in each health care profession, health care managers must assess the effects of bureaucratic imperialism in a realistic manner. The competition engendered by bureaucratic imperialism and the resultant total or partial "colonization" of an organizational unit or client group may be functional. Holden noted that conflict not only forces organizational regrouping by clarifying client loyalty and wishes but also sharpens support for the agency or unit that "wins." Furthermore, it disrupts the bureaucratic form from time to time, causing a healthy review of client need, organizational purpose, and structural pattern.

CO-OPTATION

Another method that organizations use to help ensure their survival is co-optation, an organizational strategy for adapting and responding to change. Philip Selznick described and labeled this strategy, which is viewed as both cooperative and adaptive. He defined co-optation as "an adaptive response on the part of the organization in response to the social forces in its environment; by this means, the organization averts threats to its stability by absorbing new elements into the leadership of the organization."[20] The organization, in effect, shares organizational power by absorbing these new elements. Selznick called it a realistic adjustment to the centers of institutional strength.[21]

Formal versus Informal Co-optation

In formal co-optation, the symbols of authority and administrative burdens are shared, but no substantial power is transferred. The organization does not permit the co-opted group to interfere with organizational unity of command. Normal bureaucratic processes tend to provide sufficient checks and balances on any co-opted group, just as they tend to restrict the actions of managers. Through formal co-optation, however, the organization seeks to demonstrate its accessibility to its various publics.

In health care, the co-optation process is suggested by the practice of appointing "ordinary" citizens to the board of trustees. Community mental health centers and some neighborhood health centers tend to emphasize consumer or community representation. Health planning agencies include both providers and consumers in planning for health care on a regional or statewide basis. The formalization of nursing home ombudsmen or patient care councils is still another example of this process.

Professional associations in those disciplines that have technical-level practitioners have sought to open their governing processes in response to the growing strength of the technical-level group. Increases in numbers, greater degree of training, further specialization, and a general emphasis on the democratic process and provision of rights for all members have fostered changes in these associations. Open membership, such as that recently adopted by the American Health Information Management Association, is an example of positive co-optation: the rapid developments in the wider field of information technology gave impetus to including the IT specialists in the existing health information arena. Without cooperative adaptation to such internal changes, there is a risk that additional associations will be formed, possibly weakening the parent organization.

When an organization seeks to deal less overtly with shifting centers of power and to maintain the legitimacy of its own power, co-optation may be informal in nature. For example, managers may meet unofficially with informally delegated representatives of clients, employees, or outside groups. Organizational leaders may deal regularly with some groups, but there are no visible changes in the official leadership structures. No new positions are created; committee membership remains intact. Informal co-optation may be more important than formal co-optation because of its emphasis on true power, although each form serves its unique purpose. An organization can blend formal and informal co-optation processes, since they are not mutually exclusive.

Control of Co-opted Groups

Although the co-opted group could gain strength and attempt to consolidate power, this does not happen frequently for several reasons. First, the organization has the means of controlling participation. For example, only limited support may be given to the group; these may be no physical space, money, or staff available to give to the co-opted group, or management could simply withhold support. Another possible course is to assign so much activity to the co-opted group that it cannot succeed easily. Key leaders of the co-opted group generally retain their regular work assignments but now have in addition projects and tasks relating to their special causes. Co-opted leaders also become the buffer individuals in the organization, since the group has placed its trust in them and looks for results faster than they can be produced. Such leaders may find their base of action eroded and their activity turning into a thankless task.

In a more Machiavellian approach, organizational authorities could schedule meetings at inconvenient hours or control their agenda in such a way that issues of significance to the co-opted group are too far down on the list of discussion items to be dealt with under the time constraints. Absolute insistence on parliamentary procedure may also be used as a weapon of control; a novice in the use of Robert's Rules of Order is at a distinct disadvantage when compared with a seasoned expert.

The subtle psychological process that occurs in the co-opted individual who is taken into the formal organization as a distinct outsider acts as another controlling measure. The person suddenly becomes, for this moment, one of the power holders and derives new status. Certain perquisites also are granted. Consumer representatives, for example, may find their way paid, quite legitimately, for special conferences or fact-finding trips to study a problem. The individual, in becoming privy to more data and sometimes to confidential data, may start to "see things" from the organization's point of view.

Certain subtle social barriers may make the co-opted individual uncomfortable, even though they may not be raised intentionally and may be part of the normal course of action for the group.

Individuals representing pressure groups find that their own time and energies are limited, even if they desire power. Other activities continue to demand their energies. In addition, certain issues lose popularity, and pressure groups may find their power base has eroded. Finally, the agenda items that were causes of conflict may become the recurring business of the organization. The conflict may become a routine, and the structure to deal with it may become a part of the formal organization. In the collective bargaining process, for example, the union is a part of the organization, and its leaders have built-in protection from factors that erode effective participation. Labor union officials commonly have certain reductions in workload so that they may attend to union business, space may be provided for their offices or meetings, and they may seek meetings with management as often as executives seek sessions with them. Co-optation has occurred but without a loss of identity of the co-opted group. In health care organizations, consumer participation has become part of the organizations' continuing activity through the development of a more stable process for consumer input, such as the community governing board models.

HIBERNATION AND ADAPTATION

To maintain its equilibrium, an organization must adapt to changing inputs. This adjustment may take a passive form of hibernation in which the institution enters a phase of retrenchment. Cutting losses may be the sensible option. If efforts to maintain an acceptable census in certain hospital units, such as obstetrics or pediatrics, are unsuccessful, there may be an administrative decision to close those units and concentrate on providing quality patient care in the remaining services. An organization may adjust or adapt to changing inputs more actively by anticipating them. Staff specialists may be brought in, equipment and physical facilities updated, and goals restated. Finally, the overall corporate form may be restructured as a permanent reorganization that formalizes the cumulative effects of changes. A hospital may move from private sponsorship to a state-related, affiliated status, or a health care center may become the base service unit for behavioral care programs in the area.

The relationships among the concepts of hibernation, adaptation, and permanent change can be seen in the following case history of a state mental hospital. After the state legislature cut the budget of all state mental hospitals, the institution director began to set priorities for services so that the institution could survive. The least productive departments were asked to decrease their staff. The rehabilitation department lost two aide positions. The institution director had to force the organization into a state of hibernation in order to accomplish some essential conservation of resources.

The director of rehabilitation services revised the department goals to improve the chances of departmental survival. After closing ancillary services, the director concentrated staff on visible areas of the hospital and asked them to make their work particularly praiseworthy. At the same time, the director emphasized the need to document services so that patients' progress in therapy programs could be demonstrated. The director adapted to the change in the organization.

The program changes proved successful. The director of the rehabilitation department consolidated the changes and modified the department's goals. Instead of offering periodic programs to adolescent, neurological, geriatric, and acute care patients, the staff would concentrate on acutely ill geriatric patients. The staff applied for funds that were available to treat this population. At the same time, the staff determined that the adolescent unit could benefit from their services. Although funds were shrinking, the staff serviced this unit because needs in that area were unmet. The director and the staff decided to apply for private funds to service neurological and acute care cases so that these programs could also continue. By adopting a combined strategy of hibernation and adaptation, with alternate plans for expansion, the department director was able to foster not only departmental survival but, ultimately, departmental growth.

GOAL SUCCESSION, MULTIPLICATION, AND EXPANSION

Because an organization that effectively serves multiple client groups can attract money, materials, and personnel more readily than an organization with a more limited constituency, leaders may actively seek to expand the original goals of the organization. In addition to the pressures in the organizational environment that may force the organization to modify its goals as an adaptive response, success in reaching organizational goals may enable managers to focus on expanded or even new goals. The terms *goal succession, goal expansion,* and *goal multiplication* are used to describe the process in which goals are modified, usually in a positive manner.

Amatai Etzioni described this tendency of organizations to find new goals when old ones have been realized or cannot be attained. In goal succession, one goal is reached and is succeeded by a new one.[22] The March of Dimes, with its current emphasis on the prevention of premature births and birth defects, is a case in point. Having achieved its goals of arousing public interest in infantile paralysis and raising money for research and assistance to its victims, the organization could have ceased operations. Instead, it continued to function through its network of volunteers, national leaders, and central staff to achieve a new goal: prevention of birth defects.[23]

Sometimes an organization takes on additional goals because the original goals are relatively unattainable. A church may add a variety of social services to attract members when the worship forms and doctrinal substance per se do not increase the church's membership. A missionary group may offer a variety of health care or educational services when its direct evangelical methods cannot be used. The original goal is not abandoned, but it is sought indirectly; more tangible goals of service and outreach succeed this primary goal.

Goal expansion is the process in which the original goal is retained and enlarged with variations. Colleges and universities expand their traditional educational goals to include continuing education. An acute care facility may open a long-term care hospital (25 days or longer) as an adjunct to its short-stay services. A medical center may open a specialty division just for the comprehensive care of senior citizens. The Joint Commission continues to focus primarily on inpatient acute care hospital accreditation but has expanded its standards and accreditation process to include home care, outpatient, and emergency care units. A collective bargaining unit negotiates specific benefits for its workers and takes on the administrative processing of certain elements, such as the pension fund; the basic goal of improving the circumstances of the workers is retained and expanded beyond immediate economic benefits. Another example of goal expansion may be seen in the work of the Red Cross. Organized to deal with disaster relief in World War I, it subsequently expanded its work to assist in coordinating relief from all disasters, regardless of cause. In all these examples, the basic goal is retained and the new ones derived from it; the new goals are closely related and are essentially extensions of the original goal.

Goal multiplication is also a process in which an original goal is retained and new ones added. In this case, however, the new goals reflect the organization's effort to diversify. Goal multiplication is often the natural outgrowth of success. A hospital may offer patient care as its traditional, primary goal. To this it may add the goal of education of physicians, nurses, and other health care professionals. Because excellence in education is frequently related to the adequacy of the institution's research programs, research may subsequently become a goal. The hospital may take on a goal of participating in social reform, seeking to undertake affirmative action hiring plans and to foster employment within its neighborhood. It may offer special training programs for those who are unemployed in its area or for those who are physically or mentally impaired. It may coordinate extensive social services in order to assist patients and their families with both immediate health care problems and the larger social and economic problems they face.

Similar examples can be found in the business sector. A large hotel-motel corporation, with its resources for dealing with temporary living quarters, may go into the nursing home industry or the drug and alcohol treatment facility business by offering food, laundry, and housekeeping services; it may even operate a chain of convalescent or alcohol and drug rehabilitation centers. Several real estate firms might consolidate their efforts in direct sale of homes and then offer mortgage services as an additional program. Organizations take on a variety of goals as a means of diversification; resources are directed toward satisfaction of all the goals. Such multiplication of goals is seen as a positive state of organizational growth.

ORGANIZATIONAL LIFE CYCLE

Organizational change can be monitored through the analysis of an organization's life cycle. This concept is drawn from the pattern seen in living organisms. In management and administrative literature, the development of this model stems from the work of Marver Bernstein, who analyzed the stages of evolution and growth of independent federal regulatory commissions.[24] This model of the life cycle can be applied to advantage by any manager who wishes to analyze a particular management setting.

The organization is assessed not in chronological years but in phases of growth and development. No absolute number of years can be assigned to each phase, and any attempt to do so in order to predict characteristics would force and possibly distort the model. The value of organizational analysis by means of the life cycle lies in its emphasis on characteristics of the stages rather than the years. For example, the neighborhood health centers established in the 1960s under Office of

Economic Opportunity sponsorship had a relatively short life span in comparison with the life span of some large urban hospitals that are approaching a century or more of service. Both types of organizations have experienced the phases of the life cycle, with the former having completed the entire phase through decline and—in its original form—extinction.

The phases of the organizational life cycle usually meld into one another, just as they do in the biological model. Human beings do not suddenly become adolescents, adults, or senior citizens; so, too, organizations normally move from one phase to another at an imperceptible rate with some blurring of boundaries. Finally, not every organization reflects in detail every characteristic of each phase. The emphasis is on the cluster of characteristics that are predominant at a specific time.

Gestation

In this early formative stage, there is a gradual recognition and articulation of need or shared purpose. This stage often predates the formal organization; indeed, a major characteristic of this period is the movement from informal to formal organization. The impetus for organizing is strong, since it is necessary to bring together in an organized way the prime movers of the fledgling organization, its members (workers), and its clients.

Leadership tends to be strong and committed, and members are willing to work hard. Members' identification with organizational goals is strong because the members are in the unique situation of actualizing their internalized goals; in contrast, those who become part of the institution later must subsequently internalize the institution's objectives. Members of the management team find innovation the order of the day. Creative ideas meet with ready acceptance, since there is no precedent to act as a barrier to innovation. If there is a precedent in a parent organization, it may be cast off easily as part of the rejection of the old organization. A self-selection process also occurs, with individuals leaving if they do not agree with the form the organizational entity is taking. This is largely a flexible process, free of the formal resignation and separation procedures that come later.

Youth

The early enthusiasm of the gestational phase carries over into the development of a formal organization. Idealism and high hopes continue to dominate the psychological atmosphere. The creativity of the gestational period is channeled toward developing an organization that will be free of the problems of similar institutions. There is a strong camaraderie among the original group of leaders and members.

Organizational patterns have a certain inevitability, however. If a creative new organization is successful, it is likely to experience an increase in clients that will force it to formalize policies and procedures rapidly in order to handle the greater demand for service.

Some crisis may occur that precipitates expansion earlier than planned. A health center may have a plan for gradual neighborhood outreach, for example, but a sudden epidemic of flu may bring an influx of clients before it is staffed adequately. Management must make rapid adjustments in clinic hours and staffing patterns to meet the demand for specific services and, at the same time, to continue its plan for comprehensive health screening. A center for the developmentally challenged may schedule one opening date, but a court order to vacate a large, decaying facility may require the new center to accept the immediate transfer of many patients. Routine, recurring situations are met by increasingly complex procedures and rules. Additional staff is needed, recruited, and brought into the organization, perhaps even in a crash program rather than through the gradual integration of new members.

At this point, a new generation of worker enters the organization. These workers are one phase removed from the era of idealism and deeply shared commitment to the organization's goals. The organizational structure (e.g., work flow, job descriptions, line and staff relationships, and roles and authority) is tested. For the newcomer brought in at the management level, formal position or hierarchical office is the primary base of authority. Other members of the management team, as the pioneers, know each other's strengths and weaknesses intimately, but these managers may need to test the newcomer's personal attributes and technical competence. Sometimes, because the new organization attempts to deal with some problem in an innovative manner, an individual health care practitioner is hired in a nontraditional role; not only the professional and technical competence but also the managerial competence of that individual are tested.

Communication networks are essential in any organization. During an organization's youth, it is necessary to rely on formal communication, because the informal patterns are not yet well developed, except with the core group. This lack of an easy, anonymous, informal communication network forces individuals to communicate mainly along formal lines of authority. The core group may become more and more closed, more and more "in," relying on well-developed, secure relationships that stem from a shared history in the developing organization, while the newcomers form a distinct "out" group.

The jockeying for power and position may be intense. If managers hold an innovative office, those who oppose such creative organizational patterns may exert significant pressure to acquire jurisdiction or to force a return to traditional ways.

Since there may be much innovation in the overall organizational pattern, managers have little or no precedent against which they can measure their actions.

Certain problems center on the implementation of the original plans. The planners may start to experience frustration with managers who enter the organization during this period of formalization. Perhaps the original plans need modification; perhaps the innovative, ideal approach of the original group is not working, largely because of the change in the size of the organization. The line managers find themselves in the difficult situation of seeming to fail at the task on one hand and being unable to make the original planners change their view on the other. The promise of innovation becomes empty, however, if the original planners guard innovation as their prerogative and refuse to accept other ideas.

In the youth phase of an organization, more time must be devoted to orientation and similar formal processes of integrating new individuals into the organization. Certain difficulties may be encountered in recruiting additional supervisors and professional practitioners; for example, there may be no secure retirement funds, no group medical and life insurance, and no similar benefits that are predicated on long-term investments and large membership. Salary ranges may be modest in comparison with those of more established organizations simply because insufficient time has passed for the development of adequate resources. The strong normative sense of idealism may have a negative effect on potential workers as well as a positive one; a certain dedication to the organization's cause may be expected, and it may also be assumed that personnel should be willing to work hard without being rewarded monetarily.

Bernstein stressed the increased concern for organizational survival in this youthful stage. The organization may become less innovative because it is not sure of its strength. It may choose to fight only those battles in which victory is certain. In the case of regulatory bodies, which were Bernstein's major focus, the businesses subject to regulation may be perceived as stronger than the agency itself. In a health care organization, the new unit may be treated as a stepchild of related health care institutions. A new community behavioral health center or a home care organization, for example, may have to choose between competing with older, traditional units within the parent organization and being completely independent, still competing for resources but with less legitimacy of claim. A struggle not unlike the classic parent-adolescent conflict may emerge. Thus, organizational energy may go into an internal struggle for survival rather than into serving clients and expanding goals.

If the client groups are well defined and no other group or institution is offering the same service, a youthful organization may flourish. A burn unit in a hospital may have an excellent chance of survival as an organization because of the specificity of its clients as compared, for example, with the chance of a general medical clinic's survival. A similar positive climate may foster the development of units for treatment of spinal cord injury or for rehabilitation of the hand as specialized services. In effect, a highly specialized client group may afford a unit or an organization a virtual monopoly, which will tend to place the unit or organization in a position of strength.

Middle Age

The multiple constraints on the organization at middle age are compounded by several factors. In addition to the external influences that shape the work of the organization, there are internal factors that must be dealt with, such as the organizational pattern, the growing bureaucratic form, the weight of decision by precedent, and an increasing number of traditions.

However, the organization also reaps many benefits from middle age. Many activities are routine and predictable; roles are clear; and communication, both formal and informal, is relatively reliable. These years are potentially stable and productive. There is a reasonable receptivity to new ideas, but middle age is not usually a time of massive or rapid change and disruption, even the positive disruption resulting from major innovation. The manager in an organization in its middle age performs the basic traditional management processes in a relatively predictable manner.

Periods of rejuvenation are precipitated by a variety of events. A new leader may act as a catalytic agent, bringing new vision to the organization; for example, the president of a corporation may push for goal expansion by introducing a new line of products, or an aggressive hospital administrator may push for the development of an alternate health care service model. Mergers and affiliations with new and developing types of health care institutions, such as community health centers and home care programs, may be the catalyst. Although primarily negative events, the fiscal chaos associated with bankruptcy or the loss of accreditation as a hospital may cause the organization to reassess its goals and restructure its form, thus giving itself a new lease on life.

Some external crisis or change of articulated values in the larger society may make the organization vital once again. The recent emergence of alternate modes of communal living reflects individuals' search for a mode of living that combats the alienation of urban society; organizations that provide alternative modes of living can be revitalized because of this renewed interest in shared living arrangements.

The effect of war on the vitality of the military is an obvious example of crisis as a catalytic agent that causes a spurt of new growth for an organization. The growth of consumer and environmental agencies is another organizational response to change or crisis in the larger society.

In health care, family practice has developed as a specialty in response to patients' wishes for a more comprehensive, more personal type of medical care. The hospice concept for the terminally ill has become an alternative to the highly specialized setting of the acute care hospital.

An organization may experience a significant surge of vitality because of some internal activity, such as unionization of workers. During the covert as well as the overt stage of unionization, management may take steps to "get the house in order," including greater emphasis on worker-management cooperation in reaching the fundamental goals of the organization. Service of strong client groups may become more active, both to focus attention on the institution's primary purpose and to mobilize client goodwill in the face of the potential adversary (i.e., the union). Such internal regrouping activities foster rejuvenation in the organization as an offshoot of their primary purpose, avoiding unionization or reducing its impact.

Legislation of massive scope, particularly at the federal level, may have a rejuvenating effect. The infusion of money into the health care system via Medicare and Medicaid is partly responsible for the growth of the long-term care industry, although population trends and sociological patterns for care of the aged outside of the family setting are contributing factors. The passage of the National Health Care Planning and Resource Development Act rejuvenated some of the existing health planning agencies; its gradual phasing out, of course, has had the opposite effect in some instances by forcing a decline in certain planning groups. Changes in state professional licensure laws may bring certain professional groups into a season of new vigor.

The bureaucratic hierarchy protects managers who derive authority from a position that traditionally is well defined by the organization's middle age. Planning and decision making are shared responsibilities, subject to several hierarchical levels of review. The same events that may spur rejuvenation also may hurl the organization into a state of decline, the major characteristic of the final stage: old age.

Old Age

Staid routines, resistance to change, a long history of "how we do things," little or no innovation, and concern with survival are the obvious characteristics of an organization in decline. There may be feeble attempts to maintain the status quo or to serve clients in a minimal fashion, but the greater organizational energy is directed toward efforts to survive. If the end is inevitable, resources are guarded so that the institution can fulfill its obligations to its contractual suppliers and to its past and present employees (e.g., through vested pension funds, severance pay, and related termination benefits). There may even be a well-organized, overt process of seeking job placement for certain members of the hierarchy; time and resources may be made available to such individuals. Sometimes key individuals from the dying organization attempt to develop a new organization.

Because of its dwindling resources, the organization may no longer serve clients well, and all but the most loyal clients will look for other organizations. The organization in decline cannot attract new clients; the cycle is broken. Without clients, the organization cannot mobilize financial and political resources to maintain its physical facilities, expand services, respond to technological change, or remain in compliance with new licensure or regulatory mandates. The end, which may come swiftly, may be brought about by a decision to close and a specific plan to do so in an orderly way. For example, a department store might announce a liquidation sale that ends with the closing date. Only the internal details of closing need attention. As far as clients are concerned, the organization has died.

A final closing date may be imposed on an organization; in a bankruptcy, for example, the date may be determined in the course of legal proceedings. Legislation that initially establishes certain programs may include a termination date, although the date is more commonly set when legislation to continue funding the program fails. The changes in medical care evaluation under professional standards review organizations (PSROs) and the Office of Economic Opportunity neighborhood health centers are examples in the health care field of programs that moved into a state of decline or closure when funding was no longer available through federal legislation.

The closing decision may be a more passive one; there may be a gradual diminution of services and selective plant shutdowns and layoffs, as may occur in manufacturing corporations that rely primarily on military or space contracts. Bankruptcy is costly in economic and political terms in some cases, so the decision is implemented slowly. Indeed, it sometimes seems that no one actually makes a decision in some institutions that decline. Because of its unpopularity, the decision to close certain services, such as health care services, may be made in a somewhat passive way; however, the seemingly gradual slipping away of clients and the deterioration or outright closing of urban hospitals may be accompanied by the emergence of competitive forms of health care, such as home care units, neighborhood health centers, mobile clinics, and community health centers.

Although some organizations cease to exist entirely, others may change form or come under new sponsorship. For example, some of the neighborhood health centers under specialty grant sponsorship were absorbed into other federal government systems of health clinics. Several major railroad divisions were reorganized under Amtrak. Some hospitals that had been owned and controlled by religious orders became community-based, nonprofit institutions. Some organizations seem only to change title and official sponsorship. The various types of agencies for health care planning over a decade or so have included regional medical programs, regional comprehensive health planning programs, Health Systems Agencies (HSAs), and statewide health planning agencies; the organizational structure, not the total mandate, of these agencies has changed.

The managers in the declining organization may find themselves in a caretaker role that involves such difficult activities as allaying the anxiety of workers, monitoring contradictory formal and informal information about closing, and developing a plan for closing while continuing to give a modicum of service to the remaining clients. Managers must continue to motivate the workers without a traditional reward system, even in its most limited form. Staff may be reduced, and workers may seek to use up all benefits that they may lose if the organization closes (e.g., sick days and vacation days). Line managers may be forced to deal with the hostility of the workers facing job loss. Finally, a personal decision must be made: stay to the end or leave and cut theoretical losses.

Paradoxically, this may be a time of great opportunity for managers. Middle managers may have an opportunity to participate in activities outside their normal scope as the executive team grows thin. This may be the ideal time for middle managers to try their hand at related jobs, because failure may be ascribed to the situation rather than to their inexperience or even incompetence. Valuable experience may be gained because this may also be a time of great creativity as the gestational phase begins for a new organization with its unique opportunities, challenges, and frustrations. The organizational phoenix rises—sometimes.

We now move from general survival of the total organization to the specifics of individual change strategies.

EXERCISE: BECOMING A SPLIT-DEPARTMENT MANAGER

Imagine that you are the manager of a department, the function of which is to provide service in your chosen profession. In other words, if your career is medical laboratory technology, you are a laboratory manager; if your field is physical therapy, you manage physical therapy or rehabilitation services; and so on. You are employed by a 60-bed rural hospital, an institution sufficiently small that you represent the only level of management within your function (unless your profession is nursing, in which case there will be perhaps two or three levels of management). This means that unless you are a first-line manager in nursing (for example, head nurse), you report directly to administration.

You have been in your position for about two years. Following some stressful early months you are beginning to feel that you have your job under control most of the time.

A possibility that for years had been talked about and argued throughout the local community, the merger of your hospital with a similar but larger institution (90 beds) about 10 miles away, recently became a reality. One of the initial major changes undertaken by the new corporate entity was realignment of the management structure. In addition to placing the new corporate entity under a single chief executive officer, the realignment included, for most activities, bringing each function under a single manager. Between the merger date and the present, most department managers have been involved in the unpleasant process of competing against their counterparts for the single manager position.

You are the successful candidate, the survivor. Effective next Monday you will be running a combined department in two locations consisting of more than twice the number of employees you have been accustomed to supervising.

Instructions

Generate a list of the ways in which you believe your responsibilities and the tasks you perform are likely to change because of the merger and your resulting new role. Hint: It may be helpful to make lists of what you imagine to be the circumstances before and after your appointment. For example, two obvious points of comparison involve number of employees (which implies many necessary tasks) and travel inherent in the job. See how long a list you are able to generate.

If possible (for example, within a class or discussion group), after individual lists have been generated, bring several people together, combine their lists with yours, and see if a group process can further expand the list.

Also, address the following questions:

1. What does this split-department situation do to your efficiency as a manager, and how can you compensate for this change?
2. On what specific management skill should the newly appointed split-department manager be concentrating?

NOTES

1. Eli Ginzberg, Richard B. Saltman, and Robert Brook, "Healthy Debate," *Human Resource Executive* (May 5, 1998): 58.
2. *Ibid.,* 57.
3. "Public Anger at HMOs Is Hot Political Issue." *Rochester (New York) Democrat & Chronicle,* May 17, 1998.
4. Ginzberg, Saltman, and Brook, 58.
5. "Public Anger at HMOs Is Hot Political Issue."
6. Ginzberg, Saltman, and Brook, 57.
7. Craig Gunsauley, "Unions More Willing to Deal on Managed Care for Retirees," *Employee Benefit News* 12, no. 8 (1998): 23.
8. Ginzberg, Saltman, and Brook, 59.
9. Harris Meyer, "The Right to Appeal," *Hospitals and Health Networks* 72, no. 9 (1998): 23.
10. *Ibid.*
11. Jan Greene, "Blue Skies or Black Eyes?" *Hospitals and Health Networks* 72, no. 8 (1998): 27.
12. Ginzberg, Saltman, and Brook, 57–58.
13. Mindy W. Toran, "Paradigm Lost," *Human Resource Executive* (July 1998): 52.
14. Richard Haugh, "Who's Afraid of Capitation Now?" *Hospitals and Health Networks* 72, no. 11 (1998): 22.
15. *Ibid.,* 31.
16. William Davidow and Michael Malone, *Virtual Corporation: Structuring and Revitalizing the Corporation for the Twenty-First Century* (New York: Harper-Collins, 1993).
17. Dan Rode, "On the Horizon: A National Healthcare Information Infrastructure," *Journal of the Health Information Management Association* (September 2002): 26–28.
18. Bertram Gross, *Organizations and Their Managing* (New York: The Free Press, 1968), 454.
19. Matthew Holden, Jr., "Imperialism in Bureaucracy," *American Political Science Review* (December 1966): 943.
20. Philip Selznick, *TVA and the Grass Roots* (New York: Harper Torchbooks, 1966), 13.
21. *Ibid.,* 13, 260–61.
22. Amatai Etzioni, *Modern Organizations* (Englewood Cliffs, N.J.: Prentice-Hall, 1964), 13–14.
23. David L. Sills, *The Volunteers* (Glencoe, Ill.: The Free Press, 1957), 64. Cited in Etzioni, *Modern Organizations,* 13.
24. Marver Bernstein, *Regulating Business by Independent Commission* (Princeton, N.J.: Princeton University Press, 1955).

CHAPTER 2

The Challenge of Change

CHAPTER OBJECTIVES

- Identify the impact of change on organizational life.
- Identify the manager's role as change agent.
- Review examples of successful change.
- Examine a major change having ongoing impact.
- Describe the organizational change process.
- Identify specific strategies for dealing with resistance to change.

THE IMPACT OF CHANGE

The trends and issues noted in Chapter 1 reflect the reality: change in the health care environment is continuous and challenging. Its reality is reflected in every stage of the life cycle of the organization, as well as in its attendant survival strategies. Trends and issues intensify, becoming mandates for change in patient care, the setting, the administrative support. This affects the workers at all levels. Such changes consume financial and administrative resources; they have the potential of draining emotional and physical energy away from primary goals. Thus, the managers accept the role as change agents, seeking to stabilize the organization in the face of change.

THE MANAGER AS CHANGE AGENT

Managers, as the visible leaders of their units, take on the function of change agent. This change agent role involves moving the trend or issue from challenge to stable routine. This is accomplished in several ways:

- mediating imposed change through adjusting patterns of practice, staffing, and administrative routines
- monitoring horizon events through active assessment of trends and issues
- creating a change-ready environment
- taking the lead in accepting change

REVIEW OF SUCCESSFUL CHANGE

A manager fosters a change-ready environment by reminding the work group of successful changes. This raises the comfort level of the group and provides insight into strategies for achieving desired outcomes. Four examples are provided here to illustrate the process of successful change:

- Y2K—change as opportunity
- The Patient Self-Determination Act of 1990 (PSDA)–the routinization of change
- HIPAA—extensive change via legislation
- Electronic health record—proactive change

Change as Opportunity—Y2K

Recall the transition to this new century: Y2K. The phrase alone reminds us of successful responses to an inevitable change. It also reminds us of the pre-Y2K concerns about technology-dependent systems: would they work? Faced with the possibility of massive systems failure, managers carefully defined the characteristics of this anticipated change:

1. a definitive event with an exact timetable
2. well known ahead of time (three- or four-year run-up)
3. unknown/uncertainty mixed with known technical aspects:
    a. what systems might fail; what would the resulting impact be (e.g., failure of power grids; communication disruption; financial infrastructure chaos).

During the run-up to Y2K, managers assessed the potential impact and planned accordingly. Furthermore, many managers seized the opportunity to make even bigger changes. When the cost of upgrading some existing systems was compared to adopting new systems, managers chose to spend the money and time on a comprehensive overhaul.

Funding such a major project became part of the challenge. Most chose a combination of borrowing, along with "bare bones" budgets, with deferred maintenance and elimination of discretionary projects (e.g., refurbishing) to meet this need. The end result in many organizations was the adoption of new, well-integrated computerized systems. This overall plan of upgrading was supplemented with contingency planning closer to the December 31, 1999, deadline. Managers took such practical steps as:

- eliminating all backlog (e.g. coding, billing, transcription)
- pre-registering selected patient groups (e.g., prenatal care patients)
- obtaining and warehousing extra supplies
- adjusting staffing patterns for the eve of Y2K and the days immediately following it, with workers available and trained to carry out manual backup for critical functions

Managers also took the opportunity to review and update the emergency preparedness and disaster plans for the health care organization. Again, the anticipated Y2K change was the catalytic agent for renewed efforts in these areas. Y2K came and ran its course; the change was absorbed with relative ease because of careful planning.

The Routinization of Change: The Patient Self-Determination Act of 1990

End-of-life care and related decisions have always been a part of the health care environment. However, technological change (e.g., advances in life support systems) along with definitive court cases (e.g., *Quinlan, Cruzan,* and *Conroy*) led to a renewed interest in these issues. This interest, in turn, resulted in the passage of the Patient Self-Determination Act of 1990, with implications for patient care as well as the administrative support systems. The response to this change was orderly and timely because the health care providers and the administrative teams assessed the change in a systematic manner. This strategy of absorbing change through rapid routinization into existing modes of practice included:

1. outreach to clients/patients and their families, along with the public at large, to provide information and guidance about health care proxy, advance directives, and "living wills." Information about support services such as

social service, chaplaincy, and hospice care was included as part of the regular client/patient education programs.

2. review and update of Do Not Resuscitate (DNR) orders and related protocols for full or selected therapeutic efforts

3. review of plan of care protocols for "balance of life" admissions

4. increased emphasis on spiritual and psychological considerations of patient and family, with documentation through values history or similar assessments

5. renewed involvement of the ethics committee of the medical staff to provide the health care practitioner, patient, and family with guidance. The committee also adopted review protocols to assess patterns of compliance with advance directives and end-of-life care

6. documentation and related administrative processes augmented to reflect the details of this sequence of care: e.g., documentation that an advance directive was made; movement of the document with the patient as he or she changed location; flagging the chart to indicate the presence of the directive. Existing policies and procedures were updated to reflect these additional practices

The changes stemming from this law were easily managed through systematic review and adjustment of existing, well-established routines. Because response to legislated change is often required, it is useful to examine yet another such mandate. A consideration of HIPAA reflects a different dynamic in the organizational process of responding to new requirements.

HIPAA: Extensive Change via Legislation

The Health Insurance Portability and Accountability Act of 1996, known commonly by the acronym HIPAA, crept inconspicuously upon the scene as Public Law Number 104 of the 191st Congress (PL 104-191). When it was a newly passed law its most visible portion was broadly described by the name of the law, addressing primarily "portability" of employee health insurance.

The intent of HIPAA was to enable workers to change jobs without fear of losing health care coverage. It enabled workers to move from one employer's plan to another's without gaps in coverage and without encountering restrictions based on preexisting conditions. It proclaimed that a worker could move from plan to plan without disruption of coverage.

In 1996 not a great many health care managers concerned themselves with HIPAA. Human resource managers became most aware of the new law because it concerned their benefits plans, but the burden of notification was borne mostly by the employers' health insurance carriers so there was little to do other than answering employees' questions. To many managers the employer had no concerns about HIPAA beyond ensuring health insurance portability. But HIPAA's major impact was to come later, and its arrival was a genuine eye-opener for many.

Title II in the Spotlight

This law consists of five sections. Titles I, III, IV, and V deal with employee health insurance, promote medical savings accounts, and set standards for covering long-term care. Title II is the section driving most HIPAA-related change. This section is called "Preventing Health Care Fraud and Abuse, Administrative Simplification, and Medical Liability Reform." It is referred to as just "Administrative Simplification," a term that is misleading at best; for many of the organizations that have had to comply with it, the effects have been anything but simple.

"Administrative Simplification" included several requirements designated for implementation at differing times. Compliance with the Privacy Rule, the most contentious part of HIPAA, was required by April 14, 2003. Compliance with the Transactions and Code Sets (TCS) Rule was required by October 16, 2003, and the Security Rule was set for implementation in April 2005.

Nearly all of the controversy over the intent versus the reality of HIPAA involves the Privacy Rule. In trying to strike a balance between the accessibility of personal health information by those who truly need it and matters of patient privacy, portions of HIPAA have created considerable work and expense for health care providers and organizations that do business with them, not to mention creating inconvenience and frustration for patients and others.

The Continuing Privacy Controversy

Reactions to the Privacy Rule were numerous. Patients and their advocates claimed that these new requirements were forcing a choice between access to medical care and control of their personal medical information. Government, however, claimed that the rules would successfully balance patient privacy against the needs of the health care industry for information for research promoting public health objectives, and improving the quality of care.

When HIPAA's privacy regulations first received widespread exposure, hospitals, insurers, health maintenance organizations, and others claimed that the Privacy Rule would impose costly new burdens on the industry. At the same time Congress was claiming that HIPAA's protections were immensely popular with consumers. Consumer advocates hailed the Privacy Rule as a major step toward comprehensive standards for medical privacy while suggesting that it did not go far enough.

To comply with the Privacy Rule, affected organizations were required to:

- have policies and procedures addressing the handling of patient medical information
- train employees in the proper handling of protected health information
- monitor compliance with all requirements for handling protected health information
- maintain documented proof that all pertinent information-handling requirements are being fulfilled

In many instances the HIPAA privacy requirements are causing frustration for patients and others. For example, a spouse who has to help obtain a referral or follow up on a test result cannot do so without the signed authorization of the patient (unless the patient is a minor). Anyone other than a minor or a legally incapable or incapacitated individual must give written permission for anyone else to receive any of their personal medical information.

There are a number of instances in which personal medical information can be used without patient consent. These instances, along with all patients' rights concerning personal medical information, must be delineated in the Privacy Notice that every provider organization must provide to every patient.

Effects on the Organization

All health care plans and providers must comply with HIPAA. Provider organizations include physicians' and dentists' offices; hospitals, nursing homes, and hospices; home health providers; clinical laboratories, imaging services; pharmacies, clinics and free-standing surgical centers and urgent care centers; and any others who provide health-related services to individuals. Also required to comply are other organizations that serve the direct providers of health care—for example, billing services and medical equipment dealers. All affected organizations must:

- Protect patient information from unauthorized use or distribution and from malfeasance and misuse;
- Implement specific data formats and code sets for consistency of information processing and preservation; and
- Set up audit mechanisms to safeguard against fraud and abuse.
- Also, all subcontractors, suppliers, or others coming into contact with protected patient information are required to comply with the HIPAA Privacy Rule. In addition, all arrangements with such entities must define the acceptable uses of patient information.

Depending on organization size and structure, compliance with the HIPAA Privacy Rule could involve several departments (as in a mid-size to large hospital), a few people (as in a small hospital or nursing home), or a single person (as in a small medical office). Overall, whether compliance is accomplished by separate departments or just a person or two, compliance can involve a number of activities, including information technology; health information management; social services; finance; administration; and ancillary or supporting services.

The necessary changes have been numerous and have added to workload in every affected area. Providers must now obtain written consent from patients or their legal representatives for the use or disclosure of information in their medical records. Also, providers are now legally required to disclose when patient information has been improperly accessed or disclosed.

The Privacy Rule created a widespread need for health care providers to revise their systems to protect patient information and combat misuse and abuse. Providers now must protect patient information in all forms; implement specific data formats and code sets; monitor compliance within their organizations; implement appropriate polices and procedures; provide training all in HIPAA's privacy requirements; and require the organization's outside business partners to return or destroy protected information once it is no longer needed. And it is not enough simply to do everything that is supposed to be done. There are also a number of documentation requirements as well. Even a provider organization's telecommuting or home-based program must be HIPAA compliant.

Physical Layout Considerations

The HIPAA Privacy Rule has necessitated changes in physical arrangements to ensure that no one other than the patient and caregiver or other legitimately involved person knows the nature of the patient's problem. Medical orders or information about an individual's condition must be conveyed with a guarantee of privacy. Numerous organizations had to move desks or work stations, erect privacy partitions, provide sound-proofing, and make other alterations so that no one other than those who are legally entitled to hear may overhear what passes between patient or representative and a legitimately concerned party.

The Privacy Official

Every health care provider organization must have a person designated to oversee HIPAA compliance. In a large organization this could be a full-time HIPAA coordinator; in a small organization like a medical office the task might be an additional responsibility for the office manager. This person must monitor all aspects of compliance and ensure that appropriate polices and procedures are maintained current.

The Department Manager and HIPAA

Depending on the nature of a department's activity, HIPAA's requirements could significantly affect the manager's role. For example, in addition to most managers' involvement with the Privacy Rule, someone managing in health information management (HIM) must also be concerned with the Transactions and Code Sets (TCS) Rule. A manager within information technology or information systems will be significantly concerned with the Security Rule because of its relevance for information stored or transmitted electronically.

Like other laws affecting the workplace, there is much more to compliance with HIPAA than simply putting polices, procedures, and systems in place. Some HIPAA regulations are complex, and in the most-affected areas of an organization considerable training can be required. Also, HIPAA necessitates some training for most staff regardless of department; anyone who comes into contact with protected patient information must receive privacy training. So most managers will be both trainees and trainers, learning HIPAA's privacy requirements and communicating them to employees.

Not Going Away

Some HIPAA requirements are still under scrutiny and all the dust has yet to settle, but it is clear that the law's basic privacy requirements are here to stay in one form or another. There may be more changes in how some aspects of privacy are addressed, but it is likely that the privacy rules will continue to affect every physician, patient, hospital, pharmacy, health care provider, and all other entities having contact with patient medical information in any form.

The Health Insurance Portability and Accountability Act has brought with it a considerable amount of unwelcome, unwanted, and frequently burdensome change affecting the jobs of many health care managers. Since the requirements of HIPAA are government mandates, the individual manager has no option but to comply. The manager's challenge, then, is to conscientiously approach the necessary changes in the role and incorporate them so that they are addressed as efficiently and effectively as possible. An unexpected positive outcome of the HIPAA-related actions is this: the health information management environment has been primed to undertake major efforts in expanding the electronic health record.

The Electronic Health Record: A Study in Proactive Change

Implementation of the electronic health record reflects a proactive approach to change. The application of technology to enhance the creation and use of health care information has been a welcomed advance. Health information managers have accepted this opportunity to link this challenge to their ongoing vision and mission. Yes, the technology is new, but the underlying principle is enduring: quality health information for use in patient care, research, and administrative support.

Health information practitioners have taken leadership roles in their workplaces and through their national association, the American Health Information Management Association (AHIMA), along with its state component organizations. The overall strategy is four-fold:

1. individual initiative within the workplace
2. advocacy in the public arena
3. partnership with key stakeholders
4. outreach to clients/patients

Individual Initiative

Within the workplace, individual health information managers have steadily adopted computer technology to support basic operations. Work flow and processes have been gradually converted over time, including automated master patient index, coding and reimbursement processes, digital imaging, and speech recognition dictation. The internal administrative systems have served as building blocks for the expansion of computerized systems to include the electronic health record. While individual initiative continues to be an important facet of this transition, fostering change through advocacy has been primarily an organized group effort through the national association, AHIMA.

Advocacy in the Public Arena

External forces, particularly law and regulation, impact the process. It is essential, then, that professional practitioners help shape the debate, contributing their knowledge and expertise through organized efforts. Regular interaction with lawmakers and regulatory agency officials has been central to this process. Participation in work groups, task forces, and special initiatives has been steady. Landmark events bear the imprint of such involvement, including the Center for Disease Control's Public Health Information Network to implement the Consolidated Health Informatics Standards; the Public Health Data Standards Consortium; Department of Health and Human Services' (DHHS) American Health Information Community and its initiatives toward creating a national health information network; and the Certification Commission for Healthcare Information Technology.

Partnerships with Key Stakeholders

The health information profession has long been the authoritative source of practice standards. With the advent of electronic health records, many of the questions that have arisen are variations of issues with which HIM practitioners have successfully dealt. Those experiences have prepared HIM practitioners to offer guidance in such areas as documentation content and standardization, authentication of documentation, consents, accuracy of patient information, access and authorized use of data, and data security.

AHIMA has developed a series of position papers, statements of best practices, and guidelines for these and related topics. AHIMA has strengthened its efforts through partnership with key stakeholders, as the following examples demonstrate:

- American Health Information Community (DHHS)—standards for electronic health data
- American Medical Informatics Association—data standards
- Medical Group Management Association—performance improvements and need for consistent data standards
- National Library of Medicine—data mapping (e.g., Systematized Nomenclature of Medicine [SNOMED] and International Classification of Disease, Ninth Revision [ICD-9] interface)
- Annual Corporate Partner Industry Briefing—AHIMA-sponsored exchange sessions

Through these and similar outreach efforts, AHIMA makes available valuable guidance to those involved in adopting the electronic health record. Another major initiative by AHIMA was the move toward open membership. In recognition of the important partnership with information technology specialists, clinicians, and others with a shared interest in health information, and to foster even greater teamwork, the AHIMA House of Delegates voted to eliminate associate membership, folding these members into the active membership category. An open, inclusive membership provides additional strength to the association in its efforts to foster the electronic health record initiative.

Outreach to Clients/Patients

Consumers are an important partner in the effective use of the electronic health record. AHIMA has undertaken a major initiative, the Community Education Campaign, to raise public awareness of the personal health record. Individual health information practitioners, using AHIMA-created presentations, interact at local and regional levels with consumer groups such as local chambers of commerce, health fair coordinators, specialty support groups (e.g., cancer support groups).

An important adjunct to this outreach is advocacy: clients/patients must continue to have trust in the process of revealing their personal information fully and truthfully during health care interactions. AHIMA continues to press for specific protective legislation with a non-discrimination focus: protect the patient from any discriminatory action stemming from information patient care encounters.

In summary, the electronic health record initiatives reflect the best in proactive involvement by managers in facing major change. Using the foregoing examples as background, let us now consider the theoretical aspects of organizational change.

CHANGE AND RESISTANCE TO CHANGE

Change is inevitable, but change can also be chaotic and painful. Alfred North Whitehead once said, "The art of progress is to preserve order amid change and to preserve change amid order." That statement captures the essence of change and its effects on all of life. Much change is beneficial, even necessary, but change is often upsetting and unsettling and thus must be controlled. For good or ill, change is inevitable. So, too, is resistance to change inevitable.

This section addresses the inevitability of change and how we tend to deal with change as individuals and how, as managers, we can deal with employee resistance to change. In discussing this topic it is necessary to look at individual attitudes toward change, those of both managers and employees alike, since resistance is a human reaction that can arise in anyone regardless of organizational position, and how we meet change when it is upon us and we make change work when we must.

Significant change, change that has the power to confuse, frustrate, and very nearly overwhelm, is a frequent modern concern. Broad-scale change has been a phenomenon affecting only the recent few generations, and for the most part we remain unable to shake off centuries of programming that causes us to dig in our heels and resist when change that we neither want nor welcome threatens to pull us forward.

The Collision of Constancy and Change

Humans have been thoroughly conditioned by many centuries of little or no change to expect constancy. Up until a few decades ago an individual could adopt a career and with few exceptions expect to remain in that career for a lifetime. The effects of the knowledge explosion and the industrial revolution which preceded it, however, included changes that rendered some occupations obsolete or changed them dramatically. Occupations that had existed for several generations all but vanished as machines took over work that had long been done by hand. Entire industries disappeared—for example, whaling, once an economic mainstay of the northeastern United States, shriveled and died as petroleum products replaced whale oil. Many individuals have seen their jobs and careers disappear as a consequence of change that continues to accelerate to this day.

Those working in the delivery have seen and are seeing new medical technologies arise to either replace or augment existing technologies, in some instances making it necessary for workers to learn new skills or seek new occupations. Some individuals still working in diagnostic imaging were first employed when imaging was entirely X-ray; these people have seen the addition of the CAT scan, MRI, PET scan, and other technologies. One technologist who had been employed in a hospital laboratory for 30 years observed that more than 80 percent of the tests she performed on a routine basis did not exist when she first entered the field. A professional in another field, comparing the changes in college course curricula for his field over a period of twenty years, observed that he would have to take one or two new courses each semester for the rest of his life to remain current with the pace of change in his field. And on a simpler level, for the conduct of routine business functions whether in health care or elsewhere, where have all the typewriters (and typewriter makers) gone?

People have been conditioned by centuries of little change to expect constancy or near-constancy. That, plus our natural tendency to seek equilibrium with our surroundings, conditions many of us as automatic resistors of change. We are continually attempting to preserve our equilibrium with our environment, and whenever it is disturbed we tend to take steps to reestablish that equilibrium—to return to our "comfort zone." Certainly not all people behave in the same manner, but it is likely that most people seek equilibrium with their surroundings and tend to equate security with constancy. And indeed security was once likely to be found in adopting an occupation and doing it well for life or in remaining a loyal employee of one organization for life. No longer, however, is there security in constancy; rather, today's security, to the extent we can say it exists, lies in flexibility and adaptability.

The Roots of Resistance

The principal cause of most resistance to change is the disturbance of the aforementioned equilibrium. Resistance will of course be influenced considerably by one's knowledge of where a given change is coming from. It is unlikely that you will resist a change with which you wholeheartedly agree or one that is your own idea to begin with. Such a change the individual does not resist because it is welcome and thus does not threaten one's equilibrium. Therefore, it is not change itself that individuals resist; what is resisted is *being changed*—being made to change by forces or circumstances outside of themselves.

A secondary major cause of resistance lies in our inability to mentally conceive of certain possibilities or think beyond the boundaries of what we presently know or believe. The limitations presented by what people know and what they believe can provide significant barriers to creativity and progress. Ideas that are today deemed revolutionary were not welcomed with open minds. Many people we have come to think of as innovators and visionaries were, in their day, regarded as dreamers, charlatans, or crackpots: Barely two months before the Wright brothers flew, a noted scientist publicly explained why a heavier-than-air flying machine could never work. A device called a "telephone" was branded a fraud, with an "expert" proclaiming that even if it were possible to transmit the voice over wires, the device would have no practical value. When television was new the head of a major Hollywood studio proclaimed that people would soon get tired of staring at a plywood box every night. Even in the field of medicine, change is often thought impossible: in 1837 leading British surgeon Sir John Erichson stated that the abdomen, the chest, and the brain would "forever be shut from the intrusion of the wise and humane surgeon." Note as well that many people alive today once thought that surgery on a living heart would never be possible.

To a considerable extent, then, the roots of resistance to change are within human beings themselves.

Primary Causes of Resistance

Concerning change that occurs in the workplace, we tend to be thrown off balance by changes that are thrust upon us and especially by the way in which many of these changes are introduced. Common sources of change in the work organization occur in:

- organizational structure, when departments are altered or interdepartmental relationships or management reporting relationships are changed, including the changes that result from merger, affiliation, or system formation;
- management, whether in a department, a division, or an entire organization;
- product or service lines, as services are added, dropped, or altered significantly;
- introduction of new technology, bringing with it new equipment that employees must learn to use;
- job restructuring, altering the duties of particular jobs, such as combining jobs that were formerly separate;

- methods and procedures, requiring workers to learn new ways of doing their jobs;
- the organization's policies, especially personnel policies affecting terms and conditions of employment.

Consider how much—or perhaps how little—control the average rank-and-file employee or the typical department manager can exert over the foregoing changes. In most instances the individual is essentially powerless. Managers and some employees might perhaps have a voice in restructuring jobs and altering methods and procedures, and perhaps they might be involved in selecting or recommending new equipment, but chances are they have little or no voice in the decisions necessitating such changes. It is doubtful that many employees or managers below the level of executive management have any influence on changes in products or services. And concerning the remainder of the major sources of change listed above— these significant sources of stress and resistance for managers and employees alike—rank-and-file employees and their department managers are powerless.

Organizational Changes

Depending on the extent of reorganization, structural changes within a health care organization, such as combining departments or groups or realigning departments under different executives, can engender ill feelings and generate considerable resistance. Most department managers and their employees are well aware that reorganizing under whatever name—reengineering, downsizing, whatever—often means that some people will lose their jobs, so fear and insecurity and thus resistance increase while productivity inevitably decreases. Even more likely to upset employees are the changes accompanying merger or other form of affiliation, acquisition by a larger organization, or health system formation.

Management Changes

Changes in management are among the most potentially upsetting changes employees can experience. The stress of a management change and thus the resistance to it is concentrated within the hierarchy beneath the management position that is turning over; therefore, a change in department manager will affect primarily that department while a change in chief executive officer will affect the entire organization. A change in management almost always involves exchanging a known quantity for a complete or partial unknown, and it is fear and apprehension concerning the unknown that causes most initial resistance to management changes.

Policy Changes

Major changes in the policies of the organization, especially personnel policies affecting terms and conditions of employment, are likely to spark a certain amount of employee resistance, especially if employees perceive they are losing something. In these recent years of fiscal belt-tightening it is not uncommon to see, for example, employers in health care and elsewhere shifting an increasing portion of ever-growing health insurance costs to employees, or reducing the corporate contribution to defined-contribution retirement plans or other investment plans, or reducing the sick-time benefit and combining the remainder with vacation and personal time in "paid-time-off" (PTO) plans. Such policy changes have inspired so much resistance that for some employers they have become major issues in union organizing campaigns and labor contract negotiations.

Many Causes

Resistance can arise from anywhere, resulting from almost any change within an organization, often coming from situations we might never have thought would raise objections from anyone. These recent years of turmoil in health care, with all of the fallout of "merger mania" and all of the cost-reducing and cost-saving pressures brought to bear on the country's health care delivery system, finds the health care worker—and the health care manager as well—working in an environment of intensifying change and an eroding sense of security.

Meeting Change Head-On

The health care department manager is in a uniquely difficult position relative to change impacting the health care organization. As an employee the manager is just as affected by change as the rank-and-file employees and is just as likely to feel helpless and demoralized and resistant. Yet it is up to the manager to try to minimize the negative reactions of the work group and attempt to raise the employees' morale and ensure their continued productivity. If the manager openly projects doom, gloom, and resistance, the staff will be all the more likely to become more deeply mired in doom, gloom, and resistance themselves, ensuring that morale and productivity both suffer. It can be a most difficult role for the manager to function as "cheerleader" when there seems to be nothing to cheer about. Yet the manager must make a conscious effort to rise above the doom, gloom, and resistance. Succeeding at doing so is largely a matter of attitude, including the willingness to take a moderate amount of risk.

Flexibility and Adaptability

As noted earlier, we can no longer find security in constancy, maintaining loyalty to the same ideas, concepts, and institutions for life. Rather, security, to whatever extent it exists today, is more likely found in flexibility and adaptability. The manager who remains rooted in place, with a fixed set of ideas and an unchanging concept of the job, will not be particularly successful; however, the manager who can move about, who can flex and adapt as circumstances change, stands a much greater chance of success. Also, to enhance the department's chances of success in adjusting to changing circumstances the manager must be a role model for flexibility and adaptability.

Also, a department manager may be able to help some of the employees increase their flexibility by instituting cross-training wherever possible. For cross-training to apply it is necessary that there be a number of employees distributed across multiple jobs of approximately the same skill or grade level, so cross-training is not possible in every department. When it is possible, however, there are benefits for employee, department, and organization. With people trained in multiple activities, coverage for vacations and other absences is more readily accomplished, employees get the advantages of task variety, and employees may become more secure during times of readjustment by being capable of moving into certain other jobs already trained and competent.

A Matter of Control

The department manager who becomes caught up in a sea of change should immediately learn the difference between what can be controlled and what cannot be controlled. Much energy is wasted in trying to control that which is uncontrollable. For example, you may be greatly stressed about an impending merger and subsequent combination of departments, but there is nothing you can do about it; it will happen whether you wish it or not.

Stress as a response to change both real and impending is an emotional reaction. An important early step in gaining a measure of control over your circumstances is learning to control your emotions. You may have little or no control over the changes themselves; however, you have complete control over how you respond to the changes.

Fortunately, there are usually a few factors that the individual department manager can control to some extent. Reorganizing or reengineering frequently results in the need to combine positions and restructure a number of jobs, change job descriptions, assignments, crew or team sizes, equipment, or later services. These actions usually entail changes in methods and procedures, changes that can be determined in detail within the department by the manager, often with the participation of the employees.

Addressing Resistance with Employees

A manager responsible for implementing change has three available avenues along which to approach employees regarding a specific change. The manager can (1) simply tell them what to do, (2) convince them of the necessity for doing it, or (3) involve them in planning for the change.

Tell Them

The use of specific orders or commands is one of the hallmarks of the autocratic or authoritarian leader. The boss is the boss, a giver of orders who either makes a decision and orders its implementation or relays without expansion or clarification the mandate from above.

The authoritarian approach is sometimes necessary; occasionally it is the only option available under urgent and completely unanticipated circumstances. However, in most situations the tell-them approach is the approach most likely to generate resistance, so it should be used in only those rare instances when it is the only means available.

Convince Them

In most instances, including those in which the change in question is a hard edict from top management, the individual manager has room for explanation and persuasion. At the very least there is the opportunity to try making each employee aware of the reasons for the change and the necessity for its implementation. It may be necessary for the manager to champion the cause of something clearly distasteful to all concerned (except, for example, to those mandating compliance) because it may be good for the institution overall or good for patients, or even perhaps because it is mandated by new government regulations. The employees may not like what they are called upon to do, but they are more likely to respond as needed if they know and understand why the change must be implemented.

The employees deserve all the information available, and this information often serves the manager well because it can remove the shadow of the unknown from the employees and thus lessen their resistance. Few if any changes cannot be approached by this means. The authoritarian tell-them approach should be reserved as a last resort to be used on those occasions when employees clearly cannot be "sold" on the change.

Involve Them

Whenever possible, and especially as it affects the way they do their assigned jobs, employees should become involved in shaping the details of any particular change. It has been repeatedly demonstrated that employees are far more likely to understand and comply when they have a voice in determining the form and substance of the change. For example, if new equipment is under consideration and there is sufficient lead time, it's helpful to obtain the input of the people who will have to work with the equipment once it is in place. This sort of involvement not only enhances employee cooperation, it often leads to a better decision because of the perspective of the people doing the hands-on work. When expansion or remodeling will change the characteristics of the department, employee input in the planning stages will bring the workers' perspective into determining optimal layout and work flow. Through involvement, change can become a positive force. Employees will be more likely to comply because they own part of the change; in effect, a piece of it is their idea. And there is another potential benefit to involvement as well: the employees know the details of the work in ways the manager may never know. The manager supervises a number of tasks, some of which he or she may have once done personally. However, employees regularly perform in hands-on fashion the tasks the manager only oversees. So the employees usually know the details of the work far better than the manager and are in a better position to provide the basis for positive change in task performance.

The numerous sources of management advice that promote the value of employee involvement are right; the participative or consultative approaches to management are the best ways of getting things done through employees. The most effective ways of reducing or removing the fear of the unknown make full use of communication and involvement.

Guidelines for Effective Management of Change

To secure employee cooperation and participation and successfully manage change in the workplace, it is necessary for the manager to:

- *Plan thoroughly.* Fully evaluate the potential change and examine all implications of its potential impact on the department and the total organization.
- *Communicate fully.* Completely communicate the change, starting early, ensuring that the employees are not taken by surprise. This should ideally be

two-way communication, preparing the way for employees' involvement by soliciting their comments or suggestions.

- *Convince employees.* As necessary take steps to sell employees on the value and benefits of the proposed change. When possible, appeal to employee self-interest, letting them know how they stand to benefit from the change and how it might make their work easier.

- *Involve employees when possible.* It is not possible to completely involve employees in all matters, but involvement is nevertheless possible on many occasions. Be especially aware of the value of employees as a source of job knowledge, and tap this source not only for the acceptance of change but for the development of improvements as well.

- *Monitor implementation.* As with the implementation of any decision, monitor the implementation of any change until the new way is established as part of the accepted work pattern. A new work method, dependent for its success on willing adoption by individual employees, can be introduced in a burst of enthusiasm only to die of its own weight as the novelty wears off and old habits return. New habits are not easily formed, and the employees need all the help the manager can furnish through conscientious follow-up.

True Resistance

Resistance to change will never be completely eliminated. People possess differing degrees of flexibility and exhibit varying degrees of acceptance of ideas that are not purely their own. However, involvement helps, and the manager will eventually discover, if not already having done so, that most employees are willing to cooperate and genuinely want to contribute. Beyond involvement, however, continuing communication is the key. Full knowledge and understanding of what is happening and why it is happening are the strongest forces the manager can bring to bear on the problems of resistance to change. Ultimately one will discover that it is not change that people resist so much as they resist *being changed*.

In addition to applying the foregoing strategies, managers facilitate their response to change by:

1. recommitting to the full spectrum of their role through a review of the enduring functions of the manager
2. remaining attentive to:
   a. developments in the history of management and the ways in which managers adjusted their focus from time to time

b. shifts in organizational life from informal to formal, stable organizational patterns

c. opportunities for building a strong network of internal and external relationships

The following chapter offers a fuller exploration of these concepts and strategies.

CASE: IN NEED OF IMPROVEMENT?

You are an administrative staff specialist newly employed by the hospital to act as a management engineer and address a number of issues relating to operating efficiency. Your first assignment is to analyze work methods and staffing in the central sterile supply division of materials management. The department was singled out for study because:

- The manager, a registered nurse who has held the job for more than 25 years, has requested two more processing aides although her staff is already one person larger than that of another area hospital of equivalent size.

- There has been a recent, seemingly unexplainable, upturn in the consumption of disposables.

- A number of storage shelves appear to be stocked to overflowing with infrequently used items.

- The department issues frequent rush orders to obtain needed items that have completely run out.

- Observed conditions in the department include an overcrowded storage area, a seemingly inadequate decontamination area, and a grossly oversized processing area referred to by most employees as "the ballroom."

On your initial visit to the department the first thing the manager says to you is: "So you're the one who's going to tell us what we're doing wrong?" Her tone is none too friendly.

Instructions

Develop a proposed approach to a complete study of the department, including the "sales pitch" you would use to try winning the manager's cooperation and support, specifying what should be done, why it should be done, and how you propose to address the inevitable resistance of both manager and staff.

3

Today's Concept of Organizational Management

CHAPTER OBJECTIVES

- Define management and differentiate between the art and science of management.
- Review the basic functions of management.
- Describe the major phases of the development of organizational management.
- Present the concept of the work setting as a total system.
- Introduce the concept of clientele network and describe the application of this concept to the health care setting.

THE NATURE OF MANAGEMENT: ART OR SCIENCE?

Management has been defined as the process of getting things done through and with people. It is the planning and directing of effort and the organizing and employing of resources (both human and material) to accomplish some predetermined objective. Within the overall concept of management, the function of administration can be identified. The practical execution of the plans and decisions on a day-to-day basis requires specific administrative activities that managers may assign to executive officers or administrators. Managers may find that their role includes specifically administrative activities in addition to overall management responsibilities. The workday of a typical department head in a health care institution contains a mix of broad-based managerial functions and detailed administrative actions.

Especially since the turn of the 20th century, management's scientific aspects have been emphasized. The scientific nature of management is reflected in the fact that it is based on a more or less codified body of knowledge consisting of theories and principles that are subject to study and further experimentation. Yet, management as a science lacks the distinct characteristics of an exact discipline, such as chemistry or mathematics.

The many variables associated with the human element make management as much an art as a science. Even with complex analytical tools for decision making, such as probability studies, stochastic (random) simulation, and similar mathematical elements, the manager must rely on intuition and experience in assessing such factors as timing and tactics for persuasion.

FUNCTIONS OF THE MANAGER

A manager's functions can be considered a circle of actions in which each component leads to the next. Although the functions can be identified as separate sets of actions for purposes of analysis, the manager in actual practice carries out these activities in a complex, unified manner within the total process of managing. Other individuals in the organization carry out some of these activities, either periodically or routinely, but the manager is assigned these specific activities in their entirety, as a continuing set of functions. When these processes become routine, the role of manager emerges. The traditional functions of a manager were identified by Gulick and Urwick[1] based on the earlier work of Henri Fayol.[2] Chester Barnard brought together the significant underlying premises about the role of the manager in his classic work *The Functions of the Executive*.[3]

Classic Management Functions

Management functions typically include

- *planning*—the selection of objectives, the establishment of goals, and the factual determination of the existing situation and the desired future state.
- *decision making*—a part of the planning process in that a commitment to one of several alternatives (decisions) must be made. Others may assist in plan-

ning, but decision making is the privilege and burden of managers. Decision making includes the development of alternatives, conscious choice, and commitment.

- *organizing*—the design of a pattern of roles and relationships that contribute to the goal. Roles are assigned, authority and responsibility are determined, and provision is made for coordination. Organizing typically involves the development of the organization chart, job descriptions, and statements of work flow.

- *staffing*—the determination of personnel needs and the selection, orientation, training, and continuing evaluation of the individuals who hold the required positions identified in the organizing process. (Some theorists class the staffing function within the organizing function, rather than viewing it as a separate function.)

- *directing or actuating*—the provision of guidance and leadership so that the work performed is goal-oriented. It is the exercise of the manager's influence, the process of teaching, coaching, and motivating workers.

- *controlling*—the determination of what is being accomplished, the assessment of performance as it relates to the accomplishment of the organizational goals, and the initiation of corrective actions. In contemporary management practice, the larger concepts of performance improvement and total quality management include controlling.

Figure 3–1 summarizes the classic functions of managers and their relationship to each other. In addition, managers must continually establish and maintain internal and external organizational relationships to achieve an effective working rapport. They must monitor the organization's environment to anticipate change and bring about the adaptive responses required for the institution's survival.

At different phases in the life of the organization, one or another management function may be dominant. In the early stages of organizational development, for example, planning is the manager's primary function. When the organization is mature, however, controlling functions are emphasized.

The Health Care Practitioner as Manager

In the specialized environment of a health care institution, qualified professional practitioners may assume the role of unit supervisor, project manager, or department head or chief of service. The role may emerge gradually as the number of patients increases, as the variety of services expands, and as specialization occurs

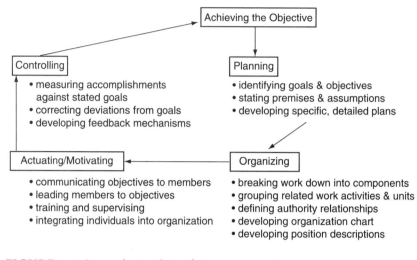

FIGURE 3–1 Interrelationship of Management Functions

within a profession. A physical therapy staff specialist, for example, may develop a successful program for patients with spinal cord injury; as the practitioner most directly involved in the work, this individual may be given full administrative responsibility for that unit. The role of manager begins to emerge as budget projections need to be made, job descriptions need to be updated and refined, and the staffing pattern needs to be reassessed and expanded.

An occupational therapist may find that a small program in home care flourishes and is subsequently made into a specialized unit. Again, this credentialed practitioner in a health care profession assumes the managerial role. The medical technologist who participates in the development of a nuclear medicine unit and the dietitian who develops a nutrition counseling program for use in outpatient clinics may also find themselves in this position.

Practitioners who develop their own independent professional practices assume the role of manager for their business enterprises. The role of the professional health care practitioner as manager is reinforced further by the various legal, regulatory, and accrediting agencies that often require chiefs of service or department heads to be qualified practitioners in their distinct disciplines. The role of manager then becomes a predictable part of the health care practitioner's tenure in an institution. Table 3–1 shows how activities in a typical workday of a department head in a health care institution reflect the functions of a manager in their classic form.

Table 3–1 The Chief of Service as Manager: Example of Daily Activities

Activity	Management Function Reflected
Readjust staffing pattern for the day because of employee absenteeism	Staffing
Review cases with staff, encouraging staff members	Controlling
to assume greater responsibility	Planning
	Leading/motivating/actuating
Counsel employee with habitual lateness problem	Controlling
	Leading/motivating/actuating
Present departmental quality assurance plan for	Planning
approval of Risk Management/Quality Assurance	Leadership
Committee	
Conduct research to improve treatment techniques	Planning
	Leadership
Dialogue with third-party reimbursement manager	Planning
about coverage for innovative services	Leadership

THE HISTORY OF MANAGEMENT

Knowledge of the history of management provides a framework within which contemporary managerial problems may be reviewed. Modern managers benefit from the experiences of their predecessors. They may assess current problems and plan solutions by using theories that have been developed and tested over time. Contemporary executives may take from past approaches the elements that have been proved successful and seek to integrate them into a unified system of modern management practice.

In an examination of the phases in management history, it must be remembered that history is not completely linear and that any period in history involves a dynamic interplay of components that cannot be separated into distinct elements. The analysis of selected processes of the various historical periods tends to obscure the fact that each period is part of a continuum of events. The specific features of management history phases given here are intended to exemplify the predominant emphasis of each period and are only highlights. The second caution is in regard to dating the various periods. The dates given here are intended as guides. There is no precise day and year when one school of thought or predominant approach began or ended. As with any study of history, the dates suggest approximate periods when the particular practices were developed and applied with sufficient regularity as to constitute a school of management thought or a predominant approach.

Scientific Management

The work of Frederick Taylor (1865–1915) is the commonly accepted basis of scientific management. Taylor started as a day laborer in a steel mill, advanced to foreman, and experienced the struggles of middle management as the workers resisted top executives' efforts to achieve more productivity. He faced the basic question: What is a fair day's work? With Carl G. L. Barth (1860–1939) and Henry L. Gantt (1861–1919), Taylor made a scientific study of workers, machines, and the workplace. These pioneers originated the modern industrial practices of standardization of parts, uniformity of work methods, and the assembly line.

Frank Gilbreth (1868–1924) and Lillian Gilbreth (1878–1972) developed a class of fundamental motions, starting with the therblig (Gilbreth spelled backwards but with the *t* and *h* transposed) as the most basic elemental motion. Lillian Gilbreth may be of particular interest to occupational therapists, since much of her later work concerned the efficiency of physically handicapped women in the management of their homes. Scientific management became an accepted, codified concept as a result of a famous case on railroad rate structures heard by the Interstate Commerce Commission. Louis D. Brandeis, who later became a Supreme Court justice, argued against rate increases by citing the probable effects of the application of "scientific management."[4] The concept emerged as the predominant approach to management during this era. It continues to be a basis for continuous improvement in productivity and cost containment.

The Behavioralists and the Human Relations Approach

Although the major figures in the development of scientific management emphasized the work rather than the worker, concern for the latter was apparent. Lillian Gilbreth, for example, was a psychologist and tended to stress the needs of the employee. Frank Gilbreth developed a model promotion plan that emphasized regular meetings between the employee and the individual responsible for evaluating the employee's work.

Unlike adherents of the scientific management approach, who considered the worker only secondarily, behavioralists focused primarily on the worker. The application of the behavioral sciences to worker productivity and interaction was exemplified in the Hawthorne Experiments conducted by Elton Mayo and F. J. Roethlisberger at Western Electric's Hawthorne Works. Through these studies, the importance of the informal group and the social and motivational needs of workers were recognized. The behavioral science and the human relations approaches may be linked because both emphasize the worker's social and psychological needs, and stress group dynamics, psychology, and sociology. Theorists associated with these approaches include Douglas MacGregor, Rensis Likert, and Chris Argyris. The Deming approach, with its emphasis on quality circles, and total quality management, with a highly participative style of management, is a contemporary example of the human relations approach. A more recent expression of this emphasis is reflected in the appreciative inquiry method of assessing the strengths of an organization.

Structuralism

Since work is done within specific organizational patterns and since the worker-superior roles imply authority relationships, the structure or framework within which these patterns and relationships occur has been studied. Structuralism is based on Max Weber's theory of bureaucracy or formal organization. Robert K. Merton, Philip Selznik, and Peter Blau, major theorists in the structuralist school of thought, gave particular attention to line and staff relationships, authority structure, the decision-making process, and the effect of organizational life on the individual worker.

The Management Process School

The special emphasis in the management process approach is on the various functions that the manager performs as a continuous process. Henri Fayol (1841–1925), a contemporary of Taylor, studied the work of the chief executive and is credited with having developed the basic principles or "laws" that are associated with management functions. His writings did not become readily available in English until 1939 when James D. Mooney and A. C. Reiley published a classification and integrated analysis of the principles of management, including Fayol's concepts.[5] Chester Barnard could be considered a member of this school of thought in that he explored the basic processes and functions of management, including the universality of these elements.

The Quantitative or Operations Research Approach

Problem solving and decision making with the aid of mathematical models and the use of probability and statistical inference characterize the quantitative or operations research approach to management. Also called the management science school, this approach includes the various quantitative approaches to executive processes and is characterized by an interdisciplinary systems approach. The urgency of the problems in World War II and in the space program speeded the development of mathematical models and computer technology for problem solving and decision making.

The Six Sigma approach to continuous quality improvement relies on statistical analysis as one of its main elements of analysis of organizational performance.

THE SYSTEMS APPROACH

Each school of management thought tends to emphasize one major feature of an organization:

1. Scientific management focuses on work.
2. Human relations and behavioralism stress the worker and the worker-manager relationship.
3. Structuralism emphasizes organizational design.
4. Management process theory focuses on the functions of the manager.
5. Management science theory adds computer technology to the scientific method.

The search for a management method that takes into account each of these essential features led to the systems approach. This focuses on the organization as a whole, its internal and external components, the people in the organization, the work processes, and the overall organizational environment.

Historical Development of the Systems Model

The systems model is generally accepted in the area of computer technology, but its use need not be limited to such an application; at its origin, it was not so restricted. A more flexible use of this approach provides the manager with a framework within which the internal and external organizational factors can be visualized. The systems approach to management emphasizes the total environment of the organization. The cycle consisting of input, transformation to output, and renewed input can be identified for the organization or for any of its divisions. The changes in organizational environment can be assessed continually in a structured manner to determine the impact of change.

Management theorists turned to biologists and other scientists to develop the idea of the organization as a total system. With this ecological approach, a change in any one aspect of the environment is believed to have an effect on the other components of the organization. The specifics are analyzed, but always in terms of the whole. The institution is considered an entity that "lives" in a specific environment and has essential parts that are interdependent.

General systems theory as a concept was introduced and defined by Ludwig von Bertalanffy, a biologist, in 1951.[6] His terminology is the foundation for the basic concepts of the general systems theory.[7] Kenneth E. Boulding developed a hierarchy of systems to help bridge the gap between theoretical and empirical systems knowledge. He noted that the general systems approach furnished a framework or skeleton for all science but that each discipline, including management science, must apply the model, add the flesh and blood of its own subject matter, and develop this analytical model further. Included in Boulding's hierarchy of systems is the concept of the open system and the idea of the social organization with role sets.[8]

Many contemporary studies of various aspects of organizations are based on the systems model. Areas of specific application include

- *cybernetics*—the science of communication and control[9]
- *data-processing systems*—systems used to guide the flow of information, usually by means of computer technology
- *rhochrematics*—the science of managing material flow, including production and marketing, transporting, processing, handling, storing, and distributing goods[10]
- *network analysis*—the process of planning and scheduling (e.g., PERT [program evaluative review technique] networks and the critical path method)
- *administrative systems*—the planned approach to activities necessary to attain desired objectives

Basic Systems Concepts and Definitions

A system may be defined as an assemblage or combination of things or parts forming a complex or unitary whole, a set of interacting units. The essential focus of the systems approach is the relationship and interdependence of the parts. The systems approach moves beyond structure or function (e.g., organization charts, departmentation) to emphasize the flow of information, the work, the inputs, and the outputs. Systems add horizontal relationships to the vertical relationships contained in traditional organizational theory.

The systems model is made up of four basic components: (1) inputs, (2) throughputs or processes, (3) outputs, and (4) feedback (Figure 3–2). The overall environment also must be considered.

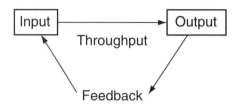

FIGURE 3–2 Basic Systems Model

The Nature of Inputs

Inputs are elements the system must accept because they are imposed by outside forces. The many constraints on organizational processes, such as government regulation and economic factors, are typical inputs imposed by outside groups. Certain inputs are needed in order to achieve the organizational goals; for example, the inputs often are the raw materials that are processed to produce some object or service. The concept of inputs may be expanded to include the demands made on the system, such as deadlines, priorities, or conflicting pressures. Goodwill toward the organization, general support, or the lack of these also may be included as inputs.

A systematic review of inputs for a health care organization or one of its departments could include

- *characteristics of clients*— average length of stay, diagnostic categories, payment status
- *legal and accrediting agency requirements*—federal conditions of participation for Medicare programs, institutional licensure, and licensure or certification of health care practitioners
- *federal and state laws concerning employers*—collective bargaining legislation, the Occupational Safety and Health Act, Workers' Compensation, Civil Rights Act
- *multiple goals*—patient care, teaching, research

The Nature of Outputs

Outputs are the goods and services that the organization (or subdivision or unit) must produce. These outputs may be routine, frequent, predictable, and somewhat easy to identify. The stated purpose of the organization usually contains information on its basic, obvious outputs. For example, a fire department provides fire protection, a hospital offers patient care, a department store sells goods, a factory produces goods, and an airline supplies transportation. Managers control routine and predictable outputs through proper planning.

Other necessary outputs are infrequent but predictable. By careful analysis of organizational data over a relatively long time period, these infrequent outputs can usually be identified. For example, hospitals or programs are reaccredited periodically, and plans can be made for the reaccreditation process because it is predictable. An organization that is tied directly to political sponsorship could take the cycle of presidential and congressional elections into account. Again, proper planning through identification and anticipation of such special periodic demands on the system leads to greater control and, consequently, stability.

Most managers face a third category: the nonpredictable outputs for which they can and must plan. Certain demands on the system are made with sufficient regularity that, although the exact number and time cannot be calculated, estimates can be made. This is an essential aspect of proper planning and controlling. In an outpatient clinic, for example, the number of walk-in and/or emergency patients is not predictable. In order to plan for these relatively random demands on the system, the manager studies the pattern of walk-in patients, their times of arrival, and the purposes of their visits. Some patient education would probably be done to help clients take advantage of orderly scheduling. Staffing patterns would be adjusted to meet the anticipated needs. The planning is designed to shift the nonpredictable to the predictable as far as possible. Other examples of nonpredictable outputs for which plans can be developed include telephone calls, employee turnover rates, and even activities required by certain kinds of seasonal disasters (e.g., tornadoes or hurricanes) or by seasonal changes in the numbers and types of clients (e.g., in a resort area).

Some outputs are unexpected, such as those that become necessary because of natural disasters or sudden economic chaos. Even in these instances, managers can anticipate and plan for Armageddon in any of its symbolic or real forms. Disaster planning, for example, is a required part of institutional health care management. The renewed emphasis on disaster planning in light of bioterrorism or other major political-social disruption has added an urgency to such planning in contemporary times.

Some outputs for health care institutions are

- maintenance of accreditation and licensure status
- compliance with special federal programs concerning quality assurance or health care planning
- provision of acute care services for medical, surgical, obstetric, and pediatric patients

- provision of comprehensive wellness and preventive health services for clients in a specific area

Outputs in health care institutions may be refined even further by adding specific time factors, quality factors, or other statements of expected performance:

- 100 percent follow-up on all patients who fail to keep appointments
- processing of specified laboratory tests within ten hours of receipt of specimen
- retrieval of patient medical record from permanent file within seven minutes of receipt of request

It may be useful to group outputs with the related inputs by formulating input/output statements. It should be noted, however, that not every input generates a direct output; there is no one-to-one relationship of inputs to outputs. It may be necessary to consider a cluster of inputs in relation to a single output. For example, the goal (output) of retrieving the medical record of a patient who enters the walk-in clinic without an appointment may require considerations (inputs) of accuracy of identification, chart availability, and delivery system procedures.

Throughputs (Withinputs)

Throughputs are the structures or processes by which inputs are converted to outputs. Physical plant, work flow, methods and procedures, and hours of work are throughputs. Inputs originate in the environment of the organization; throughputs, as the term implies, are contained within the organization. Throughputs are analyzed by work sampling, work simplification, methods improvement, staffing patterns, and physical layout analysis.

Managers may be severely limited in their ability to control inputs, but the processes, structures, organizational patterns, and procedures that constitute the throughputs are normally areas of management prerogative. For example, a chief of service cannot control patient arrivals for walk-in service in a clinic; this input is imposed on the system. The policies and procedures for processing walk-in patients, however, constitute a cluster of throughputs that can be determined by the manager. The physical space allotment for a department may be imposed; the manager must accept this input, but the final and detailed physical layout of the department is under the manager's control.

In a specialized service, the control of throughputs is directly related to the manager's professional knowledge. For example, procedures for processing patient flow within a clinic are developed by the chief of service because of that person's knowledge of patient care procedures, priorities, and the interrelationships among components of the treatment plan. The policies and procedures for the release of information from patients' health records are aspects of highly technical processes that are the domain of the professional health information specialist.

In some cases, elements that theoretically belong to the throughput category are considered inputs. These are elements that are imposed by the environment (i.e., the organization as a whole). Managers may not be able to exert direct control over some aspects of the work (e.g., in the case of physical space limitations, budget cuts, and personnel vacancies), and these elements could be listed as special inputs.

Feedback

Changes in the input mix must be anticipated. In order to respond to these changes, managers need feedback on the acceptability and adequacy of the outputs. It is through the feedback process that inputs and even throughputs are adjusted to produce new outputs. The communication network and control processes are the usual sources of organized feedback. Routine, orderly feedback is provided by such activities as market research and forecasting in business organizations, client surveys in service organizations, periodic accreditation surveys in health care institutions, periodic employee evaluations in work groups, and periodic testing and grading in an educational system. The management by objectives process, short interval scheduling, and program evaluation review technique (PERT) networks constitute specific management tools of planning and controlling that include structured, factual feedback.

If there is an absence of planned feedback, if the communication process is not sufficiently developed to permit safe and acceptable avenues for feedback, or if the feedback actually received is ignored, a certain amount of feedback will occur spontaneously. In this case, the feedback tends to take a negative form, such as a client outburst of anger, a precipitous lawsuit, a riot, a wildcat strike, a consumer boycott, or an epidemic. Spontaneous feedback could take a positive form, of course, such as the acclamation of a hero or leader after a crisis or an unsolicited letter of satisfaction from a client.

Some feedback is tacit, and the manager may assume that since there is no overt evidence to the contrary, all outputs are fine. The danger in such an assumption is that problems and difficulties may not come to light until a crisis occurs. The planning process is undermined because there are no reliable data that can be used to assess the impact of change and to implement the necessary adjustments.

Closed Systems versus Open Systems

Systems may be classified as either closed or open. An ideal closed system is complete within itself. No new inputs are received, and there is no change in the components; there is no output of energy in any of its forms (e.g., information or material). Few, if any, response or adaptation systems are needed because such a closed system is isolated from external forces in its environment and internal change is self-adjusting. Examples of closed systems include a chemical reaction taking place in a sealed, insulated container; a sealed terrarium; and a thermostat. In certain approaches to organizational theory, organizations have been viewed as closed systems—that is, the emphasis has been placed on the study of functions and structure within the organization without consideration of its environment and the consequent effect of environmental change on its processes.

An open system is in a constant state of flux. Inputs are received and outputs produced. There is input and output of both matter and energy, continual adaptation to the environment, and, usually, an increase of order and complexity, with differentiation of parts over time.

An open system constantly seeks internal balance, or homeostasis, by means of an adjustive function of stimulus-response. A change in the organizational environment (stimulus) makes it necessary to take some action (response) to maintain this balance. Notterman and Trumbull, using a laboratory model, noted three processes necessary for a system to maintain this self-regulating cycle:[11]

1. *Detection.* For regulation to take place, the disparity between the disturbed and normal (or desired) state must be detectable by the organism. Obviously, if the organism cannot sense a disturbance (perceptually or physiologically), measures cannot be taken for its correction. Equally apparent is the fact that individuals vary in both the quality and quantity of information they require in order to detect a disturbance.
2. *Identification.* The disparity must also be identified. Corrective action cannot be specific unless a given disturbance is successfully discriminated from other possible disturbances. Here again, individual differences in the form and quantity of information necessary for identification undoubtedly exist.
3. *Response Availability.* Upon detection and identification of the disturbance, the organism must be permitted by environmental, physiological, or laboratory conditions to make the correction.

The management functions of decision making, leadership, and, particularly, correction of deviation from organizational goals are necessary for the detection, identification, and proper response to changes in the organization's environment.

In the open system, the adjustment to the environmental change is made through the input-output cycle and the development of appropriate feedback mechanisms. Another major management function, then, becomes the systematic monitoring of change.

All living organisms have the capacity for maximum disorder, disintegration, and death. This tendency toward disintegration is termed *entropy*. The open system is characterized by the continual striving for negative entropy (negentropy). It tries to overcome disintegration by taking into itself more inputs or higher-level inputs (i.e., whatever it needs to produce the required outputs). Obvious examples of this include a bear storing body fat and changing its metabolism for winter hibernation or the human body building up immunity. In the management context, an organization may build a reserve of money or client goodwill against potential hard times.

Application of General Systems Theory

The systems approach enables managers to focus on the organization as a whole and to view each particular division or unit in the organization in relation to the whole. Through the systems approach, managers can cut across organizational lines to determine interrelationships in the work flow and to assess complexities in the structure and in the environment of the organization. Their attention is drawn to changes in the environment that affect the organization and its units. Managers are aided in their analysis of the organization because the input-output model frees them of personal bias toward or attachment to the existing mode of operations. Furthermore, the classic functions of a manager, which are carried out in the distinct, unique environment of a given organization, are reflected in the systems approach. Table 3–2 summarizes this interrelationship. The remainder of this presentation of management principles is developed in the context of specific functions of the manager carried out in an overall organizational environment. Since the functions of the manager are shaped and modified by the particular organizational environment, the tools for analyzing the organization will be presented first, followed by detailed discussion of individual management functions.

VIEWING THE WORK ORGANIZATION AS A TOTAL SYSTEM

There is considerable social evidence to support the basic observation that humans form groups: families, clans, neighborhoods, churches, political parties, businesses, fraternities, work groups, professional associations. The study of these groups as

Table 3–2 Relationship of Classic Management Functions and Systems Concepts

Systems Concept	Predominant Management Function
Input analysis	
Identification of constraints	
Assessment of client characteristics	Planning
Assessment of physical space	
Budget allocation analysis	
Throughput determination	
Development of policies, procedures, methods	Planning and controlling
Development of detailed departmental layout	
Specification of staffing pattern	Staffing
Methods of worker productivity enhancement	Controlling, leadership, and motivation
Output analysis	
Goal formulation	Planning
Statement of objectives	
Development of management by objectives plan	Planning and controlling
Feedback mechanisms	Controlling, communicating, and
Development of feedback processes	resolving conflict
Adjustment of inputs and outputs in light of feedback	Renewing planning cycle
Adjustment of internal throughputs	

social organizations is the proper domain of the social scientist; their study as formal organizations is the proper focus of administrative analysis.

The successful manager recognizes the impact of the organizational environment on clients, members of the organization, and the public at large as well as on the manager's specific role. An organization does not exist in a static world; rather, it is in a continual state of transaction with its environment. As an open system, the organization receives inputs from its environment—acts on them and is acted on by them, and produces outputs, such as goods and services (and even organizational survival, which can be considered an essential output). Consequently, the organizational environment consists of both internal and external components. The specific functions of the manager are modified by the organizational environment (i.e., the specific attributes of the given work setting). Classical organizational theory provides the manager with concepts to assess the organizational environment. The organizational environment may be assessed by an examination of its characteristics and components through a typology of organizations, a review of the organizational life cycle, and an analysis of the purpose and functions of organizations. The use of clientele network and systems models yields further information about the internal and external components of the organizational environment. Managers may anticipate organizational conflict when stated purposes or goals and actual practices become disparate; such an occurrence should alert managers to changes in the organizational environment so that they can develop an anticipatory response rather than a reactive response.

FORMAL VERSUS INFORMAL ORGANIZATIONS

An organization is a basic social unit that has been established for the purpose of achieving a goal. A formal organization is characterized by several distinct features:

- a common goal; an accepted pattern of purpose
- a set of shared values or common beliefs that give individuals a sense of identification and belonging
- continuity of goal-oriented interaction
- a division of labor deliberately planned to achieve the goal
- a system of authority or a chain of command to achieve conscious integration of the group and conscious coordination of efforts to reach the goal

An informal organization may be characterized by some of the features of formal organizations, but it lacks one or more of these features. Individuals who share a common value may meet regularly to foster some goal, and this group may become a recognizable formal organization. Some informal groups never develop the consistent characteristics of a formal organization, however, and simply remain informal.

Formal organizations almost inevitably give rise to informal organizations. Such informal groups may be viewed as spontaneous organizations that emerge because individuals are brought together in a common workplace to pursue a common goal, which makes social interaction inescapable. Informal organizations arise as a means of easing the restrictions of formal structures, as in the cooperative communication and coordination that may occur outside of the officially mandated channels of authority. Through an informal organization's communication network, an individual may gain valuable information that supplements or clarifies the formal communications. Also, informal groups help to integrate individuals into the organization and socialize them to accept their specific organizational roles. A manager must remain aware of the existence and composition of the informal groups in the organization so that their functioning affects the formal structure in positive rather than negative ways.

CLASSIFICATION OF ORGANIZATIONS

When an organization's managers understand and accept its nature, organizational conflict can be reduced and organizational viability increased, because the managers function in a manner consistent with the type of organization shaping the interactions. Personal conflict can be reduced. Should an individual be unwilling or unable to accept certain aspects of a particular organizational type, that individual may decide to move to a different organizational climate. For example, if an individual practitioner prefers not to function in a highly structured, bureaucratic setting, it is better to recognize this before accepting employment in a government-sponsored health care institution. An individual who believes that health care should not be "for profit" would do well to seek employment in health care settings that are not predicated on the business model. An individual may gain an insight into the climate of a particular organization through the use of organizational classifications based on prime beneficiary, authority structure, and genotypic characteristics.

Prime Beneficiary

Peter Blau and W. R. Scott presented a classification of organizations based on the prime beneficiary.[12] Their suggested model for the analysis of organizations focuses on this question: Who benefits from the existence of the organization? Four types of organizations result from the application of this criterion.[13]

1. mutual benefit associations, where the members are the prime beneficiaries; examples include a professional association, a credit union, and a collective bargaining unit
2. business concerns, where the owners are the prime beneficiaries
3. service organizations, where the clients are the prime beneficiaries
4. commonweal organizations, where the public at large is the prime beneficiary; police and fire departments are examples of commonweal organizations

Managers may formulate goals, establish priorities, and monitor activities to determine the effectiveness of the organization in meeting the needs of the prime beneficiary. Actions that do not foster such goals are eliminated and proper priorities formulated. Because the clients are the prime beneficiaries of a service organization, decisions about hours of service, the scope of services offered, and similar matters are made with the needs of clients in mind. In health care, the growing development of home care, flexible hours in outpatient care clinics, and alternatives to full hospitalization are attempts at meeting the needs of the prime beneficiaries, the patients and their families. At the same time, health care worker units involved in collective bargaining can be considered mutual benefit associations. Managers in health care settings must balance the demands made by both types of organizational forms within one organization.

Authority Structure

The organizational environment can also be classified according to the modes of authority that are operative in the institution. Managers must adopt leadership styles, develop procedures and methods for worker interaction, and determine client interactions in a manner that is consistent with the predominant authority structure. Health care organizations tend to embody more than one pattern of authority structure; for example, there are few limits on the activities of professional staff and greater limits on the activities of semiskilled and unskilled workers. The work of Amatai Etzioni provides a typology of organizations based on the authority structure predominant in the institution.[14] The classification that results from this approach may be summarized as follows:

1. predominantly coercive authority: prisons, concentration camps, custodial mental institutions, or coercive unions
2. predominantly utilitarian, rational-legal authority: use of economic rewards; businesses, industry, unions, and the military in peacetime
3. predominantly normative authority: use of membership, status, intrinsic values; religious organizations, universities, professional associations, mutual benefit associations, fraternal and philanthropic associations
4. mixed structures: normative-coercive (e.g., combat units); utilitarian-normative (e.g., most labor unions); utilitarian-coercive (e.g., some early industries, some farms, company towns, ships)

Genotypic Characteristics

Like the prime beneficiary concept, the classification of organizations by genotype is based on an analysis of their fundamental roots and purposes. Daniel Katz and Robert Kahn viewed organizations as subsystems of the larger society that carry out basic functions of that larger society. These basic functions are the focal point in this system of classification. The typology of organizations developed by Katz and Kahn is based on genotypes, or first-order characteristics: What is the most basic function that the organization carries out in terms of society?[15] These first-order, basic functions are as follows:

1. *productive or economic functions*—the creation of wealth or goods as occurs in businesses

2. *maintenance of society*—the socialization and general care of people as occurs in education, training, indoctrination, and health care

3. *adaptive functions*—the creation of knowledge as occurs in universities and
as a result of research and artistic endeavors

4. *managerial/political functions*—adjudication and coordination functions and
control of resources and people as occur in court systems, police departments, political parties, interest groups, and government agencies

The charter, articles of incorporation, and statement of purpose are official
documents of the organization that can be used to classify the organization according to this typology.

Goal statements are derived and priorities set in terms of primary function. Managers can monitor organizational change when the actual function performed differs from the stated function. When a social service agency spends a great deal of
effort determining eligibility of patients for service under a variety of government
programs, it is assuming some of the characteristics of a managerial/political organization. Sometimes this adjudication interferes with the delivery of the health
care service; managers must make decisions in the light of this conflict. If priority is given to research and education over direct patient care, the health care practitioner must again come to terms with the true nature of the organization.

CLASSIFICATION OF HEALTH CARE ORGANIZATIONS

When a health care organization is classified according to these typologies, the complexity of the setting becomes apparent. Classification by prime beneficiary offers
several possibilities. In terms of direct patient care, for example, the health care
organization can be classified as a typical service organization. On the other hand,
if it is a for-profit institution, classification as a business organization is more appropriate. If the health care organization has a mixed goal, as does a teaching hospital associated with a medical school, it can be defined as a service organization
with respect to its clients—both the physicians to be educated and the patients to
be treated. The potentially conflicting priorities of teaching and direct patient care
underlie the selection of patients for treatment, however; preference may be given
to those patients who are "interesting" cases for teaching purposes. Even when a
health care institution is not directly associated with a medical school, a variety of
clinical affiliation arrangements may be developed to meet the needs of such practitioners as occupational and physical therapists, medical technologists, social work-

ers, health information administrators, dietitians, and other groups that require clinical practice as part of their educational sequence. In developing goal statements for a department, the chief of service must keep this secondary goal in mind.

A health care organization also is a commonweal organization insofar as it protects the public interest in matters of general community health, such as the benefits of the facility's research efforts for the public at large. Health care institutions also offer a variety of free health-monitoring programs as a means of fostering health maintenance in the community.

Etzioni included the hospital as an example of normative authority structure. This point could be argued, however, depending on the focus of organizational analysis. Professional staff members tend to function in the normative mode; their codes of ethics, their professional training, and the general level of behavior expected of them modify individual participation in the organization as much as, if not more than, the formal bylaws and contractual arrangements. In this sense, the normative authority structure predominates. When the health care organization is viewed from another perspective, it seems to function more as a mixed normative-utilitarian structure. With business orientation and the increasing unionization of workers in the health care field, the utilitarian model seems to be a more appropriate category.

A coercive element is sometimes introduced into the health care setting, as when individuals are assigned to health care jobs in wartime as an alternative to military service or when hospital volunteer work is given as part of a court sentence. In such cases, a mix of normative-utilitarian-coercive authority is required and the manager must adopt a variety of leadership and motivational styles in working with the different groups in the organization. Worker or member motivation and the source of the manager's authority differ for these different groups.

In the Katz and Kahn genotypic classification, the health care organization fits two categories, again indicating the mixed mandates of such entities. As an organization concerned with restoration, the health care establishment functions to maintain society. It also performs adaptive functions when higher education and research are major goals.

CLASSIC BUREAUCRACY

Bureaucracy is such a common aspect of organizational life that it is often treated as synonymous with formal organization. The study of bureaucracy in its pure form was the work of the structuralists in management history: Max Weber, Peter Blau and W. Richard Scott, and Robert K. Merton. Weber's work is pivotal, since it presented the chief characteristics of bureaucracy in its pure form. Weber regarded the bureaucratic form as an ideal type and described the theoretically perfect organization.[16] In effect, he codified the major characteristics of formal organizations in which rational decision making and administrative efficiency are maximized. He did not include the dysfunctional aspects or the aberrations that occur when any characteristics are exaggerated, as in the popular equation of bureaucracy with "red tape." From the works of Weber and others, a composite set of characteristics or descriptive statements may be derived concerning the formal organization or bureaucracy.

1. Size
   a. large scale of operations, large number of clients, high volume of work, and wide geographical dispersion
   b. communication beyond face-to-face, personal interaction
2. Division of labor
   a. systematic division of labor
   b. clear limits and boundaries of work units
3. Specialization
   a. a result of division of labor
   b. each unit's pursuit of its goal without conflict because of clear boundaries
   c. areas of specialization and division of labor that correspond with official jurisdictional areas
   d. specific sphere of competence for each incumbent
   e. promotion of staff expertise
   f. technical qualifications for officeholders
4. Official jurisdictional areas
   a. fixed by rules, laws, or administrative regulation
   b. specific official duties for each office
5. Rational-legal authority
   a. formal authority attached to the official position or office
   b. authority delegated in a stable way
   c. clear rules delineating the use of authority
   d. depersonalization of office; emphasis on the position, not the person
6. Principle of hierarchy
   a. firmly ordered system of supervision and subordination
   b. each lower office or position under the control and supervision of a higher one
   c. systematic checking and reinforcing of compliance

7. Rules
   a. providing continuity of operations
   b. promoting stability, regardless of changing personnel
   c. routinizing the work
   d. generating "red tape"
8. Impersonality
   a. impersonal orientation by officials
   b. emphasis on the rules and regulations
   c. disregard of personal considerations in clients and employees
   d. rational judgments free of personal feeling
   e. social distance among successive levels of the hierarchy
   f. social distance from clients
9. The bureaucrat
   a. career with system of promotion to reward loyalty and service
   b. special training required because of specialization, division of labor, or technical rules
   c. separation of manager from owner
   d. compensation by salaries, not dependent on direct payment by clients
10. The bureau (or office or administrative unit)
    a. formulation and recording of all administrative acts, decisions, and rules
    b. enhancement of systematic interpretation of norms and enforcement of rules
    c. written documents, equipment, and support staff employed to maintain records
    d. office management based on expert, specialized training
    e. physical property, equipment, and supplies clearly separate from personal belongings and domicile of the officeholder

These characteristics are interwoven, each flowing from the others; for example, the growing size necessitates a division of labor, which, in turn, fosters specialization.

One of the dreams of many direct patient care practitioners is a health care delivery system that does not become bogged down in formalities. The private practice model seems to offer the solution; if the private practice or small group practice flourishes, however, the characteristics of formal organizations inevitably begin to emerge—for example, specialization and division of labor, procedures for uniformity, some form of authority structure, and a variety of rules. The wisest approach seems to involve taking the best features of formal bureaucracy and making particular efforts to avoid the negative elements, such as impersonality. Family-centered approaches to health care or the team approach are models that tend to offset the impersonalization associated with large health care organizations.

CONSEQUENCES OF ORGANIZATIONAL FORM

Managers work in specific organizational environments, and their specific functions are shaped and modified by the organizational form, structure, and authority climate. Some specific consequences concern the following organizational characteristics:

- *Size.* The more layers in the hierarchy, the greater (potentially) the limits on managers' freedom in decision making. Their decisions may be subject to review at several levels, and more decisions may be imposed from these higher levels.
- *Organizational Climate.* The degree to which clients, workers, and other managers participate in planning and decision-making processes is determined in part by the authority climate. Managers may have to modify their management or leadership style if it is inconsistent with the organization's authority structure. The basis of motivation may vary. In the highly normative setting, for example, members willingly participate; in the coercive organization, the basis of motivation tends to rest on the avoidance of punishment.
- *Degree of Bureaucracy.* A highly bureaucratic organization may be associated with great predictability in routine practices but less innovation and more resistance to change. Efforts to offset distortion caused by layering in communication may constitute a large portion of the activities of a manager in a highly bureaucratic organization.
- *Phase in the Life Cycle.* The openness to innovation and the vigorous, aggressive undertakings through goal expansion and multiplication that characterize some stages of the life cycle may permit the manager to undertake a variety of activities that are precluded by concerns for organizational survival in other phases of the life cycle.

For these reasons, managers must assess the organizational setting and their own roles. The major concepts of the clientele network, organizational life cycle, and analysis of organizational goals are tools for such assessments. Their active use fosters in the manager an awareness of the overall organizational dynamics that shape managerial practice, worker interaction, and client services.

THE CLIENTELE NETWORK

Managers must devote constant attention to the web of relationships reflecting the needs and interests of individuals and groups both internal and external to the organization. Common terms used to describe these relationships include critical partners, stakeholders, champions, super-users, or communities of interest.

A major charge given implicitly to any manager is the building of external relationships and developing a framework for partnership. This framework connects the people of the organization with one another, and with the larger communities of interest. In order to do this, the manager must identify critical relationships, develop satisfactory working relationships with the several key individuals and groups involved, and, finally, work at maintaining these relationships. With the conservation of organizational resources, time, money, and personnel as a mandate, the manager seeks to capitalize on available external sources of power, influence, advice, and support as well as to identify those areas of potential difficulty, such as competition and rivalry, erosion of client goodwill, and shifting client demand and loyalty. In an era of increasing regulation of health care, the contemporary manager in the health care setting must identify and comply with multiple sets of changing regulations and guidelines issued by federal and state government agencies as well as by the various accrediting agencies, such as the Joint Commission or the American Osteopathic Association.

Like a living organism, an organization exists in a dynamic environment to which it must continually adapt. The manager identifies these units and constructs a network of the pattern of interrelationships. Bertram Gross developed the concept of the clientele network, noting that any organization is usually surrounded by a complex array of people, units, and other organizations that interrelate with it on the basis of various roles. He called these people, units, and organizations the "publics with opinions."[17]

Wherever the concept of organization is used, a department manager could well substitute individual service or department. Although such a department or service is obviously a part of the organization, the development of the clientele network for a unit within the organization yields information about the critical relationships, clients, adversaries, and supporters of that department. Department-level managers must be aware of the unique environment of their department or service as well as the overall environment of their organization.

CLIENTS

The most obvious and immediate individuals and groups who make significant demands on the organization are the clients. Gross used the term in a broad sense—that is, to refer to those for whom goods and services are provided by the organization.[18] Immediate, visible clients in health care, both for the organization and for any department directly involved in patient care services, are the patients.

The providers of direct health care services are immediate, visible clients for certain units within the organizations. The business office, the legal staff, and the health information service offer support services to assist physicians, nurses, and social workers in the provision of patient care. Given the traditional and historical development of the modern hospital, it could be said that the physicians are a special class of clients in that the organization of the hospital or clinic gives them the necessary support personnel and services for patient care. Physicians in different specialties are clients of each other, since they depend on each other for consultative services and referrals.

Certain services may be placed into the client category vis-à-vis each other. Some service units, such as physical therapy, are income producing; because the resources obtained are used on behalf of the whole organization, other units may be considered clients of the income-producing units. The business office relies on the health information service to supply certain documentation to satisfy financial claims, and the safety committee relies on the several patient care and administrative departments to supply the information necessary to perform its function.

The use of the broadest possible definition of client alerts the manager to the subtle facets of organizational relationships. The manager who recognizes the number of distinct client groups can more effectively monitor their several and sometimes conflicting demands for services.

Although one step removed from the immediate services or goods offered by the organization, less visible clients are nonetheless legitimate users of the services or goods. By identifying these secondary clients, the manager has a key to the primary and secondary goals of the organization or unit. In the many educational programs offered within health care organizations, for example, the sponsoring institutions (e.g., a college or university), the health professionals, and the technical students are secondary, less visible clients. Hospitals traditionally have direct patient care as a primary goal, with teaching and research as secondary goals. The ordering of priorities should stem from recognition of the multilevel client demands.

The same physicians who are immediate clients in terms of their need for support services for their direct patient care activities are less visible clients in terms of their need for opportunities for education and research. The employees of the organizations are, in a sense, less visible clients, since one of the organizational outputs is the provision of jobs. Occasionally in health care the provision of jobs is an explicit goal; the neighborhood health centers sponsored by the federal government were intended not only to provide health care services but also to afford job opportunities to area residents.

The clients twice removed from the immediate goal of the organization may be termed the remote clients. Many of these individuals and groups do not even know they are being served. In addition to patient care, teaching, and research, a third goal of health care organizations is generally given as the protection of the public at large, that is, remote clients.

The manager, in assessing the stated and implied goals, may readily identify them by analyzing the needs of primary, visible clients as well as those of the less visible and remote clients. If the client demand is relatively stable, the planning, organizing, and staffing needs may be assessed in a stable manner. The net effect is efficiency in the allocation of resources of money, space, and personnel.

There is within the client group a potential capacity to control the organization. When a business has only one major purchaser of its goods or an agency has only one group to serve, the clients could easily take charge of the organization, limiting its independence. On the other hand, the organization with multiple clients must set priorities, balance conflicting demands, and maneuver so as to satisfy several groups.

The manager maintains continuous awareness of potential new clients and their needs; for example, the ever-growing leisure culture and amateur sports creates an increased need for physical therapy services. The aging of the "baby boomer" population and increased longevity lead to an increase in the need for such services as subacute care, caregiver support groups, and adult respite care. Managers reach out to such potential clients in a variety of ways such as participating in community-sponsored events (e.g., blood drives, weight loss seminars, preventive health initiatives). Managers get involved with the many support groups (e.g., kidney disease, breast cancer, arthritis), offering space for meetings and presenting educational lectures.

SUPPLIERS

Three categories of suppliers are given by Gross: (1) resource suppliers, (2) associates, and (3) supporters.[19]

Resource Suppliers

Since no organization is totally self-sufficient, it must take into itself the necessary resources, raw material, money, and goodwill that it needs to survive and function. In this sense, the organization is the client of other organizations.

Within the given organization, one department or service is the supplier of another. In assessing work flow patterns, this concept is useful in identifying which aspects of the work are within the unit's immediate control and which originate in one or several other departments. The health information service is the client of several other units in this sense. The proper gathering of patient identification information is the work of the several admissions and intake units; a health information department is dependent on these units for that part of the work flow. Resource suppliers, such as the clinic secretary, control the patient health record at the time of a patient's discharge; consequently, its timely receipt in the health information service after discharge is somewhat dependent on that unit's work flow. A centralized, computerized data processing system is dependent in the same way. The laboratory, radiology department, physical therapy department, and occupational therapy department all depend on the nursing service to bring, send, or prepare the patient so that they can proceed with their own work in a predictable manner. Essential information for the formulation of job descriptions concerning interdepartmental relationships or for the development of cross-training programs within the organization is obtained from an awareness of those organizational components that act as resource suppliers to each other.

In the same sense, the chief executive officer can be seen as a resource supplier, making the final adjudication in the allocation of space, money, and personnel to the units. The manager of the department or service should know the needs of other departments and should develop strategic alliances in the competition for scarce resources.

Resource suppliers are often external to the organization. Companies making specialty products or offering specialty services have a unique relationship to the health care organization. Such suppliers may be limited in number; in fact, there may be only one such supplier in a geographic area. The viability of such an organization is of interest and concern for the manager who relies on these products or services. Furthermore, with the implementation of such federal regulations as

HIPAA and with issues relating to risk management, the health care organization which contracts with one or another such resource supplier needs to work with that resource supplier to ensure that they, too, follow the specific regulations. These include policies, procedures, and safeguards relating to patient privacy and confidentiality. Chain of trust agreements are required for organizations dealing directly with patient care information (such as an outsourced transcription service or a medical billing service). The health care manager will attend to the quality of products and services from external sources because these become part of the services offered by the health care organization.

Managers take opportunities to partner with resource suppliers in special project development. For example, health information educators work with vendors to create virtual laboratory modules for use in educational institutions as well as for in-service training in health care settings. Another example is found in the partnerships of university-based departments of physical and rehabilitation medicine and the PALS (Promotion of Amputee Life Skills) research and training program.

Associates

Individuals or groups outside the organization who work cooperatively with the organization in a joint effort are associates of the organization.[20] Associates have a common interest and common work that unites them with the organization. The manager who recognizes the efforts of associates will actively obtain their cooperation. Through informal sharing of ideas among themselves, the various health care practitioners frequently act as associates to one another. The health information practitioners from several area hospitals may collaborate informally on a release of information policy so that there is area-wide consistency in dealing with requests for data from patient records. The AHIMA-sponsored communities of practice and related sharing of best practices is yet another example of associate activity. The medical technologists of a region may cooperate in a joint venture for blood-banking processes. The Joint Position Statement on Health Information Confidentiality, developed by the American Medical Informatics Association and the American Health Information Management Association, is yet another example of associate interaction.

Supporters

Various politically, socially, and economically powerful individuals and groups in the society may be supporters of the organization. They mobilize "friendly power" for the organization, giving it encouragement and developing a climate of goodwill toward the organization. Such supporters can coordinate major activities, such as fund-raising, public relations, and intermediate services for the organization. This type of support helps the organization to conserve its own resources for direct application to immediate goals, such as providing direct patient care. Individual organizations may quite simply lack the power to mobilize certain political or economic resources on their own behalf and may depend on a "friend in the castle" to help in these matters. The traditional pattern of appointing the political, social, and economic elite to the board of trustees in health care organizations is often an effort to mobilize such power on behalf of these organizations. Professional associations foster this relationship through regularly scheduled interaction with both state and federal lawmakers.

Occasionally, a nationally prominent figure demonstrates a particular interest in health care because of some personal experience with a particular health problem. In a sense, poliomyelitis, heart disease, and breast cancer received more attention because they affected a president or a member of his family. A leading political figure may work toward the passage of legislation on behalf of some specific health care need. A number of well-known entertainers and sports figures have supported fund-raising activities for one or another health care issues. Such individuals command resources unavailable to a single institution.

The Lions Club programs to support eye care, the Easter Seal program in fund-raising and coordination of volunteers to work with handicapped persons, and the Shriners' traditional support of health care for children with disabilities illustrate the typical activity of supporters. The traditional hospital auxiliary is yet another example of a support group. Supporters may help to coordinate activities to the mutual benefit of all participants, offsetting the destructive aspect of competition and facilitating compliance with standards set by controllers by making resources available for use by the organization.

Although an organization may not actively declare itself a supporter, the net effect of its activities may provide support. Advocacy groups for privacy in general, for example, have helped raise the social consciousness of the public toward all issues concerning privacy, thus helping health care institutions to develop guidelines for the restrictive release of information. In such situations, collaboration in the development of and lobbying for pertinent state legislation becomes possible.

ADVISERS

Although they are like supporters in some ways, advisers have more specific activities that tend to set trends for the industry. Advisers provide a particular form of resource or support through their advice. Gross stressed an important difference between supporters and advisers: The assistance and support of advisers help the organization use its resources and the support it receives from other sources.[21] Advisers stand apart from the organization and often have a more impersonal relationship with the organization than do supporters.

The advice may be in the form of overall guidelines, position papers, data analysis, sample procedures and methods, or model legislation. Examples of documents that are advisory in nature include the American Hospital Association's Guidelines on Patient Rights, the American Medical Association's Model Legislation Concerning Disabled Physicians, and the American Health Information Management Association's Coding and Reimbursement Compliance and Record Auditing guidelines.

CONTROLLERS

Those individuals or groups who have power over the organization are controllers. Health care organizations must comply with the regulations of several federal and state government agencies as well as with the mandates of the various accrediting agencies. A multi-specialty health care organization is required to meet detailed regulations from different state agencies as a condition for licensure. For example, social service agencies must meet a variety of regulations:

- adoption and foster care: Office of Children, Youth, and Families
- residential school and outpatient psychiatric clinic: Mental Health and Substance Abuse Services
- personal care home: Office of Social Programs
- skilled nursing facility: Department of Health

Table 3–3 provides a listing of organizations and agencies that have such control power. The level of detail varies greatly from the optimal standards stated by the Joint Commission to the highly detailed regulations (e.g., required room size) in a state law.

Certain controllers are internal to the organization and yet constitute a kind of separate organization. Workers as individuals are a part of the organization, but the unions that represent them stand outside the organization, exerting specific pressure on it. The governing board is an integral part of the hierarchical structure, but in some ways the board of trustees is separate from the line managers, who are controlled by the decisions made by the top-level management group. The assessment of the net effect of such controllers' input gives the manager a sense of

Table 3–3 Key Controllers

Controller	Requirements
Federal government	Conditions of participation for Medicare and Medicaid, special standards resulting from specific program funding and grants
State government	State laws and regulations for licensure of health care facilities and practitioners
Local government	Zoning codes, fire and safety requirements
Accreditation bodies	Accreditation requirements
Professional associations	Codes of conduct, professional educational requirements
Collective bargaining agreements	Detailed contract provisions
Organizational policy	Detailed provisions for each organizational unit
Various regulatory agencies	Personnel laws and regulations, such as Fair Labor Standards Act, Occupational Safety and Health Act
Third-party payers	Detailed contractual provisions concerning patient eligibility, mode of treatment covered, and similar provisions

clear boundaries for planning and decision making. However innovative an idea might be, for example, the manager must still keep management practices in line with these constraints.

Controllers may also impose conflicting regulations on the institution, such as the mandate of the federal government to maintain almost absolute confidentiality of alcohol and drug abuse records and the mandate of third-party payers to provide satisfactory evidence of treatment for reimbursement. Managers may be forced to change their managerial style as a result of certain constraints imposed by a controller (e.g., the details of a union contract may limit severely the use of the laissez-faire style of management). By means of survey questionnaires and site visits, the manager may assess the net effect of these multiple regulations on work flow, services offered, staffing patterns mandated, and job descriptions restricted and refined.

ADVERSARIES

Health care traditionally carries overtones of great compassion and deep charitable roots. Like any other organization, however, health care organizations have opponents and enemies as well as competitors and rivals. The rising cost of health care tends to make health care professionals and the organizations in which they work a source of conflict and even a target for opposition at the present time. Indeed, clients themselves at times take an adversarial stance.

Outright opponents or enemies are those individuals or groups who seek actively and aggressively to limit the organization in its activity. These opponents or enemies may have the power to bring an activity to a halt or to prohibit an activity from being started. For example, clients do not wish to have certain facilities, such as drug treatment centers or group homes for the developmentally challenged, too close to their homes. Furthermore, they may want ample parking and easy access to their hospital, but they do not want to disturb the local housing units or the business areas. Zoning codes may be enforced in order to prevent the development of alternative treatment facilities or the expansion of existing facilities. Clients may withdraw financial support as evidence of displeasure.

The concept of competition is well understood and accepted in the economic arena. Within reasonable boundaries, competition is favorable for clients because it forces providers to make products or services better or more accessible. The sharp edge of competition is also evident in health care delivery, possibly because certain factors in contemporary culture are producing shifts in client loyalty. These factors include (1) erosion of strong ethnic and religious ties to one hospital or health center; (2) the passage of the Civil Rights Act, which removed certain barriers to access; (3) urban and suburban migration patterns; and (4) the lowered birth rate.

Given a dropping inpatient census, a hospital may compete actively with a freestanding medical clinic by offering its own outpatient clinic services. In order to attract patients, one obstetrics unit may offer the latest in fetal monitoring, while another may stress family-centered childbirth. An urban medical school or medical center may offer the benefits of highly specialized techniques to offset a census drop due to the fact that certain clients seek to avoid the city. A hospital seeking financial bond approval for an expanded facility or for some special activity may engage in active outreach to increase its patient population.

Rivals, according to Gross, are those who produce different products but compete for resources, assistance, and support.[22] In the health care setting, specialty hospitals could be considered the rivals of general hospitals (e.g., a children's hospital versus a pediatrics ward in a general hospital, a lying-in hospital versus an obstetrics unit). When the emphasis in definition is placed on competition for the same resources, there is evidence of rivalry among health care institutions for scarce personnel (e.g., registered nurses for the 3 P.M. to 11 P.M. shift, trained medical transcriptionists, physicians for the emergency room).

Within an organization, one department may be cast as rival to another for needed space, additional personnel, and special funds. Managers may find that the same departments that are clients may also be supporters and rivals.

EXAMPLE OF CLIENTELE NETWORK FOR A PHYSICAL THERAPY UNIT

A tabulation method can be used to analyze a departmental clientele network. The development of such a reference tool for the internal environment of the organization provides the manager with much information concerning relationships to be developed, aspects of the work flow to be considered, and regulations and guidelines that must be satisfied. The following is the clientele network of a spinal cord treatment service in a physical therapy department:

I. Clients
  A. Immediate clients
    1. Patients on the spinal cord injury service
    2. Hospital personnel assigned to the spinal cord injury service
  B. Secondary clients
    1. Family members
    2. Hospital medical staff for inservice education and clarification of policies and procedures
    3. Physical therapy students on clinical affiliation
    4. Local hospitals requesting information on special programs dealing with treatment of the spinal cord–injured patient
  C. Remote clients
    1. Local hospitals
    2. Home health agencies
II. Suppliers
  A. Resources
    1. Physicians within the hospital who refer patients to the spinal cord injury unit
    2. Medical supply companies that supply equipment for both the patients and the department
    3. Bureau of Vocational Rehabilitation, which covers the cost of treatment and equipment
    4. Hospital transport system

B. Associates
  1. National spinal cord treatment centers
  2. Other direct patient services (e.g., nursing, occupational therapy, speech, psychology, social services)
  3. Home health agencies
  4. Professional journals
C. Supporters
  1. Hospital physicians and residents
  2. Community service organizations
  3. Auxiliary organizations serving the spinal cord service
  4. Medical supply companies
  5. County Wheelchair Sports Association
  6. Public relations department of the hospital
III. Advisers
  A. Hospital administrators
  B. Other direct patient care services within the hospital
  C. Insurance companies
IV. Controllers
  A. Accreditation agencies
    1. Joint Commission on Accreditation of Healthcare Organizations
    2. Commission on Accreditation of Rehabilitation Facilities (CARF)
    3. Accrediting Council for Graduate Medical Education for Residency Program (CGME)
  B. Federal government
    1. Medicare reimbursement regulations
    2. Equal employment opportunity
    3. Working conditions
  C. State government
    1. Licensing regulations for physical therapists
    2. Medicaid reimbursement regulations
  D. County Hospital Association
  E. Professional association codes of ethics
  F. Unions
  G. Hospital policies
V. Adversaries
  A. Opponents and enemies
    1. Consumer groups
    2. Hospital personnel resistant to change

B. Rivals and competitors
1. Other local rehabilitation centers sharing the same clientele network
2. Independent group practices specializing in rehabilitation

EXERCISE: IDENTIFYING AND DESCRIBING THE MANAGEMENT FUNCTIONS

In your own words, describe the classic management functions and their relationship to each other, including the extent to which they may or may not be interrelated. For each function, provide one specific example and explain in detail how this function, in this specific instance, relates to one or more of the other functions.

Next, describe any differences that may be encountered in addressing each function at different management levels; that is: Are there differences in the emphasis on each function for the supervisor or first-line manager as compared with the middle manager? Or for the middle manager as compared with the chief executive officer?

Finally, answer the following questions:

1. There is an old expression: *If we fail to plan, we plan to fail.* Failing to plan suggests doing nothing. Since planning is an active pursuit, how can doing nothing be indicative of "planning" to fail?
2. What is one legitimate example of organizing that the department manager may never encounter or may perhaps encounter only once in a great while? And one example of organizing that the department manager may employ multiple times in a normal workday?
3. What is the management function most closely associated with teaching, guiding, and motivating workers? Explain your answer.

NOTES

1. Luther Gulick and Lyndall F. Urwick, eds., *Papers of the Science of Administration* (New York: Institute of Public Administration, 1929).
2. Henri Fayol, *General and Industrial Administration* (Geneva, Switzerland: International Management Institute, 1929).
3. Chester Barnard, *The Functions of the Executive* (Cambridge, Mass.: Harvard University Press, 1968).
4. Louis D. Brandeis, "Scientific Management and Railroads," *The Engineering Magazine* (1911).
5. James Mooney and A. C. Reiley, *The Principles of Organization* (New York: Harper, 1939).

6. Ludwig von Bertalanffy, "General Systems Theory: A New Approach to the Unity of Science," *Human Biology* (December 1951): 303–61.

7. Ludwig von Bertalanffy, "General Systems Theory: A Critical Review," *General Systems* 7 (1962): 1–20.

8. Kenneth E. Boulding, "General Systems Theory: The Skeleton of Science," *Management Science* 2 (1956): 197–208.

9. Norbert Wiener, *The Human Use of Human Beings: Cybernetics and Society* (Garden City, N.Y.: Doubleday Anchor, 1954).

10. Stanley H. Brewer, *Rhochrematics: A Scientific Approach to the Management of Material Flows* (Seattle: University of Washington Bureau of Business Research, 1960).

11. Joseph M. Notterman and Richard Trumbull, "Notes on Self-Regulating Systems and Stress," *Behavioral Science* 4 (October 1950): 324–27.

12. Peter Blau and W. R. Scott, *Formal Organization* (San Francisco: Chandler, 1962), 42.

13. *Ibid.*, 43.

14. Amatai Etzioni, *A Comparative Analysis of Complex Organizations* (Glencoe, Ill.: The Free Press, 1961).

15. Daniel Katz and Robert L. Kahn, *The Social Psychology of Organizations* (New York: John Wiley & Sons, 1967), 11.

16. Max Weber, *The Theory of Social and Economic Organization,* trans. A. M. Henderson and Talcott Parsons; ed. Talcott Parsons (Glencoe, Ill.: The Free Press, 1947), 324–86.

17. Bertram Gross, *Organizations and Their Managing* (New York: Free Press, 1968), 114.

18. *Ibid.*

19. *Ibid.*, 119–21.

20. *Ibid.*, 121.

21. *Ibid.*, 122.

22. *Ibid.*, 130.

Planning

CHAPTER OBJECTIVES

- Define the management function of planning.
- Identify the characteristics of plans and specifically address those characteristics or features that make plans effective.
- Delineate the constraints placed upon planning and identify the boundaries to be observed in the planning process.
- Define and differentiate among the terms *philosophy, goal, objective, functional objective, policy, procedure, method,* and *rule.*
- Differentiate strategic planning as the process for determining and refining an organization's long-term objectives and determining how to allocate resources in pursuit of these objectives.

Planning is the process of deciding in the present what to do to bring about an outcome in the future. We might further qualify this description by referring to planning as the process of *tentatively* deciding what to do because we have no assurance of exactly what the future will bring.

Planning involves determining appropriate goals and deciding on the means to achieve them, making assumptions, developing premises, and reviewing alternative courses of action. It is the what, who, when, and how of alternative courses of action and of possible future actions. In planning, the manager contemplates the state of affairs desired for the future in light of what is known or can be inferred about the future. Any time we are looking ahead considering what to do in the future—whether that future is years or only minutes away—we are planning.

CHARACTERISTICS OF PLANNING

Planning is the most fundamental management function and logically precedes all other functions. Unplanned action cannot be properly controlled because there is no basis on which to measure progress; organizing becomes meaningless and ineffective because there is no specific goal around which to mobilize resources. Decisions may be made without planning, but they will lack effectiveness unless they are related to specific goals.

Planning goes beyond mere judgments, since judgments involve the assessment of a situation but do not stipulate actions to be taken. Planning concerns actions to be taken with reference to specific goals.

In planning, the ideal state is first identified. Then the plan to achieve that ideal is modified, refined, and brought to a practical level through a variety of derived elements, such as intermediate target statements, functional objectives, and operational goals. Planning includes the decision-making process, particularly in the commitment phase. Logical planning includes commitment in terms of time and actions to be taken. There is a hierarchy in the process that includes the relationship of derived plans to the master course, the linkage of short-range and long-range plans, and the coordination of division and department or unit plans with those of the organization as a whole. Finally, planning is characterized by a cyclic process in which some or many goals and specific objectives are recycled.

In a sense, some plans are never achieved completely; they are continuous. For example, the goal of health care institutions to provide quality patient care is a continuing one that invests the many derived plans with a fundamental purpose. This goal is recycled during each planning period.

PARTICIPANTS IN PLANNING

Top-level managers set the basic tone for planning, determine overall goals for the organization, and give direction on the content of policies and similar planning documents. This is not done in isolation but is based on information provided through the feedback cycle, through reports and special studies, and through the direct participation of personnel in each department or division. The manager consults the major super-users, both in the direct patient care divisions and the administrative units.

Department heads are normally responsible for the planning process in their areas of jurisdiction. They identify overall goals and policies for their department, and they develop immediate objectives, taking into account their department's particular work constraints. In some organizations, a special planning department is created, such as a program and development division or a research and development unit.

Occasionally, clients participate in the planning process; such participation is required in some externally funded programs. In health care planning, for example, provider, consumer, and business community membership are included at each level of the review process. Professional associations frequently involve their members in the planning process at local, regional, state, and national levels. Employee involvement is yet another aspect of participation. Organizations whose members belong to collective bargaining units involve employee representatives in formulating certain aspects of planning, e.g., plans to downsize or to change major patterns of staffing.

The Planning Process

Since planning is intended to focus attention on objectives and to reduce uncertainty, there must be a clear statement of goals. Once the goals to be attained have been established, premising must be developed—that is, the assumptions must be identified, stated, and used consistently. Premising includes an analysis of planning constraints and a statement of the anticipated environment within which the plans will unfold. In a health care organization, the premises reflect the level of care, the specific setting (e.g., outpatient clinic, inpatient unit, or home care), the specific number of beds per service, the anticipated number and kinds of specialty services or clinics, morbidity and mortality data for the outreach territory, and the availability of related services.

The department head states the premises on which departmental plans are based, for example, the number of inpatient beds, the readmission rate, the projected length of stay, and the interrelationship of the work flow. The following is an example of specific planning premises or assumptions based on the operation of a physical therapy service:

1. Anticipated hours of operation
   a. 6 days per week
   b. 8-hour day; evening coverage for selected patients and clinics

   2. Anticipated caseload
      a. Inpatients—100 per day
      b. Outpatients—120 per day
   3. Diagnostic categories
      a. Hemiplegics
      b. Arthritics
      c. Amputees
      d. Fractures
      e. Sports injuries
   4. Patient characteristics
      a. Adults
      b. Children
   5. Level of care
      a. Acute
      b. Subacute
      c. Convalescent
      d. Chronic

Alternate approaches to reaching the desired state are developed, and the choices to be made are stated. Commitment to one of these choices constitutes the decision-making phase. Derivative plans then are formulated, and details of sequence and timing are identified. Planning includes periodic checking and review, which leads into the control process. Review and necessary revisions of plans, based on feedback, are the final steps in the cycle of planning.

PLANNING CONSTRAINTS OR BOUNDARIES

To constrain means to limit, to bind, to delineate freedom of action. Constraints in planning are factors that managers must take into account in order to make their plans feasible and realistic. Constraints, which are both internal and external, take a variety of forms. Analysis of the organizational environment by means of the clientele network, specifically the category of "controller," leads to ready identification of planning constraints. The use of the input-output model also yields practical information about the constraints specific to an organization. The planning process itself imposes a constraint because of time factors. Sometimes a manager must settle for speed rather than accuracy in gathering the data needed for planning. The cost of data gathering and analysis is another constraint; if committees or special review groups are involved, the cost of their time must be considered.

The general resistance to change impedes the planning process so that standing plans take on the force of habit. Without a program for regular review of plans, they become static and rooted in tradition. Precedent becomes the rule, and the bureaucratic processes become entrenched. The phase in the life cycle of the organization also affects planning, as the degree of innovation that is appropriate varies with each phase.

The nature of the organization also shapes the planning process. The extent to which the organization's members participate in planning correlates with the predominant mode of authority. Highly normative organizations tend to include more member participation in their planning than do coercive ones. Ethics and values of the larger society, of the individual members, and, in health care, of the many professional organizations help shape the goal formulation and subsequent policies and practices. When health care is seen as a right and not a privilege, there may be a greater openness to innovation and a demand for outreach programs and flexible patterns of delivery of service.

Within the organization, interdepartmental relationships may be constraints. In highly specialized organizations with many services or departments, each unit manager must consider how other departments' needs and processes are interwoven with those of one's own department. Effective planning includes an assessment of such factors. The manager sometimes must accept as inputs or constraints the procedures and policies of another department.

Capital investments must also be considered. When a major commitment that involves the physical layout of the facility or some major equipment purchase has been made, the degree of flexibility in changing the process is necessarily limited.

External factors to be considered in planning include the political climate, which varies in its openness to extensive programs in health care. The era of increased federal government sponsorship, through direct provision of care, may be replaced by an era in which an attempt is made to return health care delivery to private rather than government sponsorship, or the emphasis may shift from the federal government to the state government level. The general state of labor relations and the degree to which unionization is allowed and even mandated in an industry may be imposed on the organization. The many regulations, laws, and directives constitute another set of constraints.

In health care organizations, the many legal and accrediting requirements are specific, pervasive constraints that affect every aspect of planning. Such requirements can be developed into a reference grid for the use of the manager, since compliance with these mandates is a binding element in the overall constraint on departmental functioning.

An alternate approach to the identification of constraints in any health care planning situation is the systematic recognition of the following major factors:

1. *General Setting.* The level and particular emphasis of care must be determined. For example, the goal of one institution may be acute care in specialized diagnostic categories; the goal of another may be the long-term care of the frail elderly. The critical organizational relationships that stem from the general setting should be identified (e.g., the institution's degree of independence versus its adherence to corporate and affiliation agreements and contractual arrangements). Physical location may also be a constraining factor, although an earlier decision to develop the facility in a specific location may be part of the ideal plan. For example, the decision to develop a pattern of decentralized care in order to enhance the outreach program of a community behavioral health center will serve as a constraint on many derived plans, such as work flow and staffing patterns. Information about the general setting is readily available in long-range planning documents, licensure and accreditation surveys, annual reports, and public relations materials.

2. *Legal and Accrediting Agency Mandates.* Each health care institution is regulated by a federal or state agency that imposes specific requirements for the level of care and nature of services offered. For example, a hospital is licensed by the state only after it meets certain requirements; it is approved for participation in the Medicare and Medicaid programs only after it fulfills certain conditions. Particular attention must be given to the Joint Commission's Information Management Plan in which community-wide health care planning documents are included as part of the acute care facility's overall plans. In addition, a hospital must comply with special regulations for medical care evaluation. It also must comply, at a minimum, with malpractice insurance regulations and related risk management programs as well as fire, safety, and zoning codes.

3. *Characteristics of the Clients.* The general patterns of mortality and morbidity for a given population must be considered, as well as related factors such as length of inpatient stay, frequency of outpatient services, emergency unit usage, and readmission rate. Patient sources of payment relate to the sta-

bility and predictability of cash flow. Specific eligibility for treatment may be another factor, as in certain services for veterans or programs for other specific groups. Demographic profiles for the area served, as well as the organization's internal database, are the usual sources of such information.

4. *Practitioners and Employees.* The licensure laws for health care practitioners and physicians, as well as the many federal and state laws pertaining to most classes of employees, govern the utilization of staff. These include the Labor Management Relations Act (Taft-Hartley Act), the Civil Rights Act, the Age Discrimination in Employment Act, the Unemployment Compensation and Workers' Compensation Acts, the Occupational Safety and Health Act, and the Americans with Disabilities Act. The personnel practices mandated in the accrediting agency standards and guidelines of health agencies and professional associations also must be followed. Any contractual agreement resulting from the collective bargaining process must be taken into account. The specific bylaws and related rules and regulations for medical staff and allied health care practitioners are yet another constraint on plans involving employees and professional practitioners in any role.

CHARACTERISTICS OF EFFECTIVE PLANS

Effective plans have flexibility. Plans should have a built-in capacity to change, an adaptability. A plan could include a timetable sequence, for example, that allows extra time for unexpected events before the plan becomes off schedule.

The manager seeks to balance plans so that they are neither too idealistic nor too practical or limited. Plans that are too idealistic tend to produce frustration because they cannot be attained; they may become mere mottoes. On the other hand, plans that are too modest lack motivational value, and it may be difficult to muster support for them. Clarity and vagueness must also be balanced in formulating plans. These factors help make the goals realistic. A precise goal may be a motivational tool because it provides immediate satisfaction, but there is also merit in a degree of vagueness because with some plans, especially long-range ones, it may not be possible or desirable to state goals in precise terms. Vagueness can contribute to motivation since it permits the development of detailed plans by those more directly involved in the work. Finally, vagueness can provide the necessary latitude to compromise when this is required or is a general strategy in the development of plans throughout the organization.

Anticipating Changes and Updates in Existing Plans

The effective manager monitors the planning process as an ongoing activity so that existing plans may be modified and new plans developed to meet changes in one or several planning constraints. The manager is not caught unaware but instead has an active plan to monitor potential change. Federal and state agencies as well as accrediting agencies issue their intended changes well in advance of their required implementation. The Centers for Medicare and Medicaid Services (CMS) issues its proposed rules four to six months ahead of the date for rules going into effect. Further, agencies issue annual or semiannual agendas of changes under consideration. The Office of Inspector General regularly makes known its targeted review focus for the upcoming year. This may be found in its published work plan. Professional associations routinely monitor the progress of major changes—for example, the *International Classification of Diseases, 10th modification (ICD-10)*. Plans needing modification are similarly assessed. As a manager identifies a trend or issue, he or she checks existing objectives, policies, and procedures to adjust them accordingly. An equipment recycling program may have worked well in the past, but now more particular attention is required when computers are recycled or destroyed; privacy considerations as well as environmental protection requirements need to be added as factors in such a recycling or disposal process. Another example of policy change might stem from the lessening of a previously required practice: the Joint Commission's change in requiring a unit record to permit innovation in data capture and availability for patient care.

Planning for the Unknown

In addition to planning based on well-known planning premises (e.g., the expected number of patients per year, the usual length of stay, etc.), planning for unknown events must also be accomplished. The management team typically assesses the relative unknowns and seeks to make them progressively tangible. Although complete certainty is not possible, plans for rare but probable events are not only prudent but often mandated by external agencies. The strike plan is one such example. As the contract period for a given labor union agreement concludes, it is possible that a new contract may not yet have been agreed to. The workers may strike, thereby causing work disruption. Because patient care is of primary importance, management must have a contingency plan in place well before the strike deadline. Weather-related disruptions are another instance of possible-to-probable events. Managers in hurricane-prone locations or in regions with winter storms of a crippling variety have plans in place to cover those circumstances. Managers will not know precisely how many or when such disruptions will occur, but they have anticipated them well in advance and only need to fine-tune the plan when the emergency conditions escalate.

Disaster preparedness is a prime example of planning for the unknown. The types of possible disasters (e.g., epidemic; mass casualty; bioterrorism) are identified and the plans rehearsed in great detail precisely because their incidences are so unpredictable.

Types of Plans

The planning process involves a variety of plans that develop logically from the highly abstract, as in a statement of philosophy or ideal goals, to the progressively concrete, as in operational goals and procedures. Management literature on planning consistently includes the concepts of goals and objectives as central to the planning process. The terms *goal* and *objective* are frequently used in an interchangeable manner, except in discussions of management by objectives (MBO). The MBO concept refers to specific, measurable, attainable plans for the unit, department, or organization. For the purposes of this discussion of plans, the concept of goal will be discussed in terms of overall purpose. The concept of objective will be discussed in terms of more measurable attainable plans, including unit or departmental objectives and functional objectives. Exhibit 4–1 lists the sequence of

EXHIBIT 4–1

Relationship of Types of Plans

I. Underlying Purpose/Overall Mission/Philosophy/Goal
II. Objectives
III. Functional Objectives
IV. Policies
V. Procedures
    V.1 Methods
    V.2 Rules
VI. Work Standards
VII. Performance Standards
VIII. Training Objectives
IX. Management by Objectives
X. Operational Goals

planning documents from planning state through controlling by means of operational goals.

CORE VALUES, PHILOSOPHY, AND MISSION STATEMENTS

Individuals who share a common vision and set of values come together to create a formal organization for purposes that are consistent with and derived from their common values. The statement of core values, philosophy, or mission provides an overall frame of reference for organizational practice; it is the basis of the overall goals, objectives, policies, and derived plans (see Exhibit 4–2 for a sample of a mission, vision, and values statement of a nonprofit, community-based health care center). Actual practice, as delineated in policies and procedures, should not violate the organization's underlying philosophy. As new members and clients are attracted to the organization and as the organization grows from the gestational to the youthful stage, the statement of principles may be made more explicit. A statement of core values may take one of several forms, such as a preamble, a creed, a pledge, or a statement of principle.

In addition to reflecting the values of the immediate, specific group that formed the organization, a statement of philosophy may reflect, implicitly or explicitly, the values of the larger society. To one degree or another, for example, society as a whole now accepts the burden of providing for those who need medical care. The concept of health care as a right, regardless of ability to pay, gradually emerged as an explicit value in the 1960s. Emphasis on the rights of consumers and patients emerged in a similar evolutionary pattern in the 1970s. Because free enterprise is a benchmark of the democratic way of life, a trend toward marketing and competition in health care became a feature of the 1980s and 1990s. The early 21st century is characterized by a combination of all of these considerations.

Department managers in a health care organization are guided by several philosophical premises. These may differ from, and even be in opposition to, the managers' personal values. However, as members of the executive team, the managers are expected to accept these premises. One of the goals of providing orientation and motivation is to foster acceptance of the underlying purpose of the organization. Typical philosophical premises in health care include

- the basic philosophy of the group that sponsors and/or controls the health care institution (e.g., federal or state government agency, religious or fraternal organization, business concern)

EXHIBIT 4–2

Mission, Vision, and Values of Community Hospital

Community Hospital and Health Center exists to serve the community by providing expert, affordable, and readily available evaluation and treatment of the health needs of the residents. Educational and research activities to meet community needs and improve the quality of life of the communities we serve are part of our commitment.

Vision

Our vision is to offer health services ranging from primary to specialty care, with coordination among all units, thus encouraging patient care across the continuum of care. We seek to offer cost-efficient, customized care at our facility and to coordinate care with facilities in adjacent geographic areas. We seek partnership with the business, educational, and research communities for the mutual benefit of all.

Values

Our organizations govern our actions by the following values:
- Service: excellence and compassion in all aspects of care
- Unity: team approach among the direct care providers and support staff
- Innovation: continuous learning and searching for best practices
- Adaptability: proactive toward change and supportive of others who initiate change
- Communication: openness to receive information and feedback in a nonjudgmental atmosphere

- the American Hospital Association's guidelines on patient rights and similar issues
- guidelines of accrediting agencies, such as the Joint Commission that emphasize continuity of care, patient rights, and other topics
- guidelines, codes of ethics, and position statements of professional associations (e.g., American Physical Therapy Association, American Health Information Management Association, American Occupational Therapy Association)

- values of society in general, such as concern for privacy, equal access, employee safety, and consumer/client participation in decision making
- contemporary trends in the delivery of health care, such as the shift from inpatient acute care to outpatient care and community-based outreach centers; the establishment of independent practices by health professionals (e.g., physical therapists) who formerly provided care only under the direct supervision of physicians; the emergence of technical levels in several health professions and the acceptance of the care given by technicians

Mission statements usually remain stable over the life of the organization.

Medical centers devoted to acute care as well as teaching carry out the ongoing mission of:

- educating superior physicians
- enhancing research and knowledge
- improving health care in the community and region

A specialty assisted living facility defines itself through its mission statement: to provide an assisted living residence for individuals in the early to middle stages of Alzheimer's disease and other related memory impairments, in an environment of warmth, caring, safety, with the comforts and routines of home.

The following are excerpts from statements of philosophy. One health information department has its philosophy stated in a preamble:

> Given the basic right of patients to comprehensive, quality health care, health information management (HIM), as a service department, provides support and assistance within its jurisdiction to the staff and programs of this institution. A major function of this department is to facilitate continuity of patient care through the development and maintenance of the appropriate health information systems which shall reflect all episodes of care given by the professional and technical staff in any of the components of this institution.

An educational institution adheres to the following statement of philosophy:

> One of the critical elements in an effective approach to health care is the establishment of the spirit and practice of cooperative endeavor among practitioners. Recognizing this need, the Consortium for Interdisciplinary Health Studies seeks to foster the team approach to the delivery of health care.

The following is from the statement of philosophy of a physical therapy department:

> The physical therapy department as a component of the health care system is committed to providing quality patient care and community services in the most

responsive and cost-effective manner possible. In addition, the department will participate in research and investigative studies and provide educational programs for hospital personnel and affiliating students from the various medical and health professions.

The philosophy of an occupational therapy private practice group is stated in these terms:

The Occupational Therapy Consultants, Inc. believe that humans are open systems that both influence and are influenced by the environment. Therefore, individuals are motivated to pursue goal-directed activities that reflect their values, roles, and interest. We use activities and environmental adaptations to provide positive reinforcement and a sense of mastery to our clients. We make "doing" possible.

The mission of this private practice group is as follows:

Occupational Therapy Consultants, Inc. will seek referrals from medical and nonmedical sources and offer high-quality, cost-effective services to clients and their caregivers whose roles, habits, and interests are limited by pathological, congenital, or traumatic incidents. Services, direct and consultative, will be offered in schools, homes, factories, and outpatient facilities.

The values of the organization are stated explicitly in mission and vision statements. They are embodied in subsequent management practices and documents. Note, for example, the opening clause of the sample labor union contract in Chapter 10; the shared values of fostering patient care and providing good working conditions are amplified in such a statement. Policies and practices for risk management, infection control, and in-service training are additional examples of vision and values informing day-to-day practice.

OVERALL GOALS

The goals of the organization originate in the common vision and sense of mission embodied in the statement of purpose or the underlying philosophy. They reflect the general purpose of the organization and provide the basis for subsequent management action. As statements of long-range organizational intent and purpose, goals are the ends toward which activity is directed. In a sense, a goal is never completely achieved but rather continues to exist as an ideal state to be attained.

Goals serve as a basis for grouping organizations—for example, educational organizations, health care institutions, and philanthropic or fraternal associations. Goals, like statements of philosophy, may be found in an organization's charter, articles of incorporation, statement of mission, or introduction to the official by-laws. Again, like the statement of philosophy, the overall goals may not bear a specific label; they may be identified only through common understanding. The planning process is facilitated when the philosophy and the goals are formally stated. Derivative plans may then be developed in a consistent manner and with less risk of implementing policies and procedures that violate fundamental values.

This overall goal statement for a publicly sponsored rural health agency is an example of the language and style used in stating these plans:

This agency has three primary goals:

- to provide services that will enable older adults to maintain a relatively independent lifestyle in both home and community, rather than becoming dependent upon institutional care
- to advocate for older adults in the three-county rural area
- to give priority services to those older persons with the greatest social and economic needs

OBJECTIVES

In the planning process, the manager makes the plans progressively more explicit. The move from the ideal, relatively intangible statements of mission and purpose or overall goal to the "real" plans is accomplished through the development of specific objectives that bring the goals to a practical, working level. Objectives are relatively tangible, concrete plans and are usually stated in terms of results to be achieved. The manager reviews the underlying purpose and basically answers the following question: What is my unit or department to accomplish specifically in light of these overall goals?

Achieving specific objectives tends to be a continuous process; the work of the department must satisfy these objectives over and over again. An overall goal such as "to promote the health and well-being of the community" can be accomplished only through a series of specific objectives that are met on a continuing basis. Objectives add the dimensions of quality, time, accuracy, and priorities to goals. The objectives are specific to each unit or department, while the overall goals for an organization remain the same for all units.

Objectives may be stated in a variety of ways, and different levels of detail may be used. For example, objectives may be expressed

- *quantitatively:* to maintain the profit margin of 6 percent during each fiscal year by an increase in sales volume sufficient to offset increased cost

- *qualitatively:* to make effective use of community involvement by the establishment of an advisory committee with a majority of members drawn from the active clients who live in the immediate geographical community
- *as services to be offered:* to provide comprehensive personal patient care services with full consideration for the elements of good medical care (e.g., accessibility, quality, continuity, and efficiency)
- *as values to be supported:* to ensure privacy and confidentiality in all phases of patient care interaction and documentation

Objectives for the department as a whole may include elements essential for proper delineation of all other objectives. These may be stated as objectives for the organization and need not, therefore, be repeated in the subsequent departmental statement of objectives:

- compliance with legal, regulatory, and accrediting standards and with institutional bylaws
- risk management factors, including accuracy
- privacy and confidentiality in patient care transactions and documentation
- reference to inpatient as well as outpatient/ambulatory care and other programs sponsored by the organization, such as home care or satellite clinics

Because they are intended to give specificity to overall goals, objectives are the key to management planning. Therefore, objectives must be measurable whenever possible. They must provide for formal accountability in terms of achieving the results. Furthermore, they must be flexible so that they can be adapted to changing circumstances over time. Two additional planning concepts must be used with the statements of objectives in order to make them meaningful: the statement of functional objectives and the development of policies. These related plans are both important in fleshing out departmental objectives.

FUNCTIONAL OBJECTIVES

A functional objective is a statement that refines a general objective in terms of

- specific service to be provided
- type of output
- quantity and/or specificity of output
- frequency and/or specificity of output
- accuracy
- priorities

Some elements, such as accuracy indicators, may be defined for the department or unit as a whole. A general objective's priority may be implied by its delineation in a related functional objective.

Planning data for organizing and staffing functions may be obtained by inference from statements of objectives; for example, the functional objective statement may include the stipulation that all discharge summaries shall be typed. The workload (number of discharge summaries) may be calculated based on the number of discharges per year. A priority system for processing such summaries or a designated turnaround time for such processing provides the necessary parameters for calculating the number of workers needed to meet the objective on a continuing basis. The staffing patterns for day, evening, and night shifts may be developed, again, in a way to satisfy the priority designation and turnaround time contained in the functional objective.

The relationship of the general objective and the functional objectives that support it are clearly seen in the following example drawn from the plans for a transcription/word processing unit of a health information management (HIM) service.

> *General Objective:* HIM will provide a system for dictation of selected medical reports by specified health care providers and for the transcription of these reports on a routine basis.
> *Functional Objectives:* More specifically, this system will provide for:
> 1. dictation services for attending medical staff, house officers, and associated professional staff as defined by the medical staff bylaws.
> 2. transcription of reports will be done within the following time frame:
>   a. discharge summaries within eight hours of receipt of dictation.
>   b. operative reports within four hours of receipt of dictation.
>   c. consultation reports within four hours of receipt of dictation.

This example specifies the quantity of output and the time frame and implies the priority of the objective through the designation of the time frame. A statement of accuracy is not included, because it is included in the objectives for the department as a whole. This accuracy statement, which may fall under the overall objective of risk management and quality control, may be expressed as follows:

> Health information management strives to carry out its responsibilities and activities with 100% accuracy; therefore, we strive for 100% accuracy.

The following is an example of a general objective and functional objectives from a direct patient care service:

> *General Objective:* The physical therapy department will provide evaluation and assessment procedures appropriate to the patient's condition as requested by the referring physician.

Functional Objectives: More specifically,
a. evaluations will be completed within one working day following receipt of the referral.
b. a verbal summary of findings will be submitted to the physician following the completion of the evaluation.
c. a written summary of the evaluation will be noted in the patient's chart within eight hours following the verbal report.

Excerpts from systems objectives and related functional objectives are given below. These reflect the objectives for the release of information unit of a health information service.[1]

Health information management will provide a system for the timely and accurate processing of requests and for the release of information from medical records maintained by this health care facility. Specifically, this release of information system shall be established
- to comply with all applicable state and federal laws, regulations, and accrediting standards
- to comply with the generally accepted principles of patients' rights, privacy, and confidentiality
- to comply with the Patient's Bill of Rights promulgated by the American Hospital Association, the American Psychiatric Association, the Joint Commission on Accreditation of Healthcare Organizations, federal and state regulations designating specific bill of rights statements, and the American Health Information Management Association's Code of Ethics

Health information management will develop detailed procedures for the timely, accurate, and appropriate response to requests within these basic time frames:

- emergency requests: priority response

- in-person requests from the patient or the patient's designated representative:
  1. general requests: immediate initiation of preliminary procedure; finalized response within (_____) working days of preliminary procedure
  2. requests for access to a record: immediate initiation of preliminary appointment made for review of the record (_____) days from receipt of approval for review from the attending physician

- in-person requests from non-patients: immediate initiation of preliminary prodecure; appointment made for review of record (_____) working days from receipt of approval from the attending physician, if applicable

- written requests: initial response within one working day of
                                        the request if further information, author-
                                        ization, or fees are required

                                        completed response within (_____) work-
                                        ing days after receipt of the necessary au-
                                        thorizations and/or fees

                                        return of the request completed within
                                        one working day if the request cannot be
                                        completed (for example, if the individual
                                        named in the request was not a patient of
                                        this facility)

- court orders and subpoenas: within mandated time frames

Health information management will maintain systems to
- notify Risk Management of inquiries and authorized disclosures naming the facility in potential litigation
- coordinate with Patient Billing the release of information for reimbursement purposes
- coordinate inservice training about release of information practices
  1. for HIM employees at hiring and at least yearly thereafter
  2. for employees of other departments as requested by appropriate department heads
- maintain quality control
  1. through monthly quality control reviews focusing on detecting and preventing errors
  2. through monthly quality control reviews focusing on ensuring the accuracy and timeliness of responses

POLICIES

Policies are the guides to thought and action by which managers seek to delineate the areas within which decisions will be made and subsequent actions taken. Policies spell out the required, prohibited, or suggested courses of action. The limitations on actions are stated, defined, or, at least, clearly implied. Policies predecide issues and limit actions so that situations that occur repeatedly are handled in the same way. Because policies are intended to be overall guides, their language is broad.

A balance must be achieved when policies are formulated. These comprehensive guides should be sufficiently specific to provide the user with information about the actions to take, the actions to be avoided, and when and how to respond; at the same time, however, they should be flexible enough to accommodate changing conditions. They should reinforce and be consistent with the overall goals and objectives. In addition, they should conform to legal and accrediting mandates as well as to any other requirement imposed by internal or external authorities.

Policies are relatively permanent plans, a kind of cornerstone of other, more detailed plans. Yet they must be sufficiently flexible in intent to permit change in the derived plans without necessitating a change in the policy. For example, a commitment to a centralized word processing system might be made through a policy statement on health information functions. However, no specification is made as to brand of equipment, exclusive use in in-house staffing, or external agency contract. All remain options as long as the equipment selected and the staffing pattern determined meet the policy considerations of an adequate dictation-word processing function. In the dictation-word processing policy, the essential features of the word processing system are delineated. It is easy to derive from this a decision-making matrix for the comparison and selection of one or another commercial transcription/word processing service. In this sense, a policy statement serves to preform or shape detailed decision making because the overall parameters are stated within the policy or are easily derived from it.[2]

Sources of Policy

Department or unit managers develop the policies specific to their assigned areas, but these policies must be consistent with those originated by top-level management. Policies sometimes are implied, as in a tacit agreement to permit an afternoon coffee break. An implied policy may make it difficult to enforce some other course of action, however, if the implied policy has become standard—in spite of its lack of official approval. Policies are shaped in some instances by the effect of exceptions granted; a series of exceptions may become the basis of a new policy, or at least a revision of an existing one. Certain policies may be imposed by outside groups, such as an accrediting agency or a labor union, through a negotiated contract.

A rich source of policy and related guidelines is available through national associations of the various health professionals. For example, the American Physical Therapy Association has its clinical practice series; the American Health Information Association publishes practice briefs and best practice guidelines. These sources reflect state-of-the-art practices, and the wording of these documents is carefully crafted to provide clear guidance. These suggested practices and guidelines are supported by research and field testing. Another source of wording for policy content is the official publication of a law, regulation, or standard. When these are added to a policy, appropriate citation is made and the excerpt is incorporated with the exact wording of the published law, regulation, or standard.

Wording of Policies

Policies permit and require interpretation. Language indicators, such as "whenever possible" or "as circumstances permit," are expressions typically used to give policies the flexibility needed. Policy statements in a health care institution may concern such items as definitions of categories of patients and designations of responsibility. In a health information service, policy statements may specify, for example, a standardized patient record format, the internal and external distribution of copies, the use of abbreviations, and the processing of urgent requests.

In order to decrease the sheer volume of policy statements, a glossary may be developed that includes the institutional definition of *patient* as well as definitions for terms and acronyms referring to members of the medical and professional staff and legal and accrediting bodies. Occasionally, a statement of rationale is included in a policy statement, but the manager should avoid excessive explanations; in general, the manager needs to couch policy directives in wording that predecides issues and permits actions. Another useful adjunct to the complete policy statement is the "Policy in Brief"—a short summary of major points for quick reference.

Policies are somewhat futuristic in that they are meant to remain in force, with little change, for long periods of time. In an age of rapid social and technical change, it is helpful to think in broad terms, anticipating change. It also helps to set aside the normal biases that stem from describing the way things are now.

- Edit all policies to omit sexist references (e.g., physician as "he," nurses as "she"). This is easily done by using plural pronouns.
- Edit all policies to reflect the continued growth of the nursing profession and the various health professionals who continually seek an expanded scope of practice. Include nurse practitioners, physician assistants, physical therapists, pharmacists, and similar credentialed, licensed practitioners in policy statements where applicable.
- Focus on the broad range of patient care. Although the acute care hospital is central to patient care, outpatient care, urgent care centers, and short-stay units are increasingly a part of the health care setting.
- Think "high tech," especially as technology develops in areas such as "e-health."
- Seek to avoid contradictions within policies and between policies and their related procedures. The careful development of procedures, in addition to checking against policy statements, is an essential step.[3]

The wording in the following examples, drawn from a variety of settings, tends to be broad and elastic yet gives sufficient information to guide the user. The first example is a policy for the waiver of tuition for senior citizens:

In recognition of their efforts over the years in support of education, the college will waive tuition for academic and continuing education courses for senior citizens who reside in the tricounty area. All residents at least 62 years of age who are not engaged in full-time gainful employment are eligible under this tuition waiver policy. This policy will be subject to annual budgeted funds.

This example provides a general sense of why the college is granting this waiver: in recognition of senior citizen support over the years. The outer limits of its applicability are noted: both academic and continuing education programs are included. A definition of *senior citizen* is given, and the additional eligibility factors are stated. A final parameter is included to provide flexibility should circumstances change: namely, the limitation determined by the availability of budgeted funds. With this short policy, the necessary procedures can be developed for determining eligibility, and a relatively untrained worker can make the necessary determination.

The following are typical policies for health care institutions. For employee promotion:

It is the policy of this hospital to promote from within the organization whenever qualified employees are available for vacancies. The following factors shall be considered in the selection of individual employees for promotion: length of service with the organization; above-average performance in present position; special preparation for promotion. Employees on their present job for a reasonable length of time, excluding probationary period, may request promotion during the customary period in which a job is open and posted as being available.

For admission of patients to a research unit:

Since the primary purpose of this unit is research in specialized areas of medicine, the primary consideration in selecting elective patients for admission to the research unit accommodations is given to the teaching and research value of the clinical findings. The research unit offers two types of service: inpatient and outpatient. The research unit reserves the right to assign patients to either service category, depending on the characteristics of the case and facilities available at the time.

For a physical therapy department:

The Physical Therapy Department shall be open from 8:30 A.M. to 4:30 P.M. Monday through Friday, and on weekends and holidays as required to meet patient care needs.

And following is an example of a policy regarding professional credentials:

All occupational therapy personnel will be licensed and registered.

Each applicant will submit the names of two references and the personnel officer will telephone these individuals and check on the applicant's ability to problem solve and communicate with others and his or her work habits and commitment to patient service delivery.

The director of the occupational therapy department will check to see if the applicant has passed the national certification examination and has a current state license.

Recent graduates or therapists from foreign countries may treat patients but they must be supervised by a licensed and certified occupational therapist who countersigns their patient care plans and progress notes.

Occupational therapists may not work more than six months under these conditions. If not registered and licensed within six months after hire, employment must be terminated.

A complete policy for departmental operations appears in Appendix 4–A.

PROCEDURES

A procedure is a guide to action. It is a series of related tasks, given in chronological order, that constitute the prescribed manner of performing the work. Essential information in any procedure includes the specific tasks that must be done, at what time and/or under what circumstances they must be done, and who (job title, not name of employee) is to do them. Procedures are developed for repetitive work in order to ensure uniformity of practice, to facilitate personnel training, and to permit the development of controls and checks in the workflow. Unlike policies, which are more general, procedures are highly specific and need little, if any, interpretation.

Procedures for a specific organizational unit are developed by the manager of that unit. As with other plans, departmental procedures must be coordinated with those of related departments as well as with those developed by higher management levels for all departments. For example, the procedures for patient transport to various specialized service units, such as nuclear medicine, physical therapy, or occupational therapy, are developed jointly by the nursing service and these related departments or services. In contrast, procedures relating to employee matters may well be dictated by top-level management for the organization as a whole with little, if any, procedural development done at the departmental or unit level.

Procedure Manual Format

There are three types of formats used in procedure manuals: narrative, abbreviated narrative, and playscript. The narrative format contains a series of statements in paragraph form, with special notes or explanations in subparagraphs or in footnotes. This format has the disadvantage of being difficult to refer to quickly and easily. The abbreviated narrative format illustrates procedures through the use of key steps and key points (Exhibits 4–3 and 4–4).

EXHIBIT 4–3

Abbreviated Narrative Procedure Format: Procedure for Terminal Digit Filing

Key Step

1. Terminal digit filing system

Key Points

1. Read from right to left, two digits at a time.
2. EXPLANATION: Records are filed in sections by the last two digits to the right, then the middle two digits, then the last two digits to the left. Example: if the history number is 06-52-18 find it this way:

Look here last	Look here second	Look here first
within the 18 section	within the 18 section	18
06	52	18

The last two digits (terminals) are color coded. The colors for each digit always remain the same, and once they are learned they can be used in many combinations of numbers. They help you file more accurately and quickly.

EXHIBIT 4–4

Abbreviated Narrative Procedure Format: Procedure for Interdepartmental Coordination

Key Step

1. Determine patient care need.

Key Points

1. Review medical care record.
2. Perform appropriate evaluation procedures.
3. Complete related medical documentation, including information needed for consultation.

Key Step

2. Contact appropriate department.

Key Points

1. Make verbal contact via telephone.
2. Confirm through interdepartmental request form for joint conference.

When a procedure involves several workers or departments, the playscript format may be used to advantage. Each participant in the action is identified by job title, the step is given a sequence number, key action words are stated, and action sentences are developed for the step. The playscript format is direct and specific and its focus is on "who does what and when." As each step in the procedure is analyzed and stated in terms of actor, step sequence, key action word, and action sentence, ambiguity and vagueness are avoided (Exhibit 4–5).

An alternate version of the playscript format stresses responsible party, step sequence, and action (Exhibits 4–6 and 4–7).

EXHIBIT 4–5

Playscript Format

Actor	Step Sequence	Action Words	Action Sentence
File Clerk	1	Verifies identification	Check patient identification as given in patient master file: full name, date of birth, number.
File Clerk	2	Records identification	Enter patient identification on medical report in appropriate section on form.

EXHIBIT 4–6

Alternate Playscript Format: Example 1

Responsibility	Step Sequence	Action
Patient Master File Clerk	1	Check patient's identification as given in patient master file: full name, date of birth, number.
Patient Master File Clerk	2	Enter patient identification on medical report in appropriate section on form.
Terminal Digit File Clerk	3	Obtain batches of medical reports from Patient Identification section.
Terminal Digit File Clerk	4	File each medical report in specific patient record in numeric order.

EXHIBIT 4-7

Alternate Playscript Format: Example 2

Responsibility	Step Sequence	Action
Senior Physical Therapist	1	Receives patient referral form. Enters name, date, and time received in master file.
Senior Physical Therapist	2	Assigns patient to physical therapist for evaluation.
Staff Physical Therapist	3	Arranges treatment as scheduled for patient evaluation.
Secretary	4	Requests central transportation to deliver patient and hospital chart at designated time.

Yet another version includes a set of detailed steps for each key step in the playscript sequence (Exhibit 4–8).

Leslie Matthies[4] identified the following action verbs as useful in conveying central, specific ideas for procedure statements in the playscript format:

sends	uses
shows	checks
issues	places
obtains	decides
records	receives
provides	forwards
prepares	requests

The physical format of the procedure manual is important. A procedure manual should be convenient in size, easy to read, and arranged logically. If the manual is too large or too heavy for everyday use or is difficult to read because of too many unbroken pages of type, workers tend to develop their own procedures rather than refer to the manual for the prescribed steps. The choice of a format that makes it easy to update the manual (e.g., loose-leaf binder) removes a major disadvantage or limitation regarding the manual's use: pages of obsolete procedures.

Development of the Procedure Manual

The manager who is developing a procedure manual must first determine its purpose and audience (e.g., to train new employees or to bring about uniformity of practice among current employees). The level of detail and the number and kinds

---

EXHIBIT 4–8

Alternative Playscript Format That Includes Key Steps and Detailed Steps: Example 3

Key Step	Sequence	Responsibility	Detailed Steps
Receive the incoming mail:	Step 1	Release of information clerk	• Pick up the mail from the central mail room located in room [___].
a. U.S. mail			• The mail is ready for pickup at [___] A.M.
b. interde-partmental mail			• The department mailbox is Number [___].
Perform the initial processing	Step 2	Release of information clerk	• Sort the mail by general categories: 1. loose reports received via interoffice mail: Direct these immediately to the Storage and Retrieval unit 2. mail marked "Confidential": Direct these immediately to department director's secretary 3. U.S. mail not marked "Confidential" • Open all mail except that marked "Confidential." • Staple the envelope to the back of each letter. • Date-stamp each letter in the lower right-hand area. • Do not obscure any information, such as the signature or date.

EXHIBIT 4–8 *continued*

Key Step	Sequence	Responsibility	Detailed Steps

Distribute the mail and redirect non-Department mail	Step 3	Release of information clerk	Distribution:
			• Direct loose reports to the Storage and Retrieval unit.
			• Direct "Confidential" mail to the department director's secretary.
			• Direct non-Department mail for
			  1. a staff physician to the physician's office (see the telephone directory for office room numbers)
			  2. the outpatient clinic to the clinic coordinator (see the telephone directory for the office room number)
			• If there is an obvious error by the sender, return the mail immediately to the sender (for example, if the request for information is for another area hospital).

of examples depend on the purpose and the audience. Clarity, brevity, and the use of simple commands or direct language improve comprehension. Action verbs that specify actions the worker must take help to clarify the instructions. Keeping the focus of the procedure specific and its scope limited permits the manager to develop a highly detailed description of the steps to be followed. The steps are listed in logical sequence, with definitions, support examples, and illustrations.

Methods improvement is a prerequisite for efficient, effective procedure development. Flow charts and flow process charts are useful adjuncts to the procedure manual because they require logical sequencing and make it possible to reduce the backtracking and bottlenecks in the workflow.

METHODS

The way in which each step of a procedure is to be performed is a method. Methods focus on such elements as the arrangement of the work area, the use of certain forms, or the operation of specific equipment. A method describes the preferred way of performing a task. The manager may develop methods detail as part of the training package for employee development, leaving the procedure manual free of such detail.

RULES

One of the simplest and most direct types of plan is a rule. A continuing or repeat-use plan, a rule delineates a required or prohibited course of action. The purpose of rules is to predecide issues and specify the required course of action authoritatively and officially.

Like policies, rules guide thinking and channel behavior. Rules, however, are more precise and specific than policies and, technically, allow no discretion in their application. As a result, management must direct careful attention to the number of rules and their intent. If the management intent is to guide and direct behavior rather than require or prohibit certain actions, the rule in effect becomes a policy and should be issued as such.

Like procedures, rules guide action; unlike procedures, however, rules have no time sequence or chronology. Some rules are contained in procedures (e.g., "Extinguish all smoking material before entering this facility"). Other rules are independent of any procedure and stand alone (e.g., "No Smoking"). The wording of rules is direct and specific.

- Food removed from the cafeteria must be in covered containers.
- Books returned to the library after 4:00 P.M. will be considered as returned the following day, and a late fine will be charged.
- Children under the age of twelve must be accompanied at all times by an adult who is responsible for their conduct.

PROJECT PLANNING

In addition to developing the operational plans for day-to-day functioning, managers sometimes undertake intensive project planning for major initiatives. Examples include:

- Implement an organization-wide electronic health record over a four-year period
- Form a regional health information exchange over a two-year period

- Enhance the revenue cycle processes to maximize reimbursement by collecting all the revenues to which the organization is entitled, and to accomplish this in a timely manner; systems and work flow changes to be implemented during the first three months of the new fiscal year
- Develop a leadership succession plan for the next three years in anticipation of planned retirement of (*n*) executive-level managers

Project planning is sometimes expressed primarily in terms of time frame, as in a 500-day plan to gain momentum and to demonstrate major achievements. In the 500-day plan, a rolling cycle of 200-day periods is delineated, with adjustments to the plan made at the conclusion of each phase. Planning for the next phase is fine-tuned in light of the outcomes in the preceding 200 days. The goals for such initiatives reflect actions that have the potential to yield the most results. For example, a fetal alcohol syndrome disorders clinic might focus on early intervention through emphasis on prenatal care. Other aspects of the program simultaneously unfold, but the major focus is this aspect of care.

Project planning is frequently cast in terms of strategic planning.

STRATEGIC PLANNING

In recent decades there has been steady growth in long-range planning activities. The process of strategic planning involves deciding where you want to go, how you want to be positioned, how you think you can get there, what you have to watch out for, and what it is likely to cost you. Today it is the exception to find an organization of any appreciable size that does not have someone who is wholly or largely devoted to developing long-range plans. This trend is certain to continue; there is simply too much at stake and at risk, too much capable competition at work, and too much change occurring in the environment to commit scarce resources and take chances on "shoot-from-the-hip" decisions.

Almost all management decisions made, even the most basic, have long-range implications. Whether concerned with the expansion of services, staff, or space, with developing a research program, or with instituting a student program, every decision of any appreciable scope takes months or years before it achieves its full effect. Each decision must be productive enough to pay off the investment, whether in terms of finances, services, or personnel. The effective manager must be skilled in making long-range decisions that lead to success.

It is often necessary for the manager to take chances. Success results from taking risks, taking action, and expending appropriate resources. In short, it depends on strategic planning.

What Strategic Planning Is Not

Before describing what strategic planning is, it is useful to return to some of the original thinking by the experts. Drucker suggests that it is important for the manager to know what it is not. According to Drucker:

1. It is not a box of tricks, a bundle of techniques. It is analytical thinking and commitment of resources to action. Many techniques may be used in the process—but then again, none may be needed. Strategic planning is not the application of scientific methods to business decisions. It is the application of thought, analysis, imagination, and judgment. It is responsibility, rather than technique.

2. Strategic planning is not forecasting. It is not masterminding the future. Any attempt to do so is foolish; the future is unpredictable. Strategic planning is necessary precisely because we cannot forecast.

3. Strategic planning does not deal with future decisions. It deals with the futurity of present decisions. Decisions exist only in the present. We cannot ask what the organization should do tomorrow. The question is, "what futurity do we have to build into our present thinking and doing, what time spans do we have to consider, and how can we use this information to make a rational decision now?"

4. Strategic planning is not an attempt to eliminate risk. We must understand the risks we take. We must be able to choose rationally among risk-taking courses of action rather than plunge into uncertainty on the bases of hunch, hearsay, or experience, no matter how meticulously this is measured and researched.[5]

What Is Strategic Planning?

Strategic planning is the process of determining the long-term objectives of organizations as a means of formulating strategies to accomplish these objectives. These activities and objectives lead to action today and require an appreciation of what the outcomes of strategic decisions will be in the future. Strategic planning should be viewed positively. An effective strategic plan can help the organization fulfill its mission by articulating a vision of its role, and its potential. An example of a strategic plan appears in Exhibit 4–9.

It is important to emphasize that there is no one acceptable way to engage in strategic planning. Each organization or department is unique, and any strategic plan must fit within the structure and function of the particular organization if it is to be successful.

EXHIBIT 4-9

Sample Strategic Plan

Department of Occupational Therapy
Seaview Community Hospital
Strategic Plan
June 14, 2007

I. Mission Statement

The Department of Occupational Therapy is committed to providing the highest quality of care and service to all patients and clients referred for treatment. All therapists will maintain and upgrade their clinical skills through continuing education and development.

II. Major Objectives

A. Renovate existing space to accommodate a hand rehabilitation center.
B. Recruit therapists with expertise in hand rehabilitation.
C. Develop and implement a staff development program in hand rehabilitation.

III. Action Plan

A. Renovate existing space to accommodate a hand rehabilitation center.
B. Recruit therapists with expertise in hand rehabilitation.
C. Develop and implement a staff development program in hand rehabilitation.
D. Publicize that the department is developing a hand rehabilitation center.

IV. Resources Needed

A. Funds for renovation of existing space
B. Recruitment of hand therapists
C. Consultant to assist department in developing a staff development plan
D. Public relations for new program

V. Possible Sources of Support

A. Institution's capital expense could be met through state or federal budget allocations.
B. Vacant therapy positions could be filled by hand specialists.
C. Budget items could be transferred to continuing education line.
D. Public service announcements could be placed on radio and television.

VI. Monitoring

A. Employees will be given a questionnaire to determine the extent of their satisfaction with the strategic plan and its success to date. Feedback may include suggestions for facilitating the implementation process.
B. Status and progress reports on the recruitment of hand therapists, the staff development program, and the building renovations will be required.
C. An annual review that includes the participation of all key personnel and support staff will be conducted.

Although there are a variety of ways of developing and implementing a strategic plan, there are factors that are characteristic of strategic planning in general. For example, each strategic plan should include

- a mission statement
- a definition of major objectives
- an action plan
- a description of resources needed
- a procedure for monitoring performance
- an evaluation system

Mission Statement

The mission statement should define the scope and focus of the organization's activities. It should be broad enough to encompass potential activities not currently being performed. The statement should allow for flexibility and creativity.

The mission statement can be as simple and straightforward as:

> The Department of Occupational Therapy is committed to providing the highest quality of care and service to all patients and clients referred for treatment. All staff will maintain and upgrade their clinical skills through continuing education and development.

Definition of Major Objectives

In order to fulfill its mission, the organization must decide upon a set of major objectives. The objectives should reflect what is of greatest significance for the current and future direction of the organization. The efforts of the organization will be based on its major objectives and how they fit in with its structure, purpose, and goals.

The objectives should be developed by those who will participate in achieving them. Employees will strive harder to fulfill objectives if they have had a hand in setting them.

The objectives should be clearly stated and should be measurable quantitatively and/or qualitatively. One quantitative objective might be, for example, to increase the number of pediatric patients referred to the physical therapy department. On the other hand, staff satisfaction with a new department head or a new computer filing system for medical records would be considered a qualitative objective.

It is important during strategic planning to discard objectives that are no longer productive, or objectives that have already been achieved.

Following are examples of possible major objectives:

- The Department of Occupational Therapy will develop a hand rehabilitation center that will specialize in posttraumatic injuries.
- The Department of Occupational Therapy will be staffed by therapists who are board-certified specialists in hand rehabilitation.
- The Department of Occupational Therapy will be recognized as a premier hand rehabilitation center.

Action Plan

The next stage of strategic planning is to develop an action plan that contains strategies and activities for achieving the objectives. This stage usually calls for an ability to develop new ways of doing things. Brainstorming is a common technique of searching for effective ways of achieving objectives, but intuition and luck are also necessary. The formulation of an action plan is complex, and there is usually no consensus on program strategies.

In the business arena, the action plan is referred to as the *competitive strategy*, especially as it relates to the financial objectives of the organization.

The plan should be action-oriented and should be allowed to develop over time. Few, if any, action plans can be devised overnight, and each plan should be given ample time to reach fruition. Each plan must also reflect the overall mission of the institution.

An action plan for the objective of creating a hand rehabilitation center within the department of occupational therapy might include these steps:

1. Renovate existing space to accommodate a hand rehabilitation center.
2. Recruit therapists with expertise in hand rehabilitation.
3. Develop and implement a staff development program in hand rehabilitation.
4. Through publicity, notify the hospital and local community that the department is developing a hand rehabilitation center.

Resources Needed

The resources that will be used to implement the strategic plan are, of course, essential. The statement of resources should include personnel, financial, equipment, and space requirements. The institution's policies and procedures will dictate how the resources will be described. The statement of resources should include a breakdown of activities and the necessary allocations. The strengths and the expected impact of the plan should also be presented.

To help justify the requested support, documentation might be presented that indicates how the activities relate to the institution's mission. Ideas on how to acquire federal or state grant support or private funding might also prove helpful, as might suggestions regarding the possible transfer of resources from another area within the department.

Resources needed to implement the action plan for creating a hand rehabilitation center, along with potential sources of support, might include the following:

Resource Needed	*Source of Support*
Funds for renovation of existing space	State or federal budget allocations
Hand specialists	Hiring hand specialists to fill vacant therapy positions
Consultant to assist department in devising a staff development program	Transfer of budget items from equipment to continuing education line
Public relations for new program	Public service announcements on radio and television

Procedure for Monitoring Performance

In order to effectively control the implementation of the strategic plan, it is necessary to monitor the implementation process closely. The evaluation and monitoring system can utilize several approaches. The key point is to determine how well the action plan is progressing toward its objective. The assessment may lead to reconsideration and possible refinement of the objectives, modification of the activities, alteration of the allocation of resources, refinement of roles, and reassignment of individuals.

Measuring the effectiveness of the strategic plan can be done, for example, by having the staff fill out a questionnaire or survey form or by evaluating the extent to which objectives have been achieved over a given period of time. It is important that the supervisor look for signs that implementation of the plan is obstructed or occurring too slowly.

Procedures for monitoring performance may include the following:

- *Survey Form.* Employees are given a questionnaire to determine whether they are satisfied with the strategic plan and its success to date. Feedback may include suggestions for facilitating the implementation of the plan.

- *Status Reports.* These would include periodic reports on the recruitment of hand therapists, the staff development program, and the building renovations.

Evaluation System

It is important to recognize that a strategic plan entails innovation and the breaking of new ground. Therefore, there is a need to assess the effectiveness of the plan in achieving its objectives. An evaluation of the strategic plan should thus be performed at the end of each year. The annual review should address all relevant factors, including the action plan, the institutional objectives and resources, and the problems, successes, weaknesses, and strengths of the plan. Participants should include all key personnel as well as the support staff that will be affected by the plan.

The annual evaluation may include revisions or modifications of the plan. It is best to think in terms of "augmenting" the plan instead of "revising" it. For example, if current resources are not adequate, additional resources will need to be identified.

In summary, strategic planning is indispensable for guiding toward success. It is not mere forecasting but involves a commitment to current and future courses of action. An effective plan will be productive enough to pay off the investment of time and energy.

There is a diversity of methods that can be used to develop a strategic plan. Regardless of the method, the plan should relate to the institution's mission statement, define major objectives, spell out an action plan, indicate the resources needed, and suggest a procedure for monitoring the implementation process. An annual evaluation will help to ensure that the objectives of the plan are being met.

THE PLAN AND THE PROCESS

Referring back to the beginning of the chapter, it is perhaps pertinent to offer a reminder that planning always involves tentatively deciding what might be done in a time period that is not yet here; that is, at some point anywhere from the very near to the far distant future. You plan because you do not know for certain what changes will occur in the environment; you plan because every decision carries with it some elements of risk and uncertainty.

Of course the environment will change between the time we make our tentative decisions and the time the future becomes the present, and of course we enter the overall process with less than perfect information about not only what the future will bring but often also what the present contains. Since change is continual and only partially predictable, we know at the outset that rarely will our plans be fulfilled exactly as planned. This does not, however, mean that planning is a futile activity. To the contrary, it means all the more than one might have suspected that planning is essential.

In and of themselves, plans, those collections of stated targets with dates and desired results attached, are not especially valuable. What is of inestimable value is the planning *process*, that cycle of activities in which you gather information, tentatively decide what is to be done and do it, monitor progress, alter methods as the environment changes and the unforeseen occurs, modify targets as necessary, and go through it all over again but differently. Even if your stated target remains fixed and valid but you did not attain it, the simple presence of the target gives you information you would not have had without it—you know by how much you missed, and thus know how much you must correct your approach for the next attempt.

SPACE RENOVATION AND PLANNING

Space and renovation planning present particular planning considerations for the manager. The planning constraints, for example, flow from such diverse sources as technical architectural details to federal law and regulation concerning barrier-free design for ease of access by disabled persons. Appendix 4–B provides some suggested guidelines to assist the manager in such technical planning.

EXERCISE: INTRODUCTION TO STRATEGIC PLAN DEVELOPMENT

Using the occupational therapy example provided in Exhibit 4–9 as a model, develop a hypothetical strategic plan for a department or function of your choosing. The department or function chosen should provide a professional service, and it should ideally engage in activities that are consistent with your education and experience.

Be sure to address all of the essential major components of a strategic plan. In addition, account for the following potential external (environmental) influences in your plan:

- The appearance of a new competitor offering the same service in which you are engaged within your immediate service area beginning some time within the coming 6 to 12 months or perhaps later. This competitor is definitely coming—at least its coming has been formally announced—but you do not know just when to expect its impact to be felt.

- A 50 percent likelihood of your institution merging with another provider organization of similar size 12 miles away within one and a half to four years. Exploratory merger discussions have begun between boards of directors, but considerable antagonism exists between organizations at the employee level, and vocal elements of both communities are promising to oppose any proposed merger.

Make whatever reasonable assumptions you need to make to develop your plan, and be sure to state your key assumptions.

EXERCISE: FROM INTENT TO ACTION: THE PLANNING PATH

Select a specific health care organization that you know something about. If you are or have been employed in health care, use your employing organization. (But whether it is your organization or another, there is no need to specifically identify it.) You may use a hospital, nursing home, health center, rehabilitation service, surgicenter, urgent care center, or any of a number of other health settings. Assume you are a department manager within your chosen setting.

For your chosen organization:

1. Write a *mission statement* for the organization, concise yet appropriately descriptive of why the organization exists.
2. Consistent with the organization's mission as expressed in the foregoing statement, develop a statement of *philosophy* for your department.
3. Write one major *policy* that supports the above philosophy.
4. Write two or three specific *procedures* that express aspects of the above policy as instructions for action (keeping in mind that a policy is ordinarily a statement of *what* is to be done, and a procedure consists of *how* it should be done).

NOTES

1. Joan Gratto Liebler, *Medical Records: Policies and Guidelines* (Gaithersburg, Md.: Aspen Publishers, 1997), 10: 42.
2. *Ibid.*, 10: 64–71.
3. *Ibid.*, 2: 1–25.
4. Leslie H. Matthies, *The Playscript Procedure* (New York: Office Publications, 1961), 95.
5. Peter F. Drucker, *Management: Tasks, Responsibilities, Practices* (New York: Harper & Row, 1985).

Appendix
4-A

Sample Department Policies

The following comprises a concise rendering of the basic policies governing the organization and operation of a hospital information management (formerly medical records) department. These policies relate the general activities the department will engage in for the purpose of translating its philosophy into actions. An essential next step would be the development of a procedure manual that specifies how all of these activities would be expressed in the form of procedures, literally working instructions. A complete set of procedures for a department could eventually become a fairly extensive publication. Consider that the section titled "Confidentiality, Privacy, and Data Security Considerations" alone could generate a minimum of eight separate procedures (one for each enumerated subsection).

Although the policies included here are specific to health information management, the form in which they are presented may be considered a model for the development of policies for any other function or service as well. Simply utilize the section headings in the following few pages as a gross outline for the creation of departmental policies.

HEALTH INFORMATION MANAGEMENT DEPARTMENT POLICIES

DATE ISSUED: _____

DATE REVISED: _____

MEDICAL STAFF COMMITTEE APPROVAL

NAME: _____

TITLE: _____

SIGNATURE: _____

DATE: _____

CHIEF EXECUTIVE OFFICER APPROVAL
    NAME: _____
    SIGNATURE: _____
    DATE: _____

Health information management (HIM) is a support service of [name of health care facility] whose primary purpose is to contribute to the quality of patient care through the development and maintenance of a comprehensive, centralized medical record system. This system also provides health care data and services to support and promote the related goals and activities of the health care facility: education, training, research, community health, and overall facility management and decision making.

CENTRALIZED HIM DEPARTMENT

Health information management shall be centralized in one coordinated functional unit under the direct authority of a management-level practitioner who is a specialist in health data management. This service shall be designated as health information management. The title of the organizational head of this department shall be director of HIM. This individual shall be designated as the official custodian of health information for the health care facility as a whole.

SCOPE OF SERVICE

The centralized HIM department shall provide functional support to all components of the health care facility and the various departments with respect to health information services. These functions include:

- maintaining a patient/client identification and numbering system
- creating and monitoring patient record documentation
- providing quality assurance and utilization review and studies
- performing risk management review and studies
- coordinating release of information of patient access to data, and responding to court subpoena and depositions
- providing a dictation/transcription system
- maintaining statistical abstracts and indexes
- undertaking special studies for administrative and patient care staff deliberations

- maintaining financial reimbursement support data, including diagnosis and procedure coding;
- maintaining storage and retrieval system, including chart tracking system;
- assisting in complying with legal and regulatory provisions and accrediting agency standards concerning health care data
- maintaining data security, privacy, and confidentiality processes
- providing inservice education and training for professional and support staff
- providing educational programs for students under contractual and/or affiliation agreements
- assisting in research studies

HOURS OF OPERATION AND STAFFING

The major services of the department shall be made available on a continuous basis, seven days a week, 24 hours a day. These servides include:

- a patient identification/numbering system
- access to patient care data for direct patient care purposes
- a dictation system
- transcription of priority reports needed for immediate, direct patient care

All other services shall be offered during the normal business hours of the facility, on an extended workday plan. The extended workday for the department is 7 A.M. to 6 P.M., Monday through Friday.

An appropriate combination of full-time and permanent part-time staff shall be trained to carry out the usual health information functions. In the rare event that no department employee is available to carry out an emergency request during the non–business day work period, the administrator on call shall have access to the department to arrange for retrieval of the critical information.

COMPLIANCE WITH REGULATIONS AND STANDARDS

Services and functions shall be developed and implemented in a manner consistent with five groups of regulations and standards:

1. legal and regulatory provisions affecting the facility:
   - state department of health licensure regulations
   - Medicare Conditions of Participation
   - federal and state provisions for Medicaid programs

- professional review organization mandates
- federal and state reimbursement and financing regulations

2. professional association and accrediting agency standards:
   - Joint Commission on Accreditation of Healthcare Organizations (or American Osteopathic Association)
   - American Health Information Management Association's *Code of Ethics*
3. institutional and medical staff bylaws
4. institutional policies of related departments, with particular attention given to admissions, patient billing and finance, nursing, clinic and emergency, and other departments where coordination of administrative practice and processing of patient care data are essential
5. contractual provisions with related service providers and/or reimbursement agencies and transfer agreement provisions with other health care facilities such as home care, hospice care, rehabilitation centers, and long-term care facilities

CONFIDENTIALITY, PRIVACY, AND DATA SECURITY CONSIDERATIONS

Services and functions shall be developed and implemented in such a way that confidentiality, privacy, and data security considerations are respected and fostered at all stages of health care information gathering and processing. The following eight practices help ensure that facilities will abide by these considerations:

1. *Employee orientation and training.* This area shall include:
   - mandatory completion of inservice program by all HIM employees
   - cooperation from appropriate department managers, offering of inservice education to admissions, business office, computer department, clerical support staff in outpatient clinics, emergency department, and nursing department
   - active participation in orientation of all new employees of the facility
2. *Confidentiality statement.* All HIM employees shall be required to sign the confidentiality statement (Exhibit 4A–1). This shall be placed in the employee's permanent personnel file and reviewed and updated at least annually. It shall also be updated during any year there is a significant change in the job duties of the employee.
3. *Researchers and students.* Students in education programs and researchers with access to health care data shall receive appropriate orientation and shall sign the confidentiality statement as a condition of access to the health data.

4. *Contractual services.* Appropriate provision for data security and confidentiality shall be included in any contract for service from outside vendors such as word processing, statistical abstracting, and temporary agency staffing.

5. *Centralized release of information.* All requests for release of information, regardless of the department originating or receiving the request, shall be processed in the central release of information unit of the medical record department. See release of information policy.

6. *Rules for data access and use.* Detailed rules shall be developed and enforced to limit the rules of health care data and to specify the conditions under which such data may be used. See storage and retrieval policy.

7. *Data security provisions/computer access.* Appropriate safeguards shall be adopted for computerized processes relating to health care information. See computerized data security policy.

8. *Limited access to department.*

- The following individuals who may be permitted access to health care data shall carry out an approved review of material in a supervised, restricted area that is separate from the general work area of the department.
    - patients and patient representatives, including lawyers
    - third-party review auditors from reimbursement agencies
    - students (except health care administrators and health information administrators and technicians under specific affiliation agreements)
- Visitors, including health care facility employees from other departments, shall not be permitted access to the general work area of the department except as specifically noted in designated procedures.
- Health care facility employees who are not directly and actively carrying out a necessary function (e.g., housekeeping or maintenance) shall not be admitted to the work area.
- Researchers carrying out an approved research review of data shall work in a designated area, separate from the general work area.

EDUCATION AND TRAINING

Department Employees

A systematic program of orientation, on-the-job training, specialized training, and regular in-service training shall be developed and implemented for health information employees for the following purposes:

EXHIBIT 4A–1

Confidentiality Statement

I, [name], understand that in the performance of my duties as an employee of [name of health care facility] I am required to have access to and am involved in the processing of patient care data. I understand that I am obliged to maintain the confidentiality of these data at all times, both at work and off duty. I understand that a violation of these confidentiality considerations may result in disciplinary action, including termination. I further understand that I could be subject to legal action. I certify by my signature that I have participated in the orientation and training session given on [date] concerning the privacy and confidentiality considerations of patient care.

Date   Signature

Original to be placed in the employee's permanent personnel file.
Copy to be placed in orientation and training session file.

Source: Reprinted from J.G. Liebler, *Medical Records: Policies and Guidelines*, p. 2:2, © 1990, Aspen Publishers, Inc.

- to reduce potential liability because of error
- to create a positive, motivational climate
- to enhance employee productivity and efficiency
- to enhance employee opportunity for promotion

When inservice programs reflect critical issues (e.g., fire drills, safety practices, and confidentiality), participation shall be mandatory and the program shall be offered during work hours. A variety of other offerings may be given at times when an employee may need to commit personal time and for which participation will be optional.

Management and supervisory personnel shall participate regularly in professional association meetings, conferences, and workshops as approved by the director of HIM. Appropriate budgetary support of these activities shall be made available insofar as possible.

Participation in orientation, on-the-job training, inservice offerings, and other training related to job duties shall be documented for each individual. This documentation shall become a part of the employee's permanent personnel file, and a copy shall become a part of the department inservice log. Such evidence of orientation and inservice training shall be made available when requested as part of the accreditation and/or licensure survey of the facility. Review of progress through in-service and other training shall be a part of the employee evaluation process.

Medical and Professional Staff

Health information personnel shall provide the necessary assistance in orientation and training programs for the medical and professional staff, with particular emphasis on health care data documentation, privacy and confidentiality, data security, and related matters.

Health Care Facility Personnel

Health information personnel shall provide the necessary assistance in the orientation and training of health care facility personnel in the areas of confidentiality and privacy. As time and resources permit, other program offerings may be developed and offered as part of the facility-wide training efforts.

Affiliated Programs

Active participation in the education and training of students from approved affiliated institutions (e.g., allied health and health care administration) shall be fostered in accordance with the health care facility's goal of teaching. Details of such training activities shall be specified in appropriate letters of agreement or affiliation contracts, with the approval of the chief executive officer or designee.

QUALITY ASSURANCE AND PROFESSIONAL PRACTICE STANDARDS

An active program of quality assurance review focusing on health information practices shall be undertaken by the director of health information (Exhibit 4A–2).

Major components shall include the following:

- an annual review of each function using the American Health Information Management Association's best practices guidelines or similar benchmarks

EXHIBIT 4A–2

Work Sheet for Customizing General Policies

Policy Elements	Special Considerations
Department Name	• Determine the organizational title and use it consistently throughout.
Centralized Service and Scope of Service	• Determine which departments of the facility will be covered by the policies: determine which services will be undertaken by the department.
	• Give particular attention to the impact of services to be rendered to the outpatient and emergency departments. This should include chart analyses and review, coding, and all related functions.
Hours of Operation	• Coordinate with patient care delivery; make provisions for access to critical data for off-hours.
	• Check with personnel labor relations concerning shift designations, e.g., any contractual labor agreements to be considered.
Access to Department during Nonoperating Periods	• The administrator on call is an appropriate designee; clear this with administrative officers. The director of nursing is another alternative, but this would add one more duty to individuals charged with direct patient care.
Compliance with Standards	• Refer to the work sheet done earlier in which specific state, federal, and accrediting agency provisions were noted.
Medical Staff Bylaws	• The rules and regulations section is a key area: chart content policies are an addendum to this section. Refer also to the work sheet done earlier for other medical staff issues.

continues

EXHIBIT 4A–2 *continued*

Policy Elements	Special Considerations
Contractual Provisions	• State these, and determine the requirements for providing which services to which departments; cross-reference this to the release of information because patient care data are sometimes sent with the patient directly.
Confidentiality Provisions	• See the American Health Information Management Association's guidelines for employee use.
Researchers and Students	• There is an impact on the physical layout of the department when this provision is adopted. If the present layout cannot be changed immediately, insert the phrase as far as possible and seek to have the layout changed as soon as possible.
Education and Training	• Consider the provisions of the Fair Labor Standards Act if required training is to take place after an employee's work hours.
Cross-References and Internal Consistency	• Coordinate with policies for release of information, storage and retrieval, and computerized data security.

Source: Adapted with permission from Aspen Publishers, Inc., 1997, Joan Gratto Liebler, *Medical Records: Policies and Guidelines*, 2:1–2:5.

- employee evaluation and training according to institutional practices (e.g., annual evaluation with special evaluation at the time of transfer or promotion or at the conclusion of a probationary/training period)

EXERCISE: PLANS ARE WHAT?

Consider the following statement: Plans in and of themselves are not especially useful; however, the planning *process* is invaluable.

In essay form, thoroughly explain what you believe is meant by this statement. It will be necessary to examine the statement from both directions. That is, explain the truth (or lack thereof) in the comment about plans not being especially useful, then proceed to explain the supposedly greater value of the planning process.

EXERCISE: GOALS, OBJECTIVES, AND PROCEDURES

For any department of your choosing (except for physical therapy and health information management, which are used in the chapter's examples), create a *general objective* that identifies this department's overall mission, and provide a set of three to five *functional objectives* describing how the general objective will be pursued. Then select one of your functional objectives and in outline form create at least one *procedure* that could be applied in pursuing the objective.

Appendix
4–B

Space Renovation and Planning

Most health care practitioners will, at some time in their career, participate in planning a new department or renovating an old one. This process requires knowledge of all the possible present and future uses of the space as well as an ability to make "best guesses" regarding future needs. Making changes commonly requires two to five years of work with a variety of professionals and craft specialists. To help present all the issues, we will suppose that you are working in rehabilitation as a manager and that your department head announces your department will be renovated in two years. Your participation in the planning and renovation is mandated; you are expected to improve the design of your area and increase the productivity of your staff.

The main steps for planning renovations include preparation, idea gathering, idea verification, modification of ideas, and revision of plans. After plans are finalized, your responsibilities shift and you now focus on monitoring. You supervise your staff; ensure the safety of patients, personnel, and equipment; and encourage your staff to be flexible as they try to accomplish their work in the midst of construction workers, materials and supplies, and daily inconveniences. Once the construction is complete, your job shifts again and you now test out the finished products. Follow-up is also imperative so that problems are not overlooked or forgotten.

THE PLANNING TEAM

The composition of the planning team will depend on the funding and the total allocation of support for the project, the composition of the institution's staff, and the expertise of team members. Usually the team includes representatives from facilities planning and an architect. For example, if the area to be constructed is in a hospital, the team would include the hospital administrator, appropriate department heads, the medical chief of staff, the director of nursing, an attorney, and the business manager or an accountant. An interior designer and a safety officer may also be included. It is recommended that the architect has had experience in designing similar projects and is familiar with specific characteristics of the physical environment.

PREPARATION FOR PLANNING

Before the actual design and construction phase takes place, it is helpful to address a number of preplanning factors. The scope of the preplanning stage depends on the structure and function of the area to be designed. Any present or possible future need to expand services should also be discussed among the parties involved. For example, if the health information department anticipates that after a year of operation an additional computerized data system will be required, the staff may want to know whether there is available space physically located near the department for expansion. Perhaps the department should include an additional area in the initial plans and utilize it as storage space or for another function until the time it is needed to expand services. Issues like these must be addressed before construction is started. It is likely that the costs for renovation and expansion will be higher after construction is completed.

Depending on the type and structure of the facility, general factors to be considered by the planning team before construction begins include the present and projected population trends in the area and the need for the new services based on existing services and referral sources. Information about such factors may help to support space needs and design. Other preplanning factors that should be considered include

- program purposes and goals
- location
- cost estimates
- financial resources
- equipment
- plan development

Program Purposes and Goals

Before any construction begins, it is recommended that the department define the services that will be provided. By so doing, the space needs will be better understood. The department should establish objectives and set standards that can be used to monitor and evaluate the success of the program. For example, if long-term rehabilitation services will be provided, the department should include an area for activities of daily living. If the department expects a student affiliation program, an area for students should be part of the design.

Location

The accessibility of the department must be considered prior to construction. Rehabilitation departments should be located near an elevator for easier patient transportation. The area should preferably be on the main floor near parking. In considering the location, it is important to keep in mind that the department must be accessible to and usable by the physically handicapped. The usability of bathrooms, the width of doors, and wheelchair maneuverability are some of the factors that need to be discussed with the architect as he or she begins work on the design.

Estimates

Although the exact cost for the facility may not be predictable, an approximation of the bottom-line costs may be required. The approximation should include space, equipment, and renovation expenses. Note that it is better to overestimate rather than underestimate what the final cost may be.

Financial Resources

Depending on the type of facility and the administrative structure, the manager may be requested to determine the financial resource available for construction. These resources might include state or city funding appropriations and federal or private grant support.

Equipment

Certain rehabilitation equipment (e.g., the whirlpool hubbard tank, hydraulic lift, and the shoulder wheel) is fixed equipment and must be attached to the wall beams. It is necessary to include the location of fixed equipment in the initial design of the facility. Any special specifications for equipment should also be brought to the attention of the architect. This is especially important in the case of electrical requirements. For example, certain electrical modalities (EMG, moist heating units) may require 220-volt outlets instead of the standard 110-volt outlets. Any special electrical requirements should be included in the architectural drawings prior to construction.

Plan Development

It is crucial to the success of the project to work with the architect in developing the diagrammatic scheme or drawings of the facility. Decide on major and minor needs and visualize the placement of services, furniture, and equipment. Before the plan is presented, it is helpful to prepare a preliminary drawing of the facility to show the relationship of the various areas in the department. This drawing can aid the architect in developing a working area that facilitates the maximum efficiency of traffic flow and minimizes crosswise traffic patterns. The preliminary plan should indicate how the various rooms will be divided with regard to the various functions that will be provided.

The steps in developing a plan are as follows:

1. Sketch present space and use a measuring tape to measure it. Determine the size of rooms and equipment. If you are planning new space, take the time to visit other facilities in order to measure their rooms and spatial arrangements.

2. Think about your present space and list the positive and negative factors. Include staff members in this process. The more advice you get, the better your chance of discovering all of your needs during this preliminary stage of planning.

3. Solicit ideas from other departments.

4. Visit other facilities. Note the positive and negative aspects of their space. Verify your ideas with the individuals who use the space every day.

5. Conceptualize ideas one room at a time. Keep notes on your ideas and needs.

6. Initiate a meeting with the architect or engineer who is in charge of the project. If this person does not express an interest in meeting with you, state your need to get input into the project before plans are drawn up.

7. Discuss your department's needs clearly and follow up discussions with written communications to confirm agreements.

8. Once you receive a copy of the plans, operationalize them by marking outlines of the actual equipment and cabinets on the floor with marking tape or some other form of temporary marking. Compare past and future needs and uses. Do not be afraid to ask questions or voice your discomfort with certain ideas.

The purpose of the preplanning phase is to devise a rough outline of the requirements for the space. This outline or sketch does not replace the actual design of the area.

INVENTORY OF SPACE

The space that has been made available for the new facility or department must be carefully inventoried in order to determine how the space should be apportioned. The inventory of the space should include the following:

- square footage
- size of rooms
- location of rooms
- special equipment and facilities

The amount of space (or square footage) made available to the department will influence how the space is used. The size of a room, for example, might restrict the types of services that could be provided. For example, any room designated as a location for activities of daily living (ADL) should meet minimum space requirements. If a room does not meet the requirements for ADL, it may be suitable for another function.

The location of the department within the facility is an important factor and requires careful consideration. The rehabilitation areas should be located near the elevator and, if the department provides outpatient treatments, in close proximity to parking and to the main entrance to the institution. Certain equipment may need special preparation. Computer equipment and isokinetic devices may require special wiring and will need to be placed away from areas of heavy traffic. The size of a piece of equipment may also determine where it should be placed.

ARCHITECTURAL SPECIFICATIONS

In developing the architectural plans, the following must be considered:

- the function and organization of the various components
- the spatial requirements
- the workflow patterns

Function and Organization of Components

In designing or renovating an area within a facility, adequate consideration must be given to the specific functions to be located within that area. These functions should be given a full description, including a detailed explanation of how each activity is to be carried out in the space and how each activity relates to other functions. The description should also include any special requirements that may affect the design.

During this stage of the planning process, the bulk of the responsibility belongs to the facility staff, since they are the most familiar with the unique characteristics and features of the operational programs. Depending on the scope of the project, a medical services consultant may assist the staff in preparing the description of the functional components.

The purpose of describing the functions to be performed in the work area is to furnish the architect with adequate data to begin making space allocations. The organization of the functions provides a schematic outline that can be used in establishing the spatial requirements.

Spatial Requirements

The amount of space or square footage allocated for a given work area depends on a number of considerations. The types of services to be provided, the major pieces of equipment, the storage requirements, the shape of the area, the number of personnel that will work in the area, the number of clients or patients that will be seen, the reception and secretarial support systems, among other things, need to be taken into account when determining square footage. Of prime importance in determining the space requirements are the individual circumstances for a given situation. For example, there may be a preset amount of space allocated by the facility administration for the work area. The department would then have to decide how the space would be apportioned. Regardless of the situation, judgment and experience are crucial for the design of an appropriate and effective work area.

When determining if an allotted space is sufficient, a number of factors must be considered, including the nature of the equipment that must be housed. What is the dimension of each piece of equipment and how much space and personnel are needed to safely operate it? The vendor should be able to provide this information for any piece of equipment on order.

It should also be determined how many of the staff will require a private office. In most physical therapy and occupational therapy departments, the director, assistant director, and clinical education coordinator will each require a private office, but the staff therapists will be able to share one large office space. A private office is usually between 100 and 110 square feet. The size of the office for the therapists will depend on the number of therapists. For a staff of five physical therapists, an office space of 300 square feet should be sufficient.

The criteria used to determine square footage should come from more than one source (e.g., a consultant with experience in designing similar spaces, the appropriate professional organization, and current articles). Whatever the source used to estimate square footage, it is important that the planning team carefully review the purpose of the department and the functions that will be carried out in the area.

TECHNICAL CONSIDERATIONS

The manager confers with the architect and engineer to develop the detailed specifications relating to such technical aspects as:

- electrical lighting and power needs
- humidity control
- air conditioning and ventilation
- aisle space and door clearance requirements
- floor and wall thickness
- floor load
- noise control
- privacy needs for clients and personnel

The department manager has the responsibility to call attention to any special aspect of such technical specifications.

SYSTEMATIC LAYOUT PLANNING GRID

A manager may facilitate the planning process by developing a systematic planning grid. This layout planning grid is customized for each departmental function. The key activities of the unit, internal and external contacts, special architectural needs, and similar technical details are listed. The technical consideration associated with each aspect of planning is stated. Table 4B–1 displays such a layout grid for the word processing/transcription function of a health information department.

Table 4B–1 Layout Grid for Word Processing Function—
Health Information Department

Word Processing/Transcription	
Number of Employees	Day ____ Evening ____ Night ____
Key Activities	Transcribe dictated reports
	Receive printouts from off-site transcription service
	Prepare and distribute originals and copies
	Coordinate wordflow with off-site transcription service
Contact with Clients and Patients	None
Contact with Professional Staff	Routine contact, usually by telephone, with physicians and other professionals who dictate reports
	Technical Considerations
	Total work stations: ____
	Special need: shared work space for three shifts
	Provide storage space for personal items for each worker
	No need for reception area for clients in the immediate work area
	Telephone at each workstation
	Supervisor's telephone has automatic redial capability
Interdepartmental Relationships	Coordination with chart processing: daily
	Coordination with release-of-information specialists for priority action (e.g., scheduled court or deposition appearance by ROI specialist; need for complete record)
Other Contacts	Daily contact with off-site transcription service
Privacy and Security Considerations	All material processed is confidential patient care documentation
	Night shift personnel work alone in this area of the building
	Computers and word processing equipment are "attractive" items for theft
	Holding bin for completed work designated as priority
	Word processing printer to receive off-site transmittal
	Placement of display screen so that material cannot be read by others
	Limited access to work area
	Special security alarms for safety of night shift personnel
	Equipment locks; antitheft devices on all equipment
Noise Control	Production-level word processing generates noise throughout the work periods; individual transcriptionists are generally protected from this noise because they use headphones; supervisor is exposed to this noise throughout workday
	Carpet the area
	Install sound-conditioning ceiling and walls
	Place word processing unit in separate room or surround work unit with special noise-reduction paneling
Lighting	Close work; detailed clerical work processed throughout the workday
	Overhead ambient lighting at workstation: 100 foot candles
	Direct lighting at workstaton: 100 foot candles

continues

Table 4B–1 *continued*

Word Processing/Transcription	
	Technical Considerations
Electrical Needs	Word processing unit and convenience lighting at each workstation
	Outlets for computer terminal(s) and outlets for planned expansion (4 additional workstations)
	Grounded outlets
	Power surge protection
	Minimum of 3 outlets per workstation
	No extension cords allowed
Telephone and Other Communication Devices	Needed for each workstation
	Need both internal and external access
	Workers wear headphones during most of the workday; cannot hear ringing phone; add visual signal
	Need to secure phones from unauthorized use
	Both internal and external access lines on all phones
	Equip phones with flashing light
	Equip phones with lock feature
Temperature and Humidity	Personal comfort; enhanced productivity
	Equipment considerations, especially computers
	Air-conditioned work area
	Humidity control—40% to 50%
Special Architectural Support or Weight-Bearing Considerations	Standard office equipment
	150 lbs. per sq. ft.
Work Surface Requirements	Sitting: most of work is done while sitting at desk
	Standing: sorting and distributing completed original and copies
	Mobile: none needed
Square Footage (standard allotments)	Per employee
	Per supervisor
	Aisle space
	Sorting and receiving area and remote terminal area

MONITORING AND TESTING THE CONSTRUCTION

Once plans are finalized and equipment ordered, you must wait for the construction to begin. It is best not to have employees work in any area where construction is going on. New construction is easier on the employees, the patients, and the contractors, since the new area can be segregated. If construction takes place while staff are working, you must enlist their support during this inconvenient time. Ask for a production schedule so that you can try to better organize staffing and service delivery. Protect fragile equipment from harm. Flexibility and adaptability will be needed as staff try to deal with noise, dust, strangers, and daily changes.

Monitor the installation of equipment and save instructions and guarantees.

Once construction is completed and the construction disorder is cleared away, you must test the results. Set up and test new machines and try out furniture, lights, and drawers. Report defective items to the architect.

THE AMERICANS WITH DISABILITIES ACT AND BARRIER-FREE DESIGNS

Accommodating handicapped persons to enable them to perform efficiently is both a humanitarian service and a legal requirement. It is estimated that at least 10 percent of the population have a significant physical handicap.

The Americans with Disabilities Act (ADA) provides a clear and comprehensive national mandate for the elimination of discrimination against the 43 million Americans who have physical or mental disabilities. The ADA seeks to alleviate discrimination against the disabled in employment and public accommodations and mandates that public transportation, telecommunications, and public services be accessible. The ADA also requires that newly constructed and renovated public transportation conveyances and commercial facilities be readily accessible to and usable by individuals with disabilities except where it can be shown that it is structurally impractical to meet this requirement.

Barrier-free design allows access to and free movement within a facility by persons with a wide range of disabilities. These disabilities include

- nonambulatory disabilities
- emiambulatory disabilities (e.g., the disabilities experienced by people on crutches, the grossly overweight, cardiac and pulmonary patients, stroke victims, amputees)
- disabilities involving coordination (e.g., cerebral palsy)
- sight disabilities
- hearing disabilities
- general disabilities (e.g., the disabilities associated with aging)
- temporary disabilities (e.g., disabilities associated with pregnancy)

Barrier-free design is required in both new and existing facilities of organizations that are federally sponsored or assisted by federal funds. Careful application of the criteria will be necessary if the needs of the handicapped are to be met without incurring expenses that are at great variance with the benefits received. The areas that the barrier-free design checklist covers include passenger arrival terminals, parking lots, walks, ramps, doors, entrances, corridors, public spaces, work areas, stairs, elevators, toilet facilities, drinking fountains, public telephones, controls (such as drapes, doors, windows, and light switches), identification signs, and warning or precaution areas.

Specific examples of barrier-free design include the following:

- eliminating revolving doors or providing standard doors as alternative entrances or exits
- installing time-delay doors
- placing doorknobs 36 inches from floor
- using entry and interior doors that are at least 32 inches wide
- making thresholds flush with floor
- providing ramps
- making corridors a minimum of 54 inches wide (wheelchairs need space to turn)
- providing restrooms with at least one wheelchair entry stall with grab rails
- putting controls on light switches, elevators, and fire and safety alarms that are within reach of wheelchair user
- making drapery, venetian blinds, or shade cords long enough to be reached by wheelchair user
- placing files so that access can be from front and side
- providing sturdy chairs
- providing chairs with casters for easy mobility
- providing reserved parking spaces

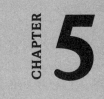

Decision Making

DEFINITION

In the planning process, the step involving the choice among alternatives is designated the decision-making phase. Decision making is choosing from among alternatives to determine the course of action. Alternatives may be limited or abundant; in any case, there must be at least two options, or there is no decision, only forced choice.

PARTICIPANTS IN DECISION MAKING

The decision-making function is an essential element of management activity at all organizational levels. The necessity to make decisions that in any way involve the use of staff or other resources is one of the defining characteristics of management regardless of organizational level. There are, however, some distinct differences in the kinds of decisions made at different levels of management.

Major decisions of significant scope or impact reside primarily with top-level management. Most of the time, however, no major decision is made by any single manager alone. The organizational hierarchy determines the pattern of participation in the decision-making process. Top-level managers usually make the pervasive, critical, nonprogrammed, root decisions such as determination of organizational goals and major policy guidelines, although they may be assisted by technical staff advisers who develop the alternatives based on research and analysis. Line managers may also be consulted. However, these decisions are ordinarily of such magnitude that the responsibility for them generally rests with the chief executive officer and governing board.

The organizational structure limits the decision-making ability of all other managers in terms of authority and responsibility for specific departments or units. Such middle managers make decisions for their own units or departments within the framework set by top management rulings. In addition, because middle managers usually have some specific technical competence, they are often key participants in decisions relating to these technical areas. Top management may defer to the technical competence of individual department heads, giving them a specific charge of making final decisions in their areas of expertise. The middle manager's decision mix, then, consists of routine, recurring decisions, and nonrecurring decisions in an area of specialized technical competence. These operational decisions are usually routinized through the development of policy and procedure to ensure smooth work flow. For example, the director of an occupational therapy department makes the routine decisions regarding vacation scheduling for department employees in accordance with overall organizational guidelines and makes certain nonprogrammed, critical decisions, such as the selection of equipment for the unit. These latter decisions are made on the basis of the director's specialized knowledge as an occupational therapist.

Rank-and-file employees are involved in decision making in both direct and indirect ways. Collective bargaining agreements may specify areas in which employees must be consulted. Sometimes their participation is limited to ratification of the contract, but their legitimate, legal claim to participation is recognized to the degree specified in the bargaining agreement. Employees are involved in the decision-making process in a continuous, although indirect, manner; all levels of management depend on the feedback provided by workers who actually perform the day-to-day activities. This feedback process may be formalized, with employees given formal recognition as participants in planning and decision making.

Clients of an organization sometimes participate in decision making. Like employees, clients may have a legitimate claim to participation because of a legislative mandate. For example, the legislation that creates or funds community mental health centers or health planning agencies often requires the presence of consumers and community members on advisory councils or even governing boards. Federal and state agencies are required to hold public hearings on certain issues, which fosters client participation in decision making. Members of professional associations also participate in the decision-making process. Although primarily limited to the role of ratifying decisions presented by an elected board or by an appointed executive officer, members of such associations can participate more actively should a group of members wish to press a claim.

The decision-making process in health care organizations has an additional dimension in that the medical staff participate in major determinations Neither clients nor employees in the usual sense of the terms, the medical staff have a tradition of involvement in hospital governance. The dual track of authority in health care organizations brings about a special situation for the chief executive officer and for line department heads who report to the administrative officer. Through the committee structure, the medical staff become involved directly in the operations of some departments. In the pharmacy, for example, decisions such as the use of brand names versus generic names in drug selection cannot be made by the pharmacist alone. The pharmacy and therapeutics committee of the medical staff must make the final decision. The day-to-day operations of the health information service are the responsibility of the health information administrator, but the health information committee may have as a charge, stated in the bylaws, the review of the health information system. Although the actions of the medical staff in these areas are generally limited to suggestions rather than mandates, a limit is imposed nonetheless on the decision-making power of these managers. Chapter 9 includes detailed discussion of participation in committees, teams, and task forces.

Chief executive officers in a health care institution hold a role similar to that of professional managers or hired administrators in an industrial or business corporation. They are not the owners, nor do they have strong kinship ties with the owners. In the case of a hospital under the control and sponsorship of a religious order or a philanthropic group, they may not necessarily be members of the sponsoring group. They must make decisions with continual reference to their unwritten mandate: What do the owners or those in authority wish them to decide? The complexities of the decision-making process become evident when the participants and their distinct roles are identified and when the difficulties imposed by the mixed authority constellation in health care organizations are recognized.

EVALUATING A DECISION'S IMPORTANCE

By its nature, decision making means commitment. The importance of a decision may be measured in terms of the resources and time being committed. Some decisions affect only small segments of the organization, while others involve the entire organization. Some decisions are irrevocable because they create new situations. The degree of flexibility that remains after the commitment has been made may also be used in evaluating the significance of a decision: Are the resulting conditions tightly circumscribed, with little flexibility permitted, or are several options still available in developing subsequent plans? Decisions regarding capital expenditures, major procedural systems, and the cost of the equipment that must be prorated over the projected life of the equipment are examples.

The degree of uncertainty—and therefore the degree of risk—associated with a decision is another dimension that must be evaluated in weighing its impact. The greater the impact in terms of time, resources, and degree of risk, the more time, money, and effort must be directed toward making such decisions. Finally, in any organization, the impact on humans is a major factor. The environmental impact and social cost must be assessed.

STEPS IN DECISION MAKING

The decision-making process consists of several sequential steps: (1) agenda building, including problem definition; (2) the search for alternatives; (3) evaluation of the alternatives; (4) commitment (i.e., the choice among alternatives); and (5) continuing assessment of decisions, which leads back to agenda building.

Agenda Building

Like planning, decision making may be viewed as a cyclic process. The first step, agenda building, flows from the feedback process. Information is gathered, clarified, and analyzed. The problem is defined and priorities are assigned. This step is critical, because subsequent decisions may be meaningless and nonproductive unless the problem has been clarified. Indeed, the wrong problem may be solved, so to speak. Without problem clarification, a manager could implement a solution—possibly one that is costly in time, effort, and personnel—only to find recurring evidence and symptoms of the original problem, which remains unidentified and therefore unsolved.

For example, in a health center, there were long delays from the time of patient arrival until the time of treatment. The nursing and physician team felt under pressure because of patient complaints about the crowded waiting room and the long waits. The first effort to find a solution resulted in a triage system through which patients were assessed promptly and assigned priorities in the treatment process. In addition, considerable effort was made to improve the time allotments and sequencing of patients in the appointment system to help create a more orderly patient flow.

Having developed the triage system, changed the staffing pattern, and revamped the appointment system, the staff was faced with the same crowded waiting room. Why? During the second analysis, the true problem was identified. Because the transportation system in the local community was inadequate, patients tended to come to the center at the beginning of the day or at the end of the noon hour, when family members were free to bring them. There was no other convenient way to get to the center. Furthermore, patients did not understand the appointment system process, nor did they believe that they would be seen at the appointed time.

When the health center, with the assistance of its community board, developed an alternate neighborhood transportation system, the problem was solved. Patient education programs concerning the appointment system were prepared, further helping to alleviate the problem.

Several management processes provide the executive with critical information for use in agenda building and problem identification. Analysis of the institution through use of the input-output model, for example, creates a systematic awareness of change in the organizational environment. Specific feedback processes, such as periodic formal reports and quality control routines, provide specific information for problem identification.

The after-action report, developed at the conclusion of a major project such as accreditation review or a demanding circumstance such as a disaster, is a rich source of information for agenda building. For example, after a major disaster, the debriefing review would focus on operational strengths: What are the reasons that the operation ran smoothly? Then lessons learned are identified (e.g., failure of certain equipment; need for greater coordination with local and regional law enforcement and medical services; need for area-wide disaster plan rehearsal).

Preparation for renegotiating a collective bargaining agreement provides an opportunity to review aspects of personnel matters, both for the group whose contract is up for renewal as well as for all employees. As with accreditation and licensure reviews, contract renegotiations provide a routine, recurring, and predicable time frame for agenda building.

Minutes of meetings of a standing committee are another source of potential agenda building: is there an item of a recurring nature? This suggests that a more effective decision is needed concerning that issue. The findings of a consultant's report (see Chapter 6 for an example) contain items for agenda building along with their priority. The findings of a licensure or accrediting agency report similarly become the basis of priority agenda.

Another tool that can be useful in the agenda-building stage of decision making is the cause-and-effect chart, frequently referred to as a "fishbone diagram." An example of such a diagram may be found in Chapter 7.

Search for Alternatives

Having defined and analyzed the problem, the decision maker searches for alternatives. It is the manager's job both to identify existing alternatives and to create new and better ones. The manager must remain open to all possible solutions to problems, taking care not to reject nontraditional approaches automatically. Alternatives may be identified quickly from past experience, but these must be accepted with caution because they may not fit the present situation. Creativity is a necessary element. An organizational climate of openness in which the development of original ideas is considered a legitimate use of the manager's time and effort fosters this approach. Coordinated time should be arranged for the management team as a whole, such as periodic team retreats during which day-to-day operations are set aside and the group assesses organizational needs and seeks creative approaches to satisfy these needs.

Chester Barnard, in his classic work on the functions of managers, stressed the importance of identifying the strategic or limiting factors that constrain the realistic development of alternatives.[1] The decision maker should confine the search for alternatives to those that will overcome these elements. This selectivity tends to prevent a waste of time and energy in developing alternatives that are infeasible and ineffective. Limiting factors that constrain decision making in health care include legal and accrediting standards, ethics, and lack of capital and trained personnel. The limiting or strategic factors change from time to time. Barnard saw the strategic factor as the point at which choice applies.[2] The solutions are narrowed to include only those that fit the organizational goals and the availability of resources. An example of a limiting factor having impact on private or group practice is the USDHHS requirement that certain electronic health record products meet the baseline requirements of the Certification Commission for Healthcare Information Technology. When the manager develops criteria for decision making, such limiting factors must be included in the decision matrix.

Evaluation of Alternatives

In order to evaluate alternatives, a manager must adopt an underlying philosophical stance and make a preliminary decision about the approach to decision making that will be taken. Depending on the philosophical stance, certain alternatives will be acceptable and others will be excluded automatically. Root and branch decision making, "satisficing," maximizing, and the use of Paretian optimality are among the fundamental types of (or approaches to) decision making that will partially determine the decisions that are actually reached.

Root and Branch Decision Making

Certain decisions are so basic to the organization's nature that their effects are pervasive and far-reaching in terms of organizational values, philosophy, goals, and overall policies. Such decisions, root decisions, invest the organization with its fundamental nature at its inception and carry it into periodic, comprehensive review of its fundamental purpose, often resulting in massive innovation. Thus, in the life cycle of an organization, root decisions may be associated with gestation, when the fundamental form and purpose of the organization are crystallized. They may occur in middle age, when new goals are developed and new organizational patterns are adopted. Finally, during old age and decline, a fundamental decision to dissolve the organization may be made. The pervasive effect of root decisions may be seen in the decision of a board of trustees to change a two-year college into a baccalaureate degree-granting institution or to convert a hospital into a multiple component health care center. By way of example, consider the decision made by a health information administrator choosing to use off-site commercial storage for hard copy records. When this change is implemented, the existing space for hard copy records will be eliminated and will not easily be recovered. Policies and procedures, budget considerations, and changes in staffing patterns also result. The decision has long-lasting implications. For these reasons, this decision ranks as a root decision. Other examples of root decisions may be noted in the major changes in some professional associations such as the recent decision of the AHIMA's decision to open active membership to all who are interested in the primary work of the association. Another example of such change is that of the American Physical Therapy Association's decision to emphasize doctoral-level preparation as the norm for its practitioners.

Charles Lindblom described root decisions and their opposite, branch or incremental decisions.[3] According to Lindblom, these incremental, limited, successive decisions do not involve a reevaluation of goals, policies, or underlying philosophy. Objectives and goals are recycled and policies are accepted without massive review and revision. Change is by degree. Only a small segment of the organization is affected.

Branch decision making is more conservative in its approach than is root decision making, with innovation inhibited. The stability of organizational life is enhanced, in many cases, when decision making is of the successive, incremental type, because the manager does not have the option of completely reviewing the organizational structure, functions, staffing patterns, equipment selection, and similar capital expenditures. Incrementalism also simplifies decision making because it tends to limit conflicts that might occur if the patterns of compromise, consensus, organizational territory, and subtle internal politics are disturbed. Incrementalism also may be the simple outcome of previous root decisions. However, the manager may overlook some excellent alternatives because they are not readily apparent in the chain of successive decisions. Incrementalism lacks the built-in safeguard of explicit, programmed review of values and philosophy.

Satisficing and Maximizing

"It might easily happen that what is second best is best, actually, because that which is actually best may be out of the question." This quotation, attributed to the philosopher-educator Cardinal Newman, expresses the idea contained in the concepts of satisficing and maximizing. In decision making, the one best solution may be determined by developing a set of criteria against which all alternatives are compared until one solution emerges as clearly preeminent. In the form of decision making known as maximizing, this one best solution is the only acceptable one.

In the form of decision making known as satisficing, a term used by Simon,[4] a set of minimal criteria is developed, and any alternative that fulfills the minimal criteria is acceptable. A course of action that is good enough is selected, with the conscious recognition that there may be better solutions. When the manager seeks several options, satisficing may be employed. As with incrementalism, satisficing obstructs absolute, rational, optimal decision making, yet it simplifies the process. In satisficing, the manager accepts the fact that not every decision need be made with the same degree of intensity.

The Pareto Principle or Paretian Optimality

Vilfredo Pareto (1848–1923) was an Italian economist and sociologist who postulated a criterion for decision making that is referred to as the Pareto principle or Paretian optimality.[5] He suggested that each person's needs be met as much as possible without any loss to another person. In this mode of decision making, certain alternatives are rejected because of the decrease in benefits for one or several groups. Decisions that result in a major gain for one individual with a concomitant major loss for another are avoided. The approach involves compromise and consensus, with each manager accepting the needs of other units of the organization as legitimate and the needs of the organization as a whole as paramount. The concessions and trade-offs in the budget process or in the labor negotiation process illustrate the balance required to satisfy the needs of many departments or groups without penalizing any one of them (or by penalizing all departments or groups in equal measure if penalization is unavoidable).

Commitment Phase

In the definition of decision making, the essential focus is choice—the specific selection from among alternatives. At some point, deliberation must be ended. If a manager does not make a decision in a timely way, someone else may make the decision. In some rare cases, managers find that alternatives are of equal merit. Should that occur, the manager can simply follow personal preference.

The commitment phase can be divided into stages: the pilot run and sequential implementation. A pilot run to test the chosen alternative helps reduce the risk attached to the decision. For example, a manufacturing company may offer a new product on trial and make further decisions based on the results. Rather than purchasing expensive equipment, managers may choose a leasing arrangement with an option to purchase. Pilot runs have two distinct limitations, however; they are costly in terms of time and money, and they are not always feasible.

In sequential implementation, managers make a basic determination and assess the results before they take the next step in the implementation process. The cycle is shortened, feedback is obtained, and alternatives are reviewed and implemented after a relatively short time. During the implementation stage, the decisions must be communicated to those who will carry out the detailed plans that flow from it.

Continuing Assessment of Decisions

The final step in the decision-making process is the continuous analysis of the decision. Through the feedback process, a new agenda is generated and new alternatives are revealed. The steps in the control process provide a link back to the planning and decision-making functions. This feedback process necessarily pervades organizational life. Planned, formal review is built into operational plans and decisions such as budget preparation, accrediting self-study processes, and labor union contract review. In addition, there is need for continuous real-time assessment of decisions that require rapid response to changing situations. An example of such a condition is an outbreak of an epidemic; disruption of service because of a protracted and polarizing labor strike is another such circumstance. In this type of situation, the classic OODA loop, or Boyd cycle, provides a method of rapid assessment and real-time adjustments to the pressing situation. This strategy was developed by Colonel John Boyd, USAF (Ret.), and has been widely used in military operations.[6] Businesses have adopted the general schematics of the OODA loop in responding to rapid change in their own and their competitors' environment. OODA is the acronym for:

- *Observe:* this is the fact-gathering stage, with emphasis on the immediate situation with its changed reality
- *Orient:* this part of the process consists of assessing one's own position in relation to the changed situation
- *Decide:* a rapid decision to commit to a new course of action in light of the changed circumstances is made
- *Action:* the new course of action is implemented without delay

The use of the OODA loop is predicated on managerial flexibility and a high degree of delegation of authority. The process is intended for use in the field, by highly skilled professionals who need to act without continual reference back to some other authority. Rapid adjustment to the plans is a key characteristic.

BARRIERS TO RATIONAL CHOICE

Managers must recognize that there are barriers to rational choice and that it may not be possible to make the perfect decision because of these subtle barriers. One set of barriers stems from human nature itself—ignorance, prejudice, and resistance to change all influence decision making. If managers do not have the necessary information or if they have it but cannot make use of it because they lack proper training in analysis, their ability to make informed decisions is circumscribed. Prejudice (i.e., preconceived opinion) is another aspect of human nature that must be taken into account. Even with sufficient factual knowledge, the value elements in decisions are inescapable. Resistance to change constitutes a third such barrier; managers may continue to make decisions based on their own past experience.

Together, these barriers constitute an overall impediment: inadequate leadership. Leaders may fail to take risks, choosing the security of incremental change. They may stifle creative thinking in themselves and their subordinates. They may so limit their zone of acceptance that change becomes difficult and decisions by precedent become the only decisions possible. They may ignore feedback, thus reinforcing their own positions and making determinations based on limited facts that are colored by their own value premises.

The internal dynamics of the decision-making process have been studied by psychologists Irving L. Janis and Leon Mann.[7] They identified four situations in which the decision maker fails to reach the ideal of "vigilant information processing":

1. If the risks involved in continuing to do whatever has been done in the past appear low, the individual is likely to go on doing it and is unlikely to collect adequate information about possible alternatives.

2. If the risks of continuing to do whatever has been done in the past appear high and if the risks of an obvious alternative appear low, the decision maker is likely to choose the obvious alternative and again is unlikely to collect adequate information about other possibilities.

3. If all the obvious alternatives seem to involve risk and if the decision maker feels that there is little chance of coming up with a better alternative, the individual is likely to engage in "defensive avoidance" by denying that a problem exists, to exaggerate the advantage of the chosen alternative, or to try to get someone else to make the decision.

4. If the decision maker feels that there is a potentially satisfactory course of action and that this alternative may disappear if there is a delay to investigate other possibilities, the individual is likely to panic, trying to pursue the obvious alternative before it is too late.

Decision makers undertake "vigilant information processing" only if they feel that all the obvious choices are risky, that there may be a better choice that is not obvious, and that there is sufficient time to seek the best possible choice.

Other barriers to rational choice flow from the organizational structure. There may be so much organizational red tape that decision making is limited to decision by precedent. Department managers may lack sufficient authority to make decisions and may be required to submit to a committee process for some decisions.

Decisions made in other departments may, in turn, affect their own, but they may have no influence in those areas. There may be a lack of sufficient coordination in decision making throughout the organization. Organizational politics (e.g., bargaining, forming alliances, and choosing "the right time") also subtly limit rational decision making.

Factors related to the social, political, and economic climate outside the organization also act as barriers. The many aspects of law and regulation governing health care set specific limits, for example. Finally, the degree of certainty under which decisions are made tends to impose limits on choice. Under conditions of high certainty, the risk involved in decision making is low and decisions may become routine. After they have been standardized through the use of policies, procedures, and rules, routine decisions may be made at lower levels of the organization. Conditions of relative uncertainty obviously increase risk, and managers attempt to evaluate alternatives in terms of probable payoff. Statistical analysis of data, market research, and forecasting are a few of the decision-making tools that may be employed in assessing comparative probability. Decisions made under great uncertainty involve the highest level of risk, and the burden for making such decisions belongs to the top echelons of the organization.

BASES FOR DECISION MAKING

Since effective decision making is critical to organizational survival, managers seek to overcome the barriers to rational choice. The bases for decision making range from intuition and serendipity to research and analysis. The manager's previous experience may be a valid basis for decisions, provided that there are no changes in the constraints, nor in the goals to be reached. Managers may draw from the experiences of other similar organizations. This "copy your neighbor" or "follow the leader" approach may provide managers with information they do not currently have. For example, another organization may have research information available, or a manager in another institution may have explored alternatives in great detail and done an analysis that others could profit from. A manager may take the philosophical attitude that it is not necessary to reinvent the wheel and that it is wise to learn from others; however, not only are these approaches based on an assumption that the managers being copied are correct in their decisions, but also they do not take into account the different constraints under which each manager operates.

The creative approach to decision making seeks to capitalize on intuition and serendipity, but the concrete analysis of information is necessary before final determinations are made. Experimentation, research, and analysis constitute the most effective base for selecting among alternatives.

DECISION-MAKING TOOLS AND TECHNIQUES

Managers have available the historical records, information about past performance, and summaries of their own and other managers' experience. In addition, managers may test alternatives through the use of decision-making tools and techniques.

Considered Opinion and Devil's Advocate

A manager may obtain the considered opinion of experts and use the technique of the "devil's advocate" to sharpen the arguments for and against an alternative. In the first instance, the manager asks staff experts or other members of the management team to assess the several alternatives and develop arguments for and against each; the resulting comparative assessment helps the decision maker to select a course of action.

When the devil's advocate technique is used, the decision maker assigns an individual or group the duty of developing statements of all the negative aspects or weaknesses of each alternative. Each alternative is then tested through frank discussion of weaknesses and error before the final decision is made. The underlying theory is that it is better to subject alternatives to strict, internal, organized criticism than to run the risk of having a hidden weakness or error exposed after a decision has been implemented. The devil's advocate does not make the decision but simply develops arguments to ensure that all aspects are considered.

The Factor Analysis Matrix

For the decision maker who must overcome personal preference to make an impartial decision, the matrix of comparative factors is an effective tool of analysis. As a first step, the decision maker develops the criteria under two major categories: essential elements (musts) and desired elements (wants). The manager begins this process by listing key factors relating to the topic. For example, in weighing alternatives to select an outsourcing service for dictation-transcription functions, the manager would consider the following:

- HIPAA-compliant encryption
- accepts dictation from land-line phone systems, PC microphone, handheld digital recording devices

- document distribution system by secure line fax, secure e-mail, remote print
- electronic edit and signature
- one-screen tracking of documentation from beginning of recording through finished document received at client site
- temporary or total outsourcing services for seasonal peak loads
- customized formatting
- 99 percent error-free guarantee
- STAT capability
- 24-hour/365-day support center
- turnaround time of 12 hours
- conformity with Medical Transcription Industry Association's billing method principles
- zero capital investment on site: use of standard Internet connections

The choices available are compared by developing a table or matrix. The factors can be assigned relative weight, as in a point scale, and the alternative with the highest point value becomes the best option. Even without the weighting factors, the matrix remains useful as a technique of factual comparison. Table 5–1 illustrates the use of the "must" and "want" categories to compare equipment for departmental use. A similar process could be used to evaluate applicants for a job; personal bias can be set aside more easily and candidates compared on the basis of their qualifications for the position (Table 5–2 and Table 5–3).

Table 5–1 Matrix of Comparison for Equipment Purchase

	Brand A	Brand B	Brand C
• Maximum cost	Acceptable	Acceptable	$14,000
• Compatibility with related equipment	Yes	Yes	No
• Minimum years of service	No	Yes	Yes
• Availability of service	Yes	Yes	Yes
• Renovation of existing space needed	No	Yes	No
x Safety features	Yes	Yes	Yes
x Trade-in value for present equipment	No	No	Yes
x Available delivery date	Yes	No	Yes
x Special training for use	No	Yes	Yes
x Lease option	No	No	Yes
• = must (required); x = want (desirable)			

Table 5–2 Matrix for Evaluation of Job Applicants

	Applicant A	Applicant B	Applicant C
Meets productivity standard at Level 1	Level 2	Level 2	Level 1
Previous experience in this type job	0	1 yr.	1 yr.
Previous experience in related clerical job	Unit Clerk	Same	None
Yrs. In organization: (policy: preference internal applicants)	3 yrs.	1 yr.	0
Willing to accept salary of $29,000	Yes	Yes	Prefers higher; wants raise within six months.
Full-time	Yes	Yes	
3 PM to 10 PM shift acceptable	Yes	Yes	Prefers day; plans to switch as soon as opening available.

Table 5–3 Matrix for Selection of Relief Therapists

Factor	Applicant A	Group 1	Group 2
Willing to work weekends/evenings	1xmonth	Yes	Bimonthly
Same person	Yes	No	Share 2 therapists
Experience	2 years	Extensive	Extensive
Continuity with staff	Yes	No	Limited
Salary	$45/hr.	$35/hr.	$65/hr.
Response to calls within:	48 hrs.	4 hrs.	2 hrs.
Reputation	Fine	Excellent	Excellent/master clinicians

The Director of OT met with the senior staff and decided that salary, continuity with staff, and response to calls were "must" areas. They decided to compromise on continuity with the staff and took a chance and hired Group 1 for a trial. They decided to give the group 60 days to work with them and to evaluate their level of performance for 30 days.

The Decision Tree

A managerial tool used to depict the possible directions that actions might take from various decision points, the decision tree forces the manager to ask the "what then" questions (i.e., to anticipate outcomes). Possible events are included, with a notation about the probabilities associated with each. The basic decisions are stated, with all the unfolding, probable events branching out from them. Decision trees enable managers to undertake disciplined speculation about the consequences, including the unpleasant or negative ones, of actions. Through the use of decision trees, managers are forced to delineate their reasoning, and the constraints imposed by probable future events on subsequent decisions become evident. Each decision tree reveals the probable new situation that results from a decision.

It is possible to use a decision tree without including mathematical calculations of probability, although computers are commonly used to calculate the probability of events when such detailed information is available. Managers in business corporations with sufficient market data about profit, loss, patterns of consumer response, and national economic fluctuations include these data in the construction of a decision tree for the marketing of a new product, for example.

Managers who lack detailed information of this type can still use decision trees to advantage. In developing a decision tree, these managers use symbols to designate points of certainty and uncertainty. For example, events of certainty may be placed in rectangles; events of uncertainty, in ovals. This technique emphasizes the relative risk in each decision track. The goal to be reached is the continual reference point. The sequence of decisions that leads to the goal with the least uncertainty emerges as a distinct track, thereby facilitating the manager's decision. For decisions in which the manager has intense personal involvement, this approach is a valuable aid in overcoming emotional barriers to objective choice.

Operations Research

During World War II, operations research was developed when the military in Britain and in the United States faced massive logistical problems. Because there was not enough time to carry out research and trial runs, conditions were simulated using models that permitted greater experimentation. Management literature contains three terms, used interchangeably at times, that reflect this process of model building to analyze decision alternatives: *operational research, operations research,* and *management science. Operational research,* the earliest term used, was shortened to *operations research* as the processes were applied to business practices.

The use of operations research, with its extensive mathematical analyses and probability calculations, became broadly feasible with the development of computer technology. By definition, operations research is an applied science in which the scientific method is brought to bear on a problem, process, or operation. It is a technique for quantitative problem solving and decision making in which mathematical models are applied to management problems. Three major steps are included in operations research techniques:

1. *Problem Formulation.* The problem is stated and preconceived notions are set aside.
2. *Construction of a Mathematical or Conceptual Model.* This is usually done through equations or formulas representing and relating critical factors that are involved in the problem under analysis.

3. *Manipulation of Variables.* This is done to develop and assess alternatives in terms of designated criteria.

Simulation and Model Building

Simulation is the representation of a process or system by means of a model. A model is a logical, simplified representation of an aspect of reality. Models range from simple (e.g., physical models) to complex (e.g., models consisting of mathematical equations). Since legal, ethical, and economic constraints limit the manipulation of reality, experimentation may be carried out on the representation of reality (i.e., the model) rather than on reality itself. Through the development of models, managers attempt to gain additional information about the uncertainties in a situation; those elements are brought into focus and assessments are made concerning the degree of chance associated with them.

Managers use several models routinely. For example, they may use a physical model of the office layout, reducing in scale the dimensions of the office space and equipment. During an inservice training session, a manager in a health-related profession may use one or several physical models, such as a model of a body organ. An organization chart is a graphic model of departmental and authority relationships. A decision tree is a schematic model of plans or decisions. Analog and mathematical models are the most complex, with mathematical models the most abstract. Some models are developed through reasoning by analogy (analog model); a problem is approached indirectly by setting up an analogous situation, solving it, and making a similar application to the original problem. The model for one problem is converted into a form suitable for a different problem.

Stochastic Simulation

A model designed to include the element of randomness is called a stochastic simulation model. *Stochastic* is derived from the Greek word meaning "guess" or "not certain." The Monte Carlo method is a form of stochastic simulation in which data are developed through the random number generator. Where the variables are uncertain, at least a sample of their values may be assigned through the development of a statistical pattern of distribution. In this way, managers may simulate such occurrences as employee absenteeism, patient arrivals, or equipment failures. The Monte Carlo technique involves factors of change and their effect on the process or system. Probability sampling is used extensively with simulation and model building.

Waiting Line and Queuing Theory

In any organization in which the demand for service fluctuates, managers must balance the cost of waiting lines with the cost of preventing waiting lines through increased service. Waiting lines or queues are a common everyday experience: customers in a grocery store, cars at a toll gate, airplanes stacked to land, patients in a clinic or emergency room, telephone requests for information. A characteristic of such queues is the randomness of demand. Waiting line or queuing theory is useful for analyzing those situations in which the units to be provided for the service are relatively predictable. The underlying premise is that delays are costly, yet too little activity on another occasion is also costly. For example, hospital emergency room resources are costly when not used; however, the cost in terms of patient pain, aggravation, and inconvenience must be taken into account if an emergency arises and there is a delay in treatment.

There are three basic components in waiting line analysis: arrivals, servicing, and queue discipline. The unit of arrival is defined (e.g., grocery orders to be rung up, planes to be landed, or patients to be examined). The pattern of arrival is studied to determine probabilities of arrival. Arrivals can be divided into three categories:

1. predetermined arrivals, such as scheduled airplane landings or scheduled patient appointments
2. random arrivals, such as emergency landings at an airport or patient arrivals at a walk-in clinic or emergency unit
3. combination of predetermined and random arrivals, such as arrivals at a clinic with both scheduled appointments and a walk-in system

Servicing is the focus of analysis of the work flow; the service is defined in terms of number of units and time needed for each pattern of distribution. Analysis of these data shows both random and constant factors that must be taken into account when procedures are developed. Various control processes are developed to smooth these internal activities. Queue discipline involves an analysis of the patterns or characteristics of the waiting line, such as the average minimum and maximum wait, the number of lines, and the manner in which units are selected for service (e.g., first come, first served; random selection; a triage system according to severity of problem or ease of processing; a priority and preference system). Through the analysis of such information, managers can make informed decisions to overcome the negative aspects of waiting lines (delay for patients) and the cost to the organization (idle equipment, overstaffing).

Gaming and Game Theory

Gaming is the simulation of competitive situations in which the element of uncertainty is introduced as a result of some other, often competing, decision maker's action. In the management field, games give reality to training situations and to the decision-making process. Unlike other forms of simulation, gaming uses human decisions, although they may be computer-assisted.

Game theory is a branch of mathematical analysis of conflict and strategy; it is associated with the concepts of zero sum games and minimax strategy. Both involve theoretical situations in which competitive conditions are central; they are based on the premises that each competitor acts rationally and seeks to maximize gain, to minimize loss, and to outwit the other competitors. Game theory remains relatively undeveloped because of the complexities that arise once the number of contestants or rules is increased.

Gaming and game theory are separate, distinct concepts, although somewhat related. These techniques of operations research are costly means of testing alternatives, yet they are less expensive than a monumental mistake. By making dry runs possible, these methods clarify the size of the risks.

HEALTH CARE PRACTITIONERS AS DECISION MAKERS

The health care practitioner in a managerial role faces decision-making situations on a daily basis. The practitioner-and-manager soon discovers, however, that he or she can experience conflict in some decision situations depending upon how these situations are viewed. Consider, for example, the potential decision to replace a specific piece of equipment and in the process upgrade the department's capability to deliver service in one particular dimension. Thinking as a practitioner, the professional may strongly desire to acquire the item knowing—or at least believing—that it is the best available for the intended use. The item, however, may cost more than the department's budget could allow, or, of even greater consequence, the item may somehow make work more difficult or more costly for two other departments. In other words, the practitioner may be inclined to respect professional practice more highly while the manager primarily recognizes broader issues, in this instance the effects on other functions. Yet this practitioner and this manager are one and the same person. This is, of course, the manifestation of the classic "two-hat" character of the first-line management role, making it essential for the professional to learn early that the perceived needs of the department must be balanced with the needs of the total organization.

Organizational decisions require the manager to concentrate on the department's relationship to the total organization. Many staff-level personnel are unable to appreciate the complex needs and demands of the organization. They are likely to hold an extremely parochial view of the organization's needs. The successful manager translates the needs of the organization into ideas that the department staff understands and appreciates. No group totally agrees with all organizational demands, but the manager should try to match the needs of personnel with the needs of the organization. To achieve this delicate balance, the manager must have a comprehensive understanding of the organization's hierarchy, resources, and personnel.

HOW BAD DECISIONS GET MADE

Sometimes a decision is simply faulty and the management team faces the question: How did such a bad decision get made? The possible answer lies in several aspects of the decision-making process. An examination of the leadership style might reveal an overly bureaucratic manner, one that excludes participant input. In another situation, the price of innovation and flexibility has become very high because any deviation from set practice carries with it both informal and formal penalties. The resulting atmosphere is one of caution and rigid adherence to prescribed practices. In yet another circumstance, the need or desire to effect an early compromise may have precluded a more thoughtful decision-making process. Finally, bad decisions sometimes stem from the no-decision option.

It has been hinted at here and there that decisions that ought to be made are sometimes subject to procrastination. Procrastination occurs for a number of reasons. Often its cause lies within the individual decision maker. Some people are simply uncomfortable with what they perceive as, perhaps, limited information, and do not wish to take a perceived undue risk. This is prevalent among managers who are uneasy in the presence of risk, and they behave as though more information will reduce or remove that uneasiness. Managers who behave in this fashion will tend to procrastinate by continuing to study a situation, thus falling victim to "analysis paralysis," in which investigation and data gathering continue and nothing is decided.

Sometimes certain decision situations are shunted aside and even literally forgotten because they are perceived as troublesome, unpleasant, annoying, or even simply too inconsequential to deserve conscious attention. The behavior fueling this form of procrastination suggests that the person who is delaying feels that ignoring the problem decision will make it go away. Once in a great while the decision situation that is ignored does indeed go away on its own. Usually, however, the situation worsens if ignored.

If, whether by procrastination or deliberate intent, one has pushed a decision situation permanently aside, the decision maker has exercised the no-decision option. Whether by conscious act or unconscious act (genuinely forgetting), the effect of the no-decision option is to decide not to decide. Therefore, exercise of the no-decision option is itself a decision, and often it is the decision of the most potentially serious and far-reaching consequences. Therefore, the no-decision option should be considered a valid alternative only under certain special circumstances (when, for example, the valid choices can be identified as do this or do nothing, and even then should be a conscious decision rather than allowing something to happen by default).

CASE: PAID TO MAKE DECISIONS?

Background

Carrie Wilson, a registered nurse with more than 10 years of active supervisory experience, was hired from outside as nursing manager for the emergency department of County Hospital. It was Carrie's style to develop insight into how to manage a given operation by putting herself where the action was and becoming totally immersed in the work. She quickly discovered, however, that her tendency to become deeply involved in hands-on work drew reactions from staff members ranging from surprise to resentment. She also discovered that her predecessor, who had been in the position for several years, had been referred to as the "Invisible Nurse." As someone said about the former manager, "I think she was a very pleasant person, but that's hard to say because we almost never saw her."

In spite of the legacy of the Invisible Nurse, Carrie provided a constant management presence and seemed determined to remain deeply involved in the work of the department. She was also determined to vastly improve the level of professionalism in the department, a quality that had struck her from the first as decidedly lacking.

In a short time Carrie had moved to reinstate and enforce a long-ignored dress code for the department, eliminate personal telephone calls during working hours except for urgent situations, curb chronic tardiness on the part of some staff members, bar food and drink and reading materials from work areas (also a reemphasis of long-ignored rules), and curb the practice of changing scheduled days of work after the time limit allowed by policy.

Carrie found her efforts frustrated at every turn. As she said to her immediate superior, "I can't understand the reaction. All I've done is insist that a few hospital rules be followed—mostly rules that have been there all along but were being ignored—and added a few twists unique to the emergency department. Just that, and yet the bitterness and lack of support and even resentment are so strong I could slice them. I'm getting all-out resistance from a few people whom I would still have to describe as good, professional nurses at heart."

Carrie's boss, the vice president for nursing service, said, "Do you suppose you may have been pushing too hard, hitting them with one surprise after another without knowing how they felt and without asking for their cooperation?"

"That's possible," answered Carrie, "but now I'm committed on several fronts and I can't back down on any of them without looking bad to the department."

"Don't think of this as a contest of wills or a game," said the vice president. "It may be necessary for you to back down temporarily in some areas or at least hold a few of your improvements up in the air for a while. It may not hurt to fall back and involve a few of your staff in looking at the apparent needs of the department."

With a touch of impatience in her voice, Carrie said, "Oh, I've heard all this stuff about participative management and staff involvement in making decisions. That may be the way for some, but that's never been my style. I'm paid to make decisions so I make them—I don't try to avoid responsibility by encouraging employees to make my decisions."

Questions

1. What are the weaknesses, if any, in Carrie's final statement about decision-making responsibility?
2. What has essentially been wrong with Carrie's approach to raising the level of professionalism in the department?
3. How has Carrie's behavior altered or otherwise affected the environment within which she expects her decisions to be implemented?
4. Ideally, how should Carrie have initially approached her plan to improve the emergency department?
5. Given the state of affairs Carrie is facing as of her conversation with the vice president, how should she go about attempting to salvage some of her ideas and proceed with the improvement of the department? Keep in mind that at this stage her actions have probably had serious effects on her chances of implementing her plans, and some of the decisions she may have already made may have to be revisited in a different fashion.

EXERCISE: THE TROUBLESOME PROFESSIONAL

Background

You are the manager of a department that provides hands-on service to both inpatients and outpatients of a large urban health care facility. One of your employees, a senior therapist named William, has been taking an increasing amount of your time and attention in ways that have filled you with growing concern. William has been in the department nearly 10 years, which is two years longer than you have been there, and at one time he seemed to have had ambitions about running the department. You feel that you have been watching William's overall reliability and effectiveness decline for the last couple of years. Specifically,

- William's performance has been noticeably deteriorating. He now arrives at work chronically late, although for years tardiness was not a problem. He is slow to start, takes numerous breaks, overstays his lunch period, and seems not interested in his patients.
- Two other employees have told you confidentially that they feel William has become alcoholic; however, even remaining alert to this possibility you have detected no signs of his being under the influence or actively using alcohol at work.
- On several occasions he has been absent from work without notification, claiming sudden illness after the fact. This has fostered ill feelings among other staff because of the last-minute staffing changes that have had to be made.
- You have discussed William's sagging performance with him every three or four weeks for the past six months. William denies any change in attitude or performance, and concerning his absences he says only that his "allergies are more troublesome than they used to be."

Instructions

Your basic assignment is to decide what you are going to do about William. The obvious choices are to do nothing or to discharge him, but there are other choices available. You are to do the following:

1. Develop at least four alternative courses of action and express these in at least one full sentence each.

2. Assess each of your alternatives in terms of whether or not it seems likely to "solve" the problem, is generally appropriate or too little or too drastic, addresses the real problem or seems to be treating only problem symptoms, and gives rise to the necessity for additional decisions.

3. Select an alternative to pursue, explain why you selected it, and outline the steps required to implement your decision.

4. Describe how you will follow up on implementation, and note your possible courses of action if your decision appears to have been inappropriate.

NOTES

1. Chester Barnard, *The Functions of the Executive* (Cambridge, Mass.: Harvard University Press, 1968), 202.
2. *Ibid.,* 205.
3. Charles Lindblom, "The Science of Muddling Through," *Public Administration Review* (Spring 1959): 79–88.
4. Herbert Simon, *Models of Man* (New York: John Wiley & Sons, 1957), 207.
5. Vilfredo Pareto, *Mind and Society* (New York: Harcourt, Brace, & Co., 1935).
6. Grant Hammond, *The Mind of War: John Boyd and American Security* (Washington, D.C.: Smithsonian Institution Press, 2001).
7. Irving L. Janis and Leon Mann, *A Psychological Analysis of Conflict, Choice and Commitment* (New York: The Free Press, 1978).

CHAPTER 6

Organizing

CHAPTER OBJECTIVES

- Define the basic management function of organizing and identify the steps in the organizing process.
- Define the key concepts of hierarchy, chain of command, splintered authority, and concurring authority.
- Identify the factors that shape the span of management.
- Differentiate between line and staff relationships and identify basic line and staff relationships.
- Describe the dual pyramid organization arrangement found in health care authority patterns.
- Identify the basic patterns of departmentation.
- Introduce the concept of the matrix organization and define the applicability of this apparently contradictory concept.
- Identify patterns of organizational flexibility: temporary agency, contractual outsourcing, and the use of independent contractors and consultants.
- Identify the principles involved in developing an organizational chart.
- Introduce job descriptions, including their uses and the elements necessary in their development.

Organizing is the process of grouping necessary responsibilities and activities into workable units, determining the lines of authority and communication, and developing patterns of coordination. It is the conscious development of the role structures of superior and subordinate, line and staff. The organizational process stems from several underlying premises:

- There is a common goal toward which work effort is directed.
- The goal is articulated in detailed plans.
- There is a need for clear authority-responsibility relationships.
- Power and authority elements must be reconciled so that individual interactions within the organization are productive and goal-directed.
- Conflict is inevitable but may be reduced through clarity of organizational relationships.
- Individual needs must be reconciled with and subordinated to the organizational needs.
- Unity of command must prevail.
- Authority must be delegated.

THE PROCESS OF ORGANIZING

The immediately identifiable aspects of the organizing process include clear delineation of the goal in terms of scope, function, and priorities. For example, will a health care institution focus on acute care for inpatients or comprehensive care, including outpatient care, even home care? Will the organization expand its services through decentralized locations and active outreach programs?

The development of a specific organizational structure must be considered. What degree of specialization will be sought? Specialization is a major feature of health care organizations; it is dictated and shaped in part by the specific licensure mandates for each health profession. The manager must assess the question of line and staff officers and units. A major organizational question concerns the division of work. What will be the pattern of departmentation? The development of the organizational chart, the job descriptions, and the statements of interdepartmental and intradepartmental work flow systems must be assessed and implemented as part of the management function of organizing. Finally, the changes in the internal and external organizational environment must be monitored so that the organizational structure can be adjusted accordingly.

In summary, the basic steps of organizing are these:

1. goal recognition and statement
2. review of organizational environment
3. determination of structure needed to reach the goal (e.g., degree of centralization, basis of departmentation, committee use, line and staff relationships)
4. determination of authority relationships and development of the organizational chart, job descriptions, and related support documents

FUNDAMENTAL CONCEPTS AND PRINCIPLES

Relationships in formal organizations are highly structured in terms of authority and responsibility. The resulting hierarchy, that is, the arrangement of individuals into a graded series of superiors and subordinates, authority holders, and rank-and-file members, constitutes one of the most obvious characteristics of formal organizations. A pyramid-shaped organization tends to result from the development of a hierarchy (Figure 6–1).

The authority and responsibility that can be observed in the hierarchy constitutes a distinct chain of command, also referred to as the scalar principle: the chain of direct authority from superior to subordinate. It was long maintained that strict unity of command—the uninterrupted line of authority from superior to subordinate so that each individual reports to one and only one superior—was fundamental to hierarchical relationships in organizations. It was seen as essential to have a clear chain of command showing who reports to whom, who is responsible for each individual's actions, and who has authority over each worker.

Unity of command is increasingly regarded as something of a theoretical ideal in that in many instances it is being abandoned in favor of split-reporting relationships in which a single subordinate reports to two or more superiors. Split-reporting relationships have been proliferating as health care organizations have merged into larger organizations or joined together in health systems. It is not at all uncommon to find, for example, a single manager over the same functions at two sites who is therefore answerable to two different site administrators. Such combinations have occurred out of economic necessity, and many of them make sense in terms of operating efficiency and optimum utilization of management capability.

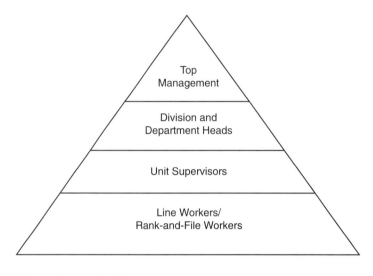

FIGURE 6–1 Pyramidal Hierachy

This efficiency can be put at risk, however, as the absence of unity of command can create a new set of problems.

The individual who reports to two superiors is put in the position of having to balance the two reporting relationships. If either superior is inflexible or overly demanding, the stage is set for subordinate burnout as the individual attempts to reconcile conflicting demands. Much of the determination of whether or not a split-reporting relationship works lies beyond the reach of the individual. Even the most highly capable subordinate can be rendered frustrated and ineffective by two superiors who have not coordinated their demands and expectations or who have each tried to have their way with the subordinate at the expense of the other.

Also, a split-reporting relationship more than doubles the communication demands on the subordinate manager. Not only does the manager have to communicate regularly with two superiors, he or she must do so in a manner that attempts to provide coordination between the needs of the two superiors.

Split reporting may generate potential conflict when managers differ in their interpretation or application of policy. For example, one manager may readily give liberal leave in bad weather or allow early closing before a holiday, while another manager may have a stricter interpretation of such practices. The employee in this situation is caught in the middle of an ambiguous situation.

Split-reporting relationships may be necessary under certain circumstances, but they should always be entered into with full awareness and consideration of the problems that may be encountered. The concept of unity of command should not be abandoned without good reason and without planning to meet the increased communication needs of the alternative arrangement.

The authority delegated to any individual must be equal to the responsibility assigned. This principle of parity—that responsibility cannot be greater than the authority given—ensures that individuals can carry out their assigned duties without provoking conflict over their right to do so. In developing policies and documents that support the organizational chart, managers must avoid contradicting this principle. At the same time, managers cannot so completely delegate authority that they become free of responsibility. This is reflected in the principle of the absoluteness of responsibility; authority may (and must) be delegated, but ultimate responsibility is retained by the manager. This, in turn, is the basis of the manager's right to exercise the necessary controls and require accountability.

Normally, managers have adequate authority to carry out the required activities of their divisions or units without recourse to the authority possessed by other managers. Two situations occur, however, in which the authority of a single manager is not sufficient for unilateral decision making or action. Occasionally, because the work must be coordinated and because there are necessary limits on each manager's authority, a problem cannot be solved or a decision made without pooling the authority of two or more managers. These problems of splintered authority are overcome in three ways: (1) the managers may simply pool their authority and make the decision or solve the problem; (2) the problem may be referred to a higher level of authority until it reaches a single manager with sufficient authority; or (3) reorganization may be done so that recurring situations of splintered authority are eliminated. Such recurring situations sometimes require adjustment in the delegation of authority.

Concurring authority is sometimes given to related departments to ensure uniformity of practice. For example, the packaging department of a manufacturing company cannot change specifications without the agreement of the production division. A computer systems manager in a health care setting may be given concurring authority on any form design changes, although this is the primary responsibility of the health information practitioner, in order to foster compatibility throughout the information processing function. Concurring authority, as a control and coordinating measure, can be a normal part of the routine check and balance system. Splintered authority and concurring authority are the natural consequences of the division of labor and specialization that make it necessary to coordinate the authority delegated to different managers.

THE SPAN OF MANAGEMENT

If authority is to be delegated appropriately, consideration must be given to the number of subordinates a manager may supervise effectively. Four terms are used to refer to this concept: span of management, span of control, span of supervision, and span of authority. Stated another way, the span of management is the number of immediate subordinates who report to any one manager. It is essential to recognize that the number of individuals whose activities can be properly coordinated and controlled by one manager is limited.

There is no ideal span of management. A span of 4 or 5 subordinates at higher levels and a span of 8 to 12 at the lower levels have sometimes been suggested. However, various modifying factors shape the appropriate span of management for any authority holder, however. These factors include the following:

- *Type of Work.* Routine, repetitive, and homogeneous work allows a larger span of management.
- *Degree of Training of the Worker.* Those who are well trained and well motivated do not need as much supervision as a trainee group; the more highly trained the group, the larger the span of management may be.
- *Organizational Stability.* When the organization as a whole, as well as the specific department, is stable, the span of control can be wider; when there are rapid changes, high turnover, and general organizational instability, a narrower span of control may be needed.
- *Geographical Location.* When the work units are dispersed over a scattered physical layout, sometimes even involving separate geographical locations, closer supervision is necessary to control and coordinate the work.
- *Flow of Work.* If much coordination of work flow is needed, there is a companion need for greater supervision and a narrow span of control.
- *Supervisor's Qualifications.* As the amount of training and experience of the supervisor increases, the span of control for that supervisor may increase also.
- *Availability of Staff Specialists.* When staff specialists and selected support services, such as a training or personnel development department, are available, a supervisor's span of management may be widened.

- *Value System of the Organization.* In highly coercive organizations, a supervisor may have a large span of management, since there is a pervasive system to help ensure conformity, even to the extent of severe punishment for deviation from the rules. In a highly normative organization, however, there may be an emphasis on participation in planning and decision making and a resultant complexity in the communication process; thus, a smaller span of management may be appropriate. In health care organizations, traditionally normative settings with respect to the professional worker, the span of management may be large because the health care professional is a specialist within an area and does not always require close supervision.

As an example, the span of management in a laboratory department is shown in the partial organizational chart of Figure 6–2. In this figure one can trace the chain of command from each supervisor in the department back up to the chief executive officer (CEO). Figure 6–3, depicting the relationships in a physical therapy department, illustrates other ways of depicting organizational relationships.

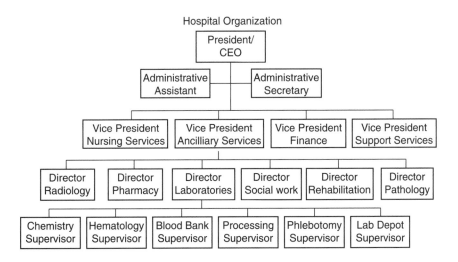

FIGURE 6–2 Partial organization chart illustrating span of management (follow from President/CEO through Vice President/Ancillary Services, and Director, Laboratories)

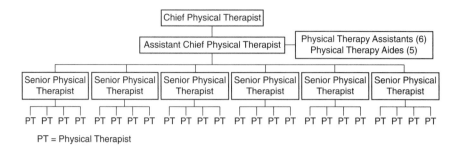

FIGURE 6–3 Physical Therapy Department Organizational Chart

LINE AND STAFF RELATIONSHIPS

The terms *line* and *staff* are key words in any discussion of organizing. In common usage, staff refers to the groups of employees who perform the work of a given department or unit. The director of nursing speaks of the nursing staff, the chief dietitian discusses the dietary staff, and the physicians who practice in a hospital are referred to as the medical staff.

In management literature, a differentiation is made between line and staff departments or officers. Line refers only to those that have direct responsibility for accomplishing the objectives of the organization, and staff refers to those that help the line units achieve the objectives. In a health care organization, direct patient care units are considered to perform line functions, and all other units are listed as staff services. The problem with this distinction becomes apparent when it must be applied to such units as the dietary, purchasing, or housekeeping departments; are these functions any less essential to the operation of a health care organization than a direct patient care unit? Some authors prefer to list such units as service departments, reserving the term *staff* for a specific authority relationship.

The concept of line and staff was inherited by management theorists from the military of the 18th and 19th centuries. An examination of a typical military encounter during this era makes it easier to conceptualize the notions of line and staff. The soldiers literally formed a line; the immediate commanding officers were those who commanded the line, that is, line officers. The actual fighting of the battle was the duty of these troops and officers. In turn, these troops and officers were assisted by staff officers and other units that provided logistical support, supplies, and information. The idea carried over as formal bureaucratic organizational theory developed in the 19th century.

The Relationship of Line and Staff Authority

The term *staff* also connotes a certain kind of authority relationship. Again, the original usage of the term was derived from the military, in which the staff assistant pattern was developed as a means of relieving commanders of details that could be handled by others. The staff officer was an "assistant to" the commander, and this assistant's authority was an extension of line authority.

Line authority is based on a direct chain of command from the top level of authority through each successive level of the organization. A manager with line authority has direct authority and responsibility for the work of a unit; the line manager alone has the right to command others to act. A staff assistant provides advice, counsel, or technical support that may be accepted, altered, or rejected by the line officer.

Functional authority is the right of individuals to exercise a limited form of authority over the specialized functions for which they are responsible, regardless of who exercises line authority over the employees performing the activities. For example, the information services staff is responsible for developing and implementing a specific computerized data collection system. The unit manager has functional authority over processing input documents, although these documents may be originated and completed by workers in other units, such as the admission office, business office, nursing service, or health information management. A human resource officer may be charged with monitoring organizational compliance with affirmative action programs or labor union contracts; the advice of such an officer could not be rejected or altered arbitrarily by a line officer.

A staff officer or manager may hold a staff position. Such an individual may be the designated officer in charge of a support department, such as the legal or personnel department. Yet this manager may also have charge of one or several workers within the unit and would exercise line authority within that unit. Organization charts, job descriptions, and similar documents should contain clear statements as to the nature of each position: whether it is a line or staff position, what kind of authority it possesses, and what its area of responsibility is.

Line and Staff Interaction

Various types of staff arrangements may be developed to channel line and staff interaction. As noted earlier, one basic mode of interaction is to designate a staff member as the personal assistant to an individual holding office in the upper levels of the organization. This position should not be confused with that of an assistant department head or assistant manager, who generally shares in direct line authority.

Managers in the upper levels of the organization may have several assistants, each carrying out highly specialized tasks. When there is only one position of assistant, this individual's work may be general, varied, and determined by the needs of the superior officer. The style of interaction may be highly personal, as when the staff assistant is seen as an alter ego of the line officer. When such a staff member indicates a point of view, a desired action, or a preferred decision, other members of the organization recognize that this individual is reflecting the opinion and wishes of the line officer.

A full department that gives specialized assistance and support frequently has a general staff. The relationship between staff and line personnel is less intimate than the assistant relationship. The work tends to be technical and highly specialized (e.g., the work of logistical staff in the military).

A third aspect of line and staff relationship is the organizational arrangement of the specialized staff. Specialized staff members (or departments in a large institution) give highly specialized counsel, such as that provided by engineers, architects, accountants, lawyers, and auditors. Finally, as noted, departments can be arranged in terms of direct line entities, assisted by support or service units.

THE DUAL PYRAMID FORM OF ORGANIZATION IN HEALTH CARE

Health care institutions are characterized by a dual pyramid form of organization because of the traditional relationship of the medical staff to the administrative staff. The ultimate authority and responsibility for the management of the institution is vested in the governing board. In accordance with the stipulations of licensure and accrediting agencies, the board appoints a chief executive officer and a chief of medical staff, resulting in two lines of authority. The chief executive officer is responsible for effectively managing the administrative components of the institution and delegates authority to each department head in the administrative component. Within the administrative units, there is a typical pyramidal organization with a unified chain of command.

The physicians and dentists are organized under a specific set of bylaws for the governance of the medical and dental staff. With governing board approval, the chief of the medical staff appoints the chief of each clinical service. Physicians and dentists apply for clinical privileges through the medical staff credentials committee and receive appointment from the governing board. A second pyramid results from this organization of the medical staff into clinical services, with each having a chief of service who reports to the chief of the medical staff.

In an effort to consolidate authority and clarify responsibility, the top administrative levels of a health care organization may be expanded to include a central officer to whom both the administrator and the chief of the medical staff report. In some institutions, however, there may be no permanent medical staff position that corresponds to the position of chief executive officer on the organizational chart. The elected president of the medical staff may fill this role when there is no organizational slot for a medical director per se. It is important to determine the precise meaning of titles as they are used in a specific health care setting. The following are titles commonly used:

- *Chief of Staff.* This is the officer of the medical staff to whom the chiefs of medical and clinical services report. The chief of staff is appointed by the governing board.
- *Chief of Service.* Each chief of service is the physician-director of a specific clinical service (e.g., chief of surgery) and is the line officer for physicians who are appointed to that specific service.
- *Department Chairperson.* The chairperson of a department is the director of a specific clinical service in an academic institution, such as a teaching hospital. (This title may be used as an alternate to chief of service in this type of setting.)
- *Medical Director.* This is a position in a line authority structure. It is sometimes seen as the counterpart of the chief executive officer for the medical staff.
- *President of the Medical Staff.* The president is the presiding officer for the medical staff and is usually elected for a year. In the absence of a full-time medical director, this individual serves as coordinating officer for the medical staff.

Although all authority flows from the governing board, there are two distinct chains of command, one in the administrative structure and one in the medical sector. Furthermore, in matters of direct patient care, the attending physician exercises professional authority; thus, a single employee not only may be subject to more than one line of authority but also may have professional authority. Line officers in the administrative unit may find that their authority is limited in some areas because of the specific jurisdiction of the medical staff committees, such as the pharmacy and therapeutics committee. The director of the physical therapy department, for example, may report to a committee of physicians of the active medical staff, which limits the authority mandate of this line manager. Because of the dual pyramid structure, much coordination is needed.

BASIC DEPARTMENTATION

The development of departments is a natural adjunct to the specialization and division of labor that are characteristic of formal organizations. Departmentation overcomes the limitation imposed by the span of management. The organization, through its departments and similar subdivisions, can expand almost indefinitely in size. Departmentation facilitates the coordination process, since there is a logical grouping of closely related activities. Basic departmentation may be developed according to any one of several patterns:

1. *By function.* Because it is logical, efficient, and natural, the most widely used form of departmentation groups all related activities or jobs together. This permits managers to take advantage of specialization and to concern themselves with only one major focus of activity. Hospital departments are usually developed according to function (e.g., the finance office and the health information management, human resources, housekeeping, maintenance, and dietary departments).

2. *By product.* All activities needed in the development, production, and marketing of a product may be grouped for purposes of coordination and control. This pattern of departmentation is used in business and industry where one or a few closely related products are grouped. It facilitates the use of research funds, the use of specialized skills and knowledge, and the development of cost control data for each product line. Functional departmentation may be an adjunct of product departmentation.

3. *By territory.* In business, the marketing process may be developed according to geographical boundaries. In service organizations, a decentralized pattern based on customer or client groupings may be appropriate. In some health care organizations, territorial departmentation is used because funding stipulations designate specific catchment areas or require coverage of certain population centers. Local needs, such as participation of clients and prompt settlement of difficulties, may be accommodated more easily through departmentation by territory. Grouping by geographical territory is a common element in outreach programs and home care services, as it fosters efficient movement of personnel to client locations.

4. *By customer.* Departmentation may be based on client needs. Specialty clinics in health care tend to follow this pattern. Government programs frequently focus on a specific client need, partly in response to the lobbying of interest groups. Specific examples of customer departmentation include special maternal and infant care programs, the Veterans Administration,

and programs for migrant workers. A university may have components such as day, evening, and weekend divisions, as well as continuing education programs, to accommodate the needs and interests of differing student populations.

5. *By time.* Activities may be grouped according to the time of day they are performed. This pattern, which is usually based on the use of shifts, is common in manufacturing and similar organizations in which the activities of a relatively large group of semiskilled or technical workers are repetitive and continue around the clock. Organizations that provide essential services throughout the day and night use this pattern, usually in conjunction with functional departmentation.

6. *By process.* Technological considerations and specialized equipment usage may lead to departmentation by process. This is similar to functional departmentation in that all the activities involving one major process or some set of specialized equipment are grouped. In health care organizations, the formation of radiology and clinical laboratory departments is an example of departmentation by process as well as by function.

7. *By number.* Departmentation may be done by assigning certain duties to undifferentiated workers under specific supervision. This form of departmentation is used when many workers are needed to carry out an activity. Its use is relatively limited in modern organizations, but it was traditional in early societies, such as tribes, clans, and armies. Organizing by sheer number may be used in such activities as house-to-house soliciting campaigns and membership drives. Unskilled labor crews may be organized in this pattern.

Orphan Activities

Certain activities may not merit grouping into a separate department, and there may be no compelling reason to place them in any specific location in the organization. Yet these orphan activities must be coordinated and interlocked with all others. The "most use" criterion is followed to resolve the question of organizational placement. The major department that most often uses or needs the service absorbs it. Other units that need the service obtain it from the major department to which it has been assigned.

Patient transportation in a hospital involves such a set of activities. These services are used by the physical therapy, occupational therapy, and radiology departments, among others, but overall coordination is assigned to the inpatient nursing units because one central placement is needed for these groups of workers. As another example, in small nursing homes one worker often performs several activities on a limited basis, such as general maintenance activities, running errands, and transporting patients to appointments with private physicians. The individual with these responsibilities may report to a central manager, such as the director of nursing, since the director or a delegate is present on all shifts. This arrangement provides coordination and control of the activities.

Deadly Parallel Arrangements

In an alternative organizational pattern, the higher levels of management establish dual organizational units for the purposes of control or competition. As a control device, the parallel arrangement permits comparison of costs, productivity, and similar parameters. Competition may be enhanced, if this is desired as a means of motivation, because productivity and performance can be compared.

SPECIFIC SCHEDULING

The determination of specific coverage of key functions through specific scheduling, usually by shift, is an essential aspect of organizing. Exhibit 6–1 provides an example of the development of coverage based on work flow. A mix of full-time and part-time workers and overlapping shifts at times of high volume demand in the work flow are essential considerations in developing this particular plan.

FLEXIBILITY IN ORGANIZATIONAL STRUCTURE

Managers, in their role as change agents, continually seek ways to respond to change in the external and internal organizational environment. It may be necessary to adjust traditional organizational patterns because of advances in modern technology, the increase in workers' technical and professional training, the need to offset employee alienation, and the need to overcome the problems inherent in decentralized, widely dispersed units.

In general, functional departmentation has been predominant, and there has been a strong emphasis on unity of command. When technical advice or assistance was needed, staff roles were developed to assist the line managers. When intraorganizational communication and cooperation among several units were needed, the committee structure was employed. Three alternative temporary or permanent

EXHIBIT 6-1

Specific Scheduling by Shift: Health Information Services

Planning Premises

1. Clinic days and hours

   Monday through Friday 8:00 A.M. to 7:00 P.M.

   Scheduled appointments and walk-ins

   Saturday and Sunday 8:00 A.M. to 4:00 P.M.

   Primarily walk-ins; occasional scheduled appointments

2. Tasks and deadlines (based on operational goals for department)

   Pull and deliver charts for appointments for chart availability one hour before clinic opening.

   Pull and deliver charts for walk-ins within 15 minutes of call for chart.

   Refile charts within two hours of return by clinic (pick up and return of charts scheduled every two hours).

   File late and continuing care reports within two hours of receipt.

3. Special task

   Search for charts unavailable or not found on first attempt. Perform this task at 8:00 A.M., 12:00 P.M., and 2:00 P.M. weekdays.

4. Full-time equivalents (FTEs) needed

   Eight (8) (to be full-time employees)

5. Number of floaters needed to provide vacation, holiday, and sick-time coverage

   Two (2) FTEs, to consist of four (4) part-time positions assigned as needed based on vacation, holiday, and sick-time experience.

Monday Through Friday

7:00 A.M. to 3:00 P.M. Shift 2 FTEs

   Search for charts missing or not found on initial attempt

   Pull and deliver charts for walk-ins throughout shift

   Pick up and return charts to file, two-hour rotation

   Pull charts for next day's clinic appointments

continues

EXHIBIT 6-1 *continued*

9:00 A.M. to 5:00 P.M. Shift 2 FTEs
    Pick up and return charts to file, two-hour rotation
    Pull charts for next day's clinic appointments
    Process late and continuing care reports
    Search for charts missing or not found on initial attempt (for late afternoon and early evening clinic appointments)
    Pull and deliver charts for walk-ins 3:00 P.M. to 5:00 P.M.
3:00 P.M. to 11:00 P.M. Shift 2 FTEs
    Pull and deliver charts for evening clinic walk-ins
    Pick up and return charts to file, two-hour rotation
    Process late and continuing care reports
    Carry out quality control audit of files

Saturday and Sunday

8:00 A.M. to 4:00 P.M. Shift 1 FTE per day
    Pull and deliver charts for walk-ins
    Pick up and return charts to file, two-hour rotation
    Process late and continuing care reports
    Carry out quality control audit of files

organizational patterns allow managers to retain the benefits of these traditional practices and to reduce some of their disadvantages: (1) the matrix approach, (2) temporary departmentation, and (3) the task force. These approaches may supplement the traditional organizational structure or, in the case of the matrix approach, supplant it.

Matrix Organization

Matrix organization, a design that involves both functional and product departmentation, is used predominantly to provide a flexible and adaptable organizational structure for specific projects in, for example, research, engineering, or product development. This pattern is also called grid or lattice work organization and project or product management. The matrix of organizational relationships involves a chief for the technical aspects, an administrative officer for the managerial aspects, and a project coordinator as the final authority. This dual authority structure is a predominant characteristic of the matrix organization and stands in distinct contrast to the unity of command in the traditional organizational pattern.

Workers are essentially borrowed from functional units and temporarily assigned to the project unit. Rather than designating line and staff interactions, the developers of the matrix pattern seek to create a web of relationships among technical and managerial workers. Multiple reporting systems are developed and communication lines are interwoven throughout the matrix.

Participants in the matrix organizational pattern tend to be highly trained, self-motivated individuals with a relatively independent mode of working. These functional personnel are grouped together according to the needs dictated by the phase of the project that has been undertaken. In the matrix arrangement, workers receive direction from the technical or the administrative chief as appropriate, but it is assumed that they have the ability to develop the necessary communication and work patterns without specific direction in every aspect. The project coordinator has the traditional responsibilities of guiding the technical and administrative groups and of developing the basic channels of communication and lines of coordination; however, there may be none of the detailed stipulations that are commonly associated with the highly bureaucratic traditional organizational pattern. In the health care organization, a matrix organization frees nurses, physical therapists, occupational therapists, and other direct patient care professionals from some of the relatively rigid elements of formal organization.

Temporary Departmentation

The temporary department or unit reflects a management decision to create an organizational division with a predetermined lifetime to meet some temporary need. This lifetime may be imposed by an inherent, self-limiting element, such as funding through a defense contract or private research grant. Although the predominant organizational structure may be modified periodically, there is an implicit assumption that the basic unit will remain substantially unchanged for the life of the organization. The use of the term *temporary* may be somewhat misleading: temporary departmentation usually reflects an organizational pattern that will exist for more than a few months, since an activity limited to only a few months' duration would be placed under the category of special project or task force rather than temporary departmentation. Several years may be involved, although there is no set rule.

The development of a new product, i.e., the calculation of comparative cost data, product development, and marketing, may be placed under a temporary department assigned to carry out the necessary research development and marketing within a specific time period. A team of workers with the necessary specialized knowledge may be assembled under the jurisdiction of the temporary department, deadlines set, necessary accounting processes developed, and related functions delineated.

In businesses and institutions with defense contracts or research grants, temporary departmentation provides the necessary organizational structure without interference with the establishment's normal efforts. Equipment is purchased and workers hired with special funds designated for that purpose. These workers are not necessarily subject to the same pay scale, fringe benefits, union contracts, and similar regulations as are regular employees. The manager must make it clear to these workers that their jobs are temporary, limited to the life of the contract or grant. There should also be a clear understanding about worker movement into the main organizational unit: Is this employee eligible for such movement with or without having accrued seniority and similar benefits? Patients who receive full or partial subsidy for their care in a health care institution under a special research grant or project should be informed about the limited scope of the project, and their options for continuity of care about the life of the project should be explained.

Temporary Agency Services

Staffing flexibility may also be achieved or enhanced through the use of temporary help from agencies that specialize in supplying trained personnel to cover short-term needs. "Short-term" in this sense is ordinarily construed as a period not exceeding six months. The employees engaged under an arrangement with a temporary help agency are employees of the agency, not the utilizing organization. There are several advantages to the use of agency "temps." The organization is spared the effort and expense of recruiting, hiring, training, and separating employees who will be in the work force for perhaps only a few weeks. Also, in most instances of the employment of temps, these employees come trained in the basics of the job and require only specific departmental orientation. Although the organization pays something of a premium in that the rate for a temp includes the person's pay and benefits and the agency's profit, the temp alternative is often more economical than paying overtime premium to regular staff to cover the need. There are in health care, however, some marked exceptions to this claim of economy; professional staff such as registered nurses, physical therapists, and a number of others are always more costly as temporaries than regular staff. Presently the reasons for engaging professional temps have little or nothing to do with "short-term needs"; the key reasons for today's use of professional temps are the shortage of adequate staff and the attendant difficulties experienced in recruiting critically needed personnel.

It should be stressed that temporary help arrangements need to be limited to a period of less than six months. Federal law requires that anyone working for an organization for a period exceeding six months must be considered an employee for purposes of earning credit toward retirement. Some non–health care organizations' past practices—often involving laying off employees and hiring them back as "temporaries" at lower rates of pay and with fewer benefits and the inability to accrue retirement credit—were seen as a deliberate strategy to avoid certain costs. In any event, however, a temporary engagement that has extended beyond the six-month guideline should be examined closely for alternative ways of meeting the need. The key criterion for the appropriate use of temporary staff is the short-term nature of the need. In the health care setting especially, the prolonged use of temps to meet a continuing need is never as economical as engaging permanent staff.

Outsourcing

Outsourcing is simply the process of having certain services that could be provided internally performed by agencies or individuals external to the organization. Outsourcing has been an actively used alternative in manufacturing industries for many years. It is common in manufacturing for a company to rely on external suppliers to provide them with various components made to their specifications. In fact, what we now know as outsourcing probably began in manufacturing in the manner just described, although the label "outsourcing" is considerably newer than the activity itself.

Many of the decisions favoring outsourcing are made for economic reasons. Quite simply, if a service can be obtained externally for less than the cost of providing it internally, outsourcing may be considered a preferred alternative (providing, of course, that the external source meets all of the organization's quality requirements).

Often the economic decision favoring outsourcing is driven by volume considerations. Should there not be enough of a particular activity required to justify hiring and staffing to perform it (for example, some specialized task requiring just a few hours each week), outsourcing may be the logical alternative.

Outsourcing decisions may also hinge upon the presence or absence of particular skills or capabilities. For example, a large health care organization may have its own in-house legal counsel, whereas a smaller organization will outsource all of its legal work to an external law firm. Or perhaps a hospital that is having difficulty keeping up with medical transcription because of position vacancies or abnormally high volume of dictation will farm out some of its transcription work to an external service.

Contracted Services

The general heading of outsourcing includes the use of contract management services and the use of independent contractors. Under contract management the entirety of a particular service associated with the organization is managed by or perhaps provided in full by an external organization that specializes in that service. Probably the two most common hospital and nursing home services provided under contract management are food service and housekeeping, although in one setting or another essentially every conceivable service has been contracted out by some health care organizations. Contract management may involve management alone or the complete provision of the service. At one particular hospital, for example, an external firm supplies the management of food service while the rank-and-file food service workers remain hospital employees, but at the same hospital housekeeping is provided by an external firm utilizing its own staff with no involvement of hospital employees.

The use of so-called independent contractors has received considerable government attention over the past couple of decades. Generally, to qualify under Internal Revenue Service (IRS) guidelines as an independent contractor and thus be paid as a supplier rather than as an employee, a worker is required to demonstrate a level of independence not commonly found in an employer-employee relationship, as evidenced by the following principal factors:

- The worker personally invests in the facilities and equipment that are used in performing the services.
- The worker can expect to either make a profit or experience a loss from the activity (other than because of simple nonpayment for services provided).
- The worker provides services for two or more unrelated clients or customers within the same period of time.
- The worker makes services available to any or all potential clients or customers on a regular and consistent basis.

It is the presence of the foregoing conditions that the IRS will look for in assessing the nature of the relationship in which an external service is provided. Using an independent medical transcriptionist as an example, if Ms. Jones acquired her own equipment and offers transcription services to a number of organizations including Hospital A, chances are Ms. Jones will be considered an independent contractor. If, however, Ms. Jones is performing transcription for Hospital A only, working in her home using equipment largely or completely provided by Hospital A, Ms. Jones will be considered an employee of Hospital A. And as an employee

Ms. Jones must be on the payroll of Hospital A with all that that implies (various personnel expenses for the hospital, and withholding taxes and such for Ms. Jones).

The use of independent contractors may generate cost savings because of the elimination of personnel expense associated with training, physical space requirements, unemployment compensation, and other aspects of direct employment. However, the health care organization department that makes use of independent contractors must have consistently applied guidelines governing such working relationships. Exhibit 6–2 provides a set of sample guidelines for contract specifications for independent contractors using, for illustrative purposes, guidelines applied in arrangements with an outsourced dictation-transcription service.

EXHIBIT 6–2

Guidelines for the Use of Contractual Services

Contracts with incorporated contractual services shall be approved by Human Resource Division and shall include the following elements as a minimum:

- HIPAA-compliant confidentiality and security measures
- Accept dictation from land-line phone systems, PC microphones, handheld digital recorders
- Document distribution by secure line fax, secure e-mail, remote print
- Electronic editing and signature
- Tracking system of document from beginning of recording through document received
- Customized format
- 99 percent error free guarantee
- STAT capability
- 24-hr/365-day support center
- Turn around time of (n) hours
- Conform with Medical Transcription Industry Association billing method principles

Telecommuting

If our hypothetical Ms. Jones of the foregoing section does all or most of her work at home, serving only Hospital A and using some Hospital A hardware and software, she may be considered a telecommuting employee.

Telecommuting is an employment arrangement in which a person who is on the organization's payroll works a regularly scheduled amount of time each week at home or some other external location with the support of the appropriate equipment and services. As a flexible work-style option telecommuting is a significant step beyond what is often called "flextime." The telecommuter works in a setting other than the traditional office or shop and is supervised by means other than management provided by an immediately present supervisor.

Sometimes existing informally by arrangement between manager and employee, telecommuting is not a radically new idea. Many outside salespersons as well as consultants of various kinds have done it for years, working out of offices in their homes and visiting the company's headquarters just occasionally. In recent years, however, telecommuting possibilities have been significantly expanded and enhanced by advances in computers and telecommunications technology.

Whether full-time or part-time, telecommuters are regular employees on the payroll of the organization. They are decidedly not independent contractors or freelancers who are paid per piece or per job and excluded from employee benefits, and they do not conform to the criteria by which the IRS defines independent contractors.

There is a temptation to sometimes regard telecommuting as simple, consisting of just having an employee work at home rather than at the office, but effective telecommuting is considerably more involved. Many employees might wish to work in telecommuting situations, but it is the organization and not the employee that sets the criteria. Telecommuting is never appropriate for employees whose primary duties involve direct interaction with clients or customers on site, and it is inappropriate for people who work on team undertakings that require regular employee interaction. And even if a particular job's duties would seem to lend themselves to telecommuting, such an arrangement should never be considered for employees who have yet to prove themselves as reliable self-starters.

Telecommuting cannot be a hit-or-miss proposition. It requires a consistent policy delineating the rules for its use, specifying:

- *Where* the telecommuter can work: whether just at home or at other sites as well
- *Work status:* whether full-time or part-time

- *When* one can work: whether the employee sets the hours, the organization sets the hours, or the employee is allowed to flex around required "core" hours
- *Technology* required: whether what's needed is determined by the telecommuter or designated by the business

In developing a telecommuting policy it is best to secure the input of not only affected managers but some of the likely telecommuters, as well. The telecommuting policy should require that any such arrangement be described by specific objectives, detailed results expected, and how accomplishments are measured.

For certain kinds of activities telecommuting has been practiced for years. For example, traditional telecommuting arrangements have included data entry, customer billing, and medical transcription. However, most jobs that are performed independent of other people and that do not require high-cost specialized equipment are possibilities for telecommuting. Many jobs can lend themselves to telecommuting as long as the arrangement can satisfactorily serve the needs of all concerned.

The individual in a telecommuting situation stands to benefit from reduced travel time and fewer transportation concerns, comfort of work environment and dress, freedom from interruptions, possibly flexible hours, and in some instances relief from child care concerns. Some professional and technical employees find that on telecommuting days they are more available for telephone consultation than when they are in a busy office environment. The organization frequently gains productive efficiency and is often able to reduce expenses and save energy and in general reduce the strain on facilities and services. In fact, some organizations have adopted telecommuting as a means of avoiding the addition of more space. Telecommuting can also aid in recruiting and retaining employees.

Telecommuting is not likely to succeed with the occasional employee who is unable to cope well with isolation from coworkers and the absence of traditional supervision. And the manager who is constantly—or, at the other extreme, never—checking up on the unseen employee will not do well with telecommuting employees. Managers inexperienced with telecommuting often fear they will not be able to monitor employee activities sufficiently, perhaps feeling they cannot effectively manage people who are not under their full-time direct supervision. Thus the manager of telecommuters must necessarily manage by results, using goals, objectives, and quotas.

Before going forward with any telecommuting arrangement:

- Check with your counterparts at other organizations of comparable size and complexity about their experiences with telecommuting.

- Be certain the desired arrangement is consistent with the organization's personnel and business systems (time reporting, payroll, etc.).
- If unionized employees are potentially involved, sound out the union concerning their stand on telecommuting and bring them into the process early.

Needless to say, a great many employees would be likely to jump at the opportunity to work at home. However, telecommuting should never be adopted simply because some employees want to do it. Telecommuting should be seriously considered only if doing so would seem to make good business sense.

THE ORGANIZATIONAL CHART

The management tool used for depicting organizational relationships is the organizational chart. It is a diagrammatic form, a visual arrangement, that depicts the following aspects of an institution:

1. major functions, usually by department
2. relationships of functions or departments
3. channels of supervision
4. lines of authority and of communication
5. positions (by job title) within departments or units

There are numerous reasons for using organizational charts:

- Since an organizational chart maps major lines of decision making and authority, managers can review it to identify any inconsistencies and complexities in the organizational structure. The diagrammatic representation makes it easier to determine and correct these inconsistencies and complexities.
- An organizational chart may be used to orient employees, since it shows where each job fits in relation to supervisors and to other jobs in the department. It shows the relationship of the department to the organization as a whole.
- The chart is a useful tool in managerial audits. Managers can review such factors as the span of management, mixed lines of authority, and splintered authority; they can also check that individual job titles are on the chart so it is clear to whom each employee reports. In addition, managers can compare current practice with the original plan of job assignments to determine if any discrepancies exist.

Certain limitations are inherent in the rather static structure presented by organizational charts, and these limitations can offset some of the advantages of using the charts:

- Only formal lines of authority and communication are shown; important lines of informal communication and significant informal relationships cannot be shown.
- The chart may become obsolete if not updated at least once a year (or whenever there is a major change in the organizational pattern).
- Individuals without proper training in interpretation may confuse authority relationship with status. Managers whose positions are placed physically higher in the graphic representation may be perceived as having authority over those whose positions are lower on the chart. The emphasis must be placed on the direct authority relationships and the chain of command.
- The chart cannot be properly interpreted without reference to support information, such as that usually contained in the organizational manual and related job descriptions.

Types of Charts

There are two major kinds of organizational charts: master and supplementary. The master chart depicts the entire organization, although not in great detail, and normally shows all departments and major positions of authority. A detailed listing of formal positions or job titles is not given in the master chart, however. Each supplementary chart depicts a section, department, or unit, including the specific details of its organizational pattern. An organization has as many supplementary charts as it has departments or units.

The supplementary chart of a department usually reflects the master chart and shows the direct chain of command from highest authority to that derived by the department head. The master chart usually shows the major functions, while the supplementary charts depict each individual job title and the number of positions in each section, as well as full-time or part-time status. Additional information, such as cost centers, major codes, or similar identifying information, sometimes appears on the charts.

General Arrangements and Conventions

The conventional organizational chart is a line or scalar chart showing each layer of the organization in sequence (Figure 6–4). In another arrangement, the flow of authority may be depicted from left to right, starting with major officials on the extreme left and with each successive division to the right of the preceding unit. The advantage of this form stems from its similarity to normal reading patterns. A circular arrangement, in which the authority flows from the center outward, is

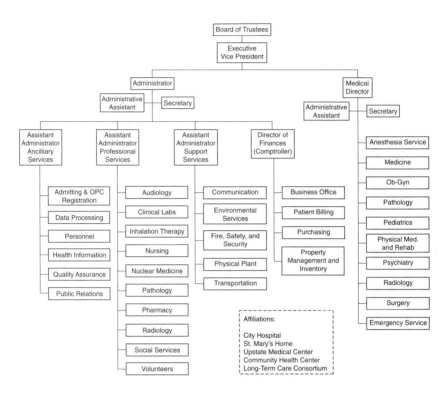

FIGURE 6–4 Master Organizational Chart of a Hospital

sometimes used; its advantage is that it shows the authority flow reaching out and permeating all levels, not just flowing from top to bottom.

Certain general conventions are followed when an organizational chart is drawn. Ordinarily line authority and line relationships are indicated by solid lines, and staff positions are indicated by broken or dotted lines. In Figure 6–5, the position of health information consultant has a staff relationship to the administrator, which is, accordingly, shown by a broken line. Sometimes the staff relationship is indicated by a small *s* with a slash mark setting it off from the job title. Occasionally, a special relationship is indicated by surrounding an entire unit or even another organization with broken lines and leaving it unconnected to any line or staff unit. Such a unit is included in the organizational chart to call attention to the existence of a related, auxiliary, or affiliated organization. This technique is used in Figure 6–4 to indicate the relationship of the teaching institutions affiliated with the hospital.

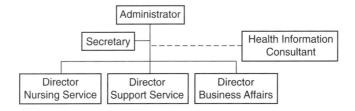

FIGURE 6–5 Special Relationships: Consultant in Advisory Role

Preparing the Organizational Chart

If the chart is prepared during a planning or reorganization stage, the first step is to list all the major functions and the jobs associated with them. The major groupings by function then are brought together as specific units, for example, all jobs dealing with the file area or with patient identification systems, all jobs dealing with physical medicine and rehabilitation, or all jobs dealing with data processing and computer activities. If there is a question about the proper placement of one or several functions, managers can derive significant information by asking the following questions:

- If there is a problem, who must be involved to effect a solution?
- Do the supervisors at each level have the necessary authority to carry out their functions?
- If a change in systems and procedures is needed, who must agree to the changes?
- If critical information must be channeled through the organization, who is responsible for its transmission throughout each unit of the organization?

As an aid in developing the organizational chart, it is useful to prepare a simple tabulation showing the following information:

1. job title
2. reporting line: supervised by whom (title)
3. full-time or part-time
4. day, evening, or night shift
5. line or staff position

The inclusion of the incumbent's name is optional for this worksheet preparation, although names may be useful in a subsequent managerial audit of the department in which the manager is comparing present practice with the original plan.

The use of names as the basic means of developing the chart could be misleading, however, as it may block managers' thinking, causing them to describe organizational relationships as they are rather than as they should be. It may be best to show names only on a staffing chart that is prepared after the organizational chart has been developed.

After obtaining the necessary information about work relationships, shifts, supervisory needs, and span of management factors, managers develop the final chart, using the general conventions for depicting organizational relationships. A support narrative or a section of the organization's manual can be developed to give additional information.

THE JOB DESCRIPTION

The duties associated with each job should be determined by the needs of the department. Frequently, jobs evolve as duties become assigned to an employee. These jobs are accumulations of tasks rather than products of prior planning. Some form of control is necessary to keep assignments within intended limits. In order to provide this control of the various work assignments, the duties and responsibilities of each job should be set forth in written form. This helps to ensure that employees' concepts of their duties will be consistent with those of the manager and with the needs of the department.

In every formal organization, there are job descriptions to cover all jobs. In order to fill the various positions with the appropriate employees, it is necessary to match the jobs available in the department with the individuals. This can only be done with the help of job descriptions, which are written objective statements defining duties and functions. Each job description includes responsibilities, experience, organizational relationships, working conditions, and other essential factors of the position.

Job Analysis

Preceding the development of a job description there should be a thorough job analysis that serves as a single source for the various uses to be made of information concerning a specific job. In addition to providing all of the information necessary for the development of the job description, the job analysis serves a variety of other uses that include performing a job evaluation (establishing an appropriate pay grade for the job), developing recruiting specifications, conducting employee orientation and education, and planning for staffing requirements.

Managers in many organizations will recognize what is described herein as a job analysis as the instrument they presently refer to as the job description. As a job description it is liable to be lengthy, perhaps running to several pages. It undoubtedly contains more information than is needed in an efficient job description or, for that matter, more than is needed for any single use of job information. A complete job analysis surely fits the bill as a job description; however, the problem is that it overfills this particular need. Using this complete rendering of job information as a job description results in unnecessarily voluminous job description files and often poses difficulties for performance appraisal systems that are appropriately based on duties as enumerated in a job description.

The specific advantage of the use of a job analysis is that a single job analysis can sometimes serve as a "master" for a family of jobs. Consider, for example, a job analysis of perhaps six pages in length for "Registered Nurse (RN)." This thorough job analysis would be written to be descriptive of all registered nurse positions in the organization, with all duties or groupings of duties described in general terms. Related to this master job analysis there may be any number of one- or two-page job descriptions addressing the specific variations of registered nurse, such as RN, Emergency Department; RN, Medical/Surgical; RN, Operating Room; and so on. Surely ten or a dozen one- or two-page job descriptions are far more efficient and much easier to use than ten or a dozen six-page documents filled with duplicative information, much of which is not immediately relevant to the uses of a job description.

At one time or another all of the information gathered via a thorough job analysis will be relevant to some important application. But as far as the job description is concerned, every reasonable effort should be made to present the information it contains in a concise manner. The concise job description is generally of greater immediate value as a working document than the complete job analysis.

Job Description Content and Format

The format of a job description should present the information in an orderly manner. Since there is no standard format, job descriptions vary with the type of facility and with the size and scope of the department. The following format is suggested as a guide:

- Job Title. The job should be identified by a title that clarifies the position. The inclusion in the job title of such words as *director, supervisor, senior, staff,* or *clerk* can help to indicate the duties and skill level of the job. Examples of job titles that indicate such specificity are: Physical Therapist—Vestibular and Balance Program Coordinator; Health Information—Coding and Reimbursement Clinical Specialist.

- Immediate Supervisor. The position and title of the immediate supervisor should be clearly identified.
- Job Summary. A short statement of the major activities of the job should indicate the purpose and scope of the job in specific terms. This section serves principally to identify the job and differentiate the duties that are performed from those of other jobs.
- Job Duties. The major part of the job description should state what the employee does and how the duties are accomplished. The description of duties should also indicate the degree of supervision received or given.
- Job Specifications. A written record of minimum hiring requirements for a particular job comes from the job analysis procedure. The items covered in the specifications may be divided into two groups:
  1. The skill requirements include mental and manual skills, plus personal traits and qualities, needed to perform the job effectively:
     - minimum educational requirements
     - licensure or registration requirements
     - experience expressed in objective and quantitative terms, such as years
     - specific knowledge requirements or advanced educational requirements
     - manual skills required in terms of the quality, quantity, or nature of the work to be performed
     - communication skills, both oral and written
  2. The physical demands of a job may include the following:
     - physical effort required to perform the job and the length of time involved in performing a given activity
     - working conditions and general physical environment in which the job is to be performed
     - job hazards and their probability of occurrence

Exhibit 6–3 is a typical job description for a clerical position.

In some institutions, the job specifications are organized as a separate record because the information is not used for the same purpose as the information contained in the job description. The specifications receive the most usage in connection with the recruitment and selection of employees, since this part of the job description defines the qualifications that are needed to perform the job. Job evaluations and the establishment of different wage and salary schedules are other functions that depend on the data contained in the job specifications.

Job Rating and Classification

Before employees are selected and hired, the organization develops a job classification. This classification is based on the results of the job rating process. In job rating, each set of functions within each unit of the organization is analyzed using some set of common denominators. In health care, these variables include complexity

EXHIBIT 6–3

Excerpts from Typical Job Description: Clerical Position

Job Summary

This is a clerical position in the health information service of an acute care facility affiliated with a medical school and a research institution. This full-time, day shift position is under the direct supervision of the Assistant Health Information Administrator; incumbent performs duties with relative independence, referring exceptions to policy and procedure to supervisory personnel within the department.

Job Duties

1. Receives visitors to the department; processes their requests by routing them to appropriate supervisors; assists requestor as needed; schedules appointments.
2. Takes dictation from transcribing machine and from rough draft and transcribes according to prescribed format.

Job Specifications

1. Fluency in English language, both oral and written expression.
2. Ability to create final copy, from both dictation and handwritten copy, error-free minimum of 70 words per minute.
3. Minimum of high school diploma or its equivalent and at least one year of secretarial experience or successful completion of postsecondary secretarial school.

Note flexibility in requirement 3; this fosters a nondiscriminatory approach to hiring, giving flexibility to the manner in which an individual may qualify for the position.

of duties; error impact; contacts with patients, families, and other individuals both within and outside of the organization; degree of supervision received and nature of duties ranging from unskilled to highly technical and professional. Mental and physical demands as well as working conditions may also be assessed because these variables may make a job different from seemingly similar positions in the organization.

When developing a job description, it is useful to compare the draft of the description with the job rating scale specific to the organization. From this "dry run," changes in actual wording may result so that the final expression of job duties and related conditions matches the categories or factors to be assessed. Without such a correlation between the job rating scale and the job description's wording, inequities could be fostered. Similar jobs could receive different ratings based on a lack of proper wording in a particular job description.

Ideally, the overall job rating process contains safeguards against discrepancies; ideally, the personnel manager makes such job rating information available to unit managers. It is still the duty and prerogative of line managers to take active steps in these matters and anticipate the job rating process.

In addition to the overall job classification, the wage and salary and fringe benefit package may be predicated on information gained in the job description or job rating process. Another key to success in developing useful job descriptions is to assess the written document for its adequacy in conveying information about the factors used in job rating and wage and salary considerations.

Two additional outcomes of the job classification that concern the manager are the determinations made for exempt and nonexempt positions under the Fair Labor Standards Act (FLSA) and the applicability of a union contract in terms of jobs included in a particular bargaining union. In both of these cases, information about supervisory activity is critical. Thus there is another benchmark against which to measure the adequacy of the job description: Does it contain sufficient information to justify inclusion—or exclusion—of a job in terms of overtime pay and related FLSA provisions? Is the nature of the job clearly delineated in terms of rating as skilled or unskilled, technical or professional, for purposes of union contract applicability?

Recruitment

Certain steps in the recruitment process involve information derived from the job description. Internal job posting may involve the placement of the complete job description in a specified location, such as on an employee bulletin board. Potential transfer employees essentially participate in a self-selection or rejection process as they read this job description. They can take the opportunity to assess such practical aspects of a job as shift work or weekend coverage requirements in terms of their availability to work such hours.

The physical, mental, or technical demands of the job also may sway the potential transfer employee to reconsider applying for a position. Then, too, the job description may have the effect of encouraging applicants. Does the job description contain enough information to help prospective employees make such a preliminary determination?

Those involved in the preliminary selection interviews, usually members of the human resources department, need sufficient information about all the jobs in the institution to carry out initial screening. The unit managers must convey, through the job description, key points of information about duties, responsibilities, and qualifications. It is important to note that the unit manager is the individual most familiar with the work of the unit. This information must be conveyed in a way that it can be understood by persons who are not involved in the unit or department on a daily basis.

Awareness of the wide audience who will use the job descriptions will help the manager write them in understandable form. The unit manager may find it useful to try out the wording of a job description on another manager. Does the wording convey enough information for this person, familiar with the health care setting but not necessarily familiar with the details of the specific department, to form a basic idea of the job?

The Final Selection Process

A major use of the job description occurs during the selection process as the candidate is matched to the job. During the selection interview, information about the duties, responsibilities, and qualifications is conveyed. One sensitive overlay to the selection process, which includes all aspects of the interview, testing, and physical examination, is strict avoidance of discriminatory practices, even inadvertent discrimination.

When the job, as summarized in the job description, is the focus of the interview, it is easier to avoid the pitfalls of interviewing that could suggest discriminatory practices. Thus with a job description that spells out such expectations as weekend coverage, shift work availability, and similar requirements, the manager and prospective employee can deal with that set of expectations without the manager probing in any way into such questions as days of religious observance, arrangements for child care, and other topics that are off limits for direct inquiry. The emphasis is on the job as it is described.

Job qualifications and mental, physical, and technical demands become the objective measures of candidate suitability when they are derived from job duties. These in turn foster a positive climate of compliance with nondiscriminatory practices.

For example, if the job duties include frequent routine interaction with patients in need of emergency care and the patient population involved is non–English speaking, a qualification of fluency in a specific language is not discriminatory. If the unit manager can tie each qualification to one or more job duties, the likelihood of discriminatory practices in the employment selection process is diminished. Sometimes it may seem that one is stating the obvious, such as ability to read, write, speak English (or some other language) with ease, hear, see, and lift—so why spell these out? These elements are specified in detail when they are true requirements. The purpose of the job description, with its explicit requirements, is to provide all parties with necessary information about the job so that there is no misunderstanding later.

Another method to use in making a dry run of the job description that helps the manager determine the level of detail needed under the foregoing conditions is working with human resources management using a sample of applications that have been received over some period of time. How does the manager's job description hold up? On what basis would the manager hire, or not hire, a particular individual in light of the job description as it is written?

Employee Development and Retention

At each point of employee development, activities focus on the work to be done within each job. Orientation and training programs take on greater meaning as they are tailored to specific job duties and qualifications. Training outcomes can be stated in terms of the trainee's ability to perform the duties. This is another step toward objective evaluation of candidates.

Job descriptions also provide a focus for performance evaluations. Has the worker accomplished the duties and responsibilities made known in the job description? Error correction, retraining, and, if necessary, disciplinary action are carried out in the context of the job for which the individual was hired. In cases of grievance, emphasis will be given to the worker's accomplishment of the job duties, with the presumption that these have been made known to the worker. A comprehensive, up-to-date job description is a valuable management document in such cases.

Finally, in cases of illness or injury under review by such agencies as Workers' Compensation or the Occupational Safety and Health Administration (OSHA), the basic determination of job relatedness is made using the job description. Below is a summary of uses of the job description. How would the manager's current descriptions hold up when scrutinized in relation to each of these applications?

Summary of Uses of the Job Description

The job description

- fosters or contributes to overall compliance with legal, regulatory, contractual, and accrediting mandates
- serves as a basis for job rating, job classification, and wage and salary administration
- serves as a basis for determining exemption or inclusion under provisions of the Fair Labor Standards Act and collective bargaining agreements
- provides information to prospective employees and to employer representatives during the recruitment and selection process
- serves as a basis for orientation and training programs at the time of initial selection, transfer, or promotion
- serves as a basis for performance evaluation, error correction, retraining requirements, and grievance determinations
- provides information to determine eligibility for claims under Workers' Compensation, OSHA, and similar programs

Jobs, like the organizational structure of a hospital, are dynamic in nature. Changes in the size and nature of the organization, the introduction of new equipment, or the employment of new treatment techniques—to mention only a few factors—have a definite influence on the duties and requirements of jobs. Thus, the manager and the employees of a department must review the description of each job on a periodic, regular schedule (at least once a year). The document should be dated when it is first prepared, redated when it is reviewed, and again redated when it is revised. An up-to-date accurate job description is essential when the human resources department recruits applicants for a job or when the manager hires new employees, appraises the performance of existing employees, and attempts to establish an equitable wage and salary pattern within the department.

See Exhibits 6–4 to 6–7 for examples of job descriptions and job duty delineations.

EXHIBIT 6–4

Job Description for Release of Information Specialist

JOB TITLE: Release of Information Specialist
RESPONSIBLE TO: Director, Health Information Service

Responsibilities

Under the general direction of the director, Health Information Service, this specialist is responsible for processing requests for release of information from the official medical records of this facility. All work is carried out in accordance with the department's approved policies and procedures.

Job Setting and Conditions

This is an advanced-level clerical position in the Health Information Service of this [n]-bed facility. The position is full-time, day shift. Normal working days and hours are Monday through Friday, 8:30 A.M. to 4:30 P.M., with a paid 45-minute lunch period. Adjustments to the normal schedule are required when the employee travels to and from court or other site of legal proceedings to give testimony in response to subpoenas and court orders.

Job Duties

In accordance with department policies and procedures, this specialist carries out these 13 major and closely related duties and responsibilities:

1. Processes requests for release of information from the official records maintained by this facility
2. Receives and processes all incoming written requests for such release
3. Receives visitors to the unit to process these requests and inquiries
4. Answers the unit telephone to process these requests and inquiries
5. Reviews each request to determine
   a. need for authorization
   b. adequacy of authorization
6. Prepares responses appropriate to each request

EXHIBIT 6–4 *continued*

7. Calculates, collects, and transmits fees associated with the release of information
8. Photocopies material from the original medical record and prepares abstract summaries
9. Accepts, processes, and responds to subpoenas and court orders
10. Maintains the release of information log used to track the status of each request
11. Operates the office equipment normally used in the routines of daily work, such as photocopy and facsimile equipment, and computers
12. Promotes public relations through prompt and courteous service
13. Fosters respect for patient privacy by maintaining confidentiality in all phases of the work

Education and Experience

- The trainee should have a high school diploma or the equivalent.
- The trainee should have had advanced clerical training, which includes typing and computer skills, basic filing and bookkeeping, basic office procedures, and basic medical record terminology and practice.
- The trainee should have had relevant experience in clerical duties sufficient for individual development to the level of independent functioning with minimal direction.
- A trainee is acceptable provided the individual meets the established work standards within [n] weeks of completion of the mandatory training program for this job.

Skills

- fluent in English
- able to process final copy, error free, within prescribed deadlines
- able to maintain alphabetical and numerical files with no errors
- able to maintain fee collection system with no errors

continues

EXHIBIT 6–4 *continued*

Physical and Mental Demands

- ability to withstand the pressure of continual deadlines and receipt of work with variable requirements
- ability to concentrate and maintain accuracy in spite of frequent interruptions
- ability to be courteous, tactful, and cooperative throughout the working day
- ability to use judgment in carrying out all phases of the work
- ability to maintain confidentiality with regard to all phases of the work
- acute visual and auditory senses
- ability to communicate clearly in English in both oral and written forms of expression
- ability to sit for long periods; move about the facility; stoop and lift light loads such as packets of mail, medical records, and packages
- ability to use standard office equipment including computers, photocopy and facsimile machines, and reader-printers

Special Requirements

- Ability to drive a car to and from area courts and law offices in the [*n*-county] area for the purpose of responding to subpoenas and depositions.
- Ability to maintain flexible working hours when required to travel to and from, and participate in, legal proceedings requiring the presentation of medical records and/or the provision of testimony.

DATE:

REVISIONS:

Reprinted from permission from Aspen Publishers, Inc. Joan Gratto Liebler, *Medical Records: Policies and Guidelines*, 1997; 10:90.

EXHIBIT 6-5

Job Description for Registered Nurse

Job Title	Department
Registered Professional Nurse	Emergency Department
Emergency Department	
Reports To	Revised
Nursing Manager	
Emergency Department	

Job Objectives

To assume responsibility for the delivery of patient care through the nursing process of assessment, planning, implementation and evaluation, diagnosing and treating human response to actual or potential health problems through such services as case finding, health teaching, health counseling, and provision of care supportive to or restorative of life and well-being, and executing medical regimens prescribed by a licensed or otherwise legally authorized physician or dentist.

Job Responsibilities

In addition to the duties of the basic RN job description are the following:

1. Counts narcotics and orders from pharmacy if needed.
2. Checks crash carts and emergency equipment (defibrillator, pacemaker, etc.) and documents.
3. Receives report from previous shift.
4. Reevaluates and assesses patients and sets priorities.
5. Receives new patients—assesses and obtains vitals, initiates appropriate treatment, sets priorities. Performs nursing assessment on all patients, obtaining subjective data through patient interview and eliciting objective data through physical assessment techniques.
6. Documents—date, time, assessment, vitals and history on chart and nurse's notes.
7. Initiates physician orders and obtains specimens.
   a. Starts IV
   b. Draws blood
   c. Obtains EKG
   d. Provides O_2 therapy

continues

EXHIBIT 6–5 *continued*

    e. Monitors cardiac status

    f. Medicates

    g. X-rays (orders)

8. Observes and evaluates patient's status continuously and documents.
9. Communicates significant patient status change to physician and charge.
10. Instructs and teaches patients/families in regard to treatments, Rx, and discharge follow-up document.
11. Transcribes physician orders on admitted patients.
12. Initiates lab requisitions as necessary.
13. Orders medication supply.
14. Cleans units between patients.
15. Transfers admitted patients to receiving units and gives report.
16. Maintains admission log (ECU).
17. Gives report to oncoming shift.
18. Performs many clerical functions in the absence of clerical support.
19. Responds to "Blue Alerts" in X-ray, OPD, physical medicine, and labs.
20. Responds anywhere on hospital grounds for accidents, injuries, and emergencies when summoned by Public Safety.
21. Responds to radiation, hospital, and community disaster.
22. Complies with all policies and procedures of the department and the hospital.
23. Performs all functions of phlebotomy, IV therapy, and EKG service.
24. Functions in the absence of Social Service, making appropriate arrangements and referrals.
25. Classifies all admitted patients every shift.
26. Possesses knowledge and expertise associated with performing or assisting with the following:

    Medical

      Pediatric and Adult

    Cardiac

      Identification of cardiac arrhythmias

      Cardiac lead placement

      Mechanical operation of cardiac monitors

EXHIBIT 6–5 *continued*

Defibrillation and cardioversion
Insertion of pacemaker
Hemodynamic Monitoring and Fluid Monitoring
Insertion and monitoring of arterial lines
Calibration of arterial monitor
CVP insertion and monitoring
Calibration of IVAC
MAST trousers

Respiratory

Insertion—extubation and monitoring of ET tubes and EOAs
Administration of respiratory treatment (ex. D30, O_2, ventimask, coup tent ventimask, coup tent ventilators)

Therapeutic and Diagnostic Procedures

Peritoneal dialysis—fluid exchange
Thoracentesis
Peritonealcentesis
Lumbar puncture
Lavage—poisons and overdoses

Surgical—Adult and Pediatric

Lacerations—suturing, cleansing, and dressing
Abscesses—incision and drainage, dressing
Burns—treatment and dressings
Eye burns (chemical and trauma)—irrigation, dressing
Penetrating chest wounds—thoracotomy
Peritoneal tap
Insertion of NG tubes
Declotting dialysis shunts
Management of arterial and venous bleeding
Insertion of chest tubes—pneumo- and hemothorax

Orthopedic

Cervical fracture—stabilization; traction techniques
Limb fracture—stabilization; casting, pinning, splinting, traction
Sprains—ace wraps, splinting, crutch walking
Hip fracture—stabilization; alignment

continues

EXHIBIT 6–5 *continued*

Gynecologic
Vaginal fetal delivery
Spontaneous abortion
Rape examination—collection of evidence
Pelvic exams
Culdecentesis
Hemophiliac
Preparation and administration of blood products
Psychiatric
Restraining and confinement procedures

Preparation and Training

Graduation from accredited RN program. Licensed as an RN by New York State.

Consequence of Error

Probable errors may be difficult to detect such as improper use or setup of treatments or procedures. Most work is not directly verified or checked. Constantly relating to general public affecting outside image of hospital. Extensive responsibility in life/death/health issues.

Level of Supervision

Employee and supervisor, in consultation, develop deadlines, projects, and work to be done where supervisor sets objectives; 21–50 percent of work is reviewed by first level of supervision.

Experience

1–3 years of previous work experience.

Confidential Data

Has full and complete access to confidential data such as patient medical records and histories, personnel matters, and legal matters where utmost integrity is required to safeguard the patient, hospital, and employee.

Mental/Visual Demand and Physical Effort

Flow of work frequently produces a high level of mental/visual fatigue associated with constant reprioritizing, uncontrollability of patient census, and legal ramifications of actions. Seven or more hours standing or walking 95 percent of the time.

EXHIBIT 6–5 *continued*

Pushing/pulling 3–4 hours. Lifts and transports patients (95–300 pounds) frequently. Repetitive use of both hands. Grasping simple/light to firm/strong of both hands. Fine dexterity required with cardiac monitors, vents, IVACs, EKG machine.

Directs Work of Others and Number of Employees Supervised

Helps orient, train, develop, coach, direct, and measure performance by LPN, ED, Tech., volunteers, observers (EMT, nursing students).

Environment

Undesirable working conditions. Exposure to infectious disease, chemicals, virus, odors, noise, and exhaust fumes from ambulances. Temperature change due to ambulance entrance.

EXHIBIT 6–6

Job Description for Physical Therapist

Job Title Staff Physical Therapist	Department Physical Medicine and Rehabilitation
Reports To Physical Therapy Supervisor	Revised

Job Objectives

Designs, implements, and performs or supervises physical therapy treatment programs based on physician referrals or prescriptions. Provides periodic teaching programs to other professionals and to the public. Provides supervision for physical therapy students during their affiliations at General Hospital.

continues

EXHIBIT 6–6 *continued*

Job Responsibilities

I. Perform a complete initial evaluation. Consult the medical record and obtain the pertinent medical history.

  A. Perform initial evaluation within next working day of receiving inpatient requisition as dated on arrival in department.

  B. Pertinent past medical history is obtained 100 percent of the time as documented in the initial note.

  C. Perform appropriate tests and evaluation skills for every patient according to accepted standards.

II. Conduct reevaluations of patient. Modify or change treatment programs if the initial program is not meeting set goals. Set new goals if appropriate.

  A. Reevaluations are performed at least once a week with objective findings documented in the chart.

  B. Treatments are changed if no improvement is noted with 3–5 treatments as judged by reevaluation.

  C. New goals are established with patient as per department policy.

III. Plan and implement an appropriate initial treatment program. Set appropriate goals. Provide written home instruction and assistive equipment, if needed.

  A. Plan and implement appropriate initial treatment program 100 percent of the time according to established practices.

  B. Specific, objective, quantifiable, appropriate goals are set in 100 percent of initial evaluations as per documentation in the patient chart.

  C. Organized home exercise programs are provided to the patient when professionally deemed necessary as documented in the patient chart.

  D. Assistive equipment is provided for the patient when professionally deemed necessary as documented in the patient chart.

IV. Demonstrate good and safe patient techniques.

  A. Safe patient care techniques are observed 100 percent of the time according to department policies and procedures.

EXHIBIT 6–6 *continued*

V. Maintain a high level of productivity.
   A. An average of 25 treatments on outpatient rotations, 18 treatments on inpatient rotation is performed on a daily basis as documented by periodic productivity surveys.
   B. Patient waiting time is minimized to 15-minute wait from set appointment time as observed by supervisor and input from the office staff.
VI. Be certain that the patient has an appropriate written referral.
   A. Patients have an appropriate written referral at the time of initial treatment as per chart review.
VII. Maintain complete records of patients' evaluations, treatment, progress, and discharge status. Forward this information to appropriate professionals.
   A. For outpatients, documentation of evaluations, treatment, and progress is performed at each session as per chart review.
   B. For inpatients, documentation of evaluations, treatment, and progress is performed at least 2–3 times per week as per chart review.
   C. Progress notes contain ( ) percent of necessary information according to peer review standards.
   D. Documentation is performed at least prior to the patient's next scheduled appointment as observed by supervisor and other staff.
   E. Progress/discharge notes are sent at the time of the patient's appointment or within two weeks of notification that a patient has completed therapy as observed by the supervisor.
VIII. Include required forms in patients' charts.
   A. Medicare forms/compensation forms are completed within 48 hours of initial evaluation as observed by supervisor and feedback from other staff.
   B. PRI forms are completed and inserted in the charts every Tuesday as observed by supervisor.
IX. Charge patients according to treatment and time spent.
   A. Charges are completed within 24 hours according to schedule of patients treated.

continues

EXHIBIT 6–6 *continued*

X. Work as part of the rehab team to meet patient needs.
A. Counsel and teach patients and their families.
B. Contact the physician for changes in treatment programs.
C. Interact with other involved health professionals—PM&R members, nurses, social workers, prosthetists.
D. Aid in discharge planning by contacting appropriate personnel/attending discharge planning rounds as indicated by feedback from personnel.
E. Provide counseling and education to patients and families as professionally indicated as observed by supervisor and feedback from patients/family members.
F. Tactfully handle counseling with concern for patient's well-being, as indicated by feedback from patients and family members.
G. Provide changes in treatment programs/discussion of patient's condition as indicated by chart documentation.

XI. Attend at least one continuing education course/seminar outside the hospital. Give inservices on new material to the rest of the department.
A. Attend at least one continuing education course/seminar outside the hospital per year as documented by course completion certificate.
B. Present inservices on completion of all outside courses/seminars according to department policy.

XII. Attend scheduled hospital and departmental rounds and inservices.
A. Attend all inservices scheduled during usual work hours as documented by attendance records.
B. Attend hospital rounds as indicated according to department scheduling.

XIII. Participate in at least one special hospital, departmental, or community project, including standing committees, public education/patient education seminars, audits. Write programs for department, handouts, home exercise programs, evaluation forms.

XIV. Assist with the supervision and guidance of new personnel, assistants, students, and volunteers as assigned. Report progress or problems as appropriate.

XV. Assist in maintaining treatment area and equipment. Assist other therapists as needed.

EXHIBIT 6–6 *continued*

   A. Maintain the treatment area at least once a day as observed by
      the supervisor and other staff.
   B. Assist other therapists, as needed, as observed by the supervisor
      and other staff.
   C. Be flexible with scheduling within the workday to allow for unex-
      pected needs as observed by the supervisor and other staff.
XVI. Assist with new programs and procedures.
   A. Assist with implementation of new programs/procedures as indi-
      cated by established practice as observed by the supervisor.
   B. Incorporate new ideas and procedures into treatment programs
      as indicated by established practice as documented in the
      patient chart.

Preparation and Training

Master's degree or certificate
degree in physical therapy or
related field. Licensed to practice
in New York State.

Consequence of Error

Probable errors may be serious
involving improper treatment or
procedures.

Experience

Three to six months of previous
experience. Usually gained through
educational field experience.

Confidential Data

Has full and complete access to
patient records and financial
information.

Level of Supervision

Employee and supervisor together
develop deadlines, project and
review assignments. From 5 to
20 percent of work reviewed by
second-level supervisor.

Directs Work of Others and/or Number of Employees Supervised

Assists with supervision of Physical
Medicine Assistants, Physical
Therapy students, and volunteers
5 percent.

Mental/Visual Demand and Physical Effort

Flow of work frequently produces a
high level of mental/visual fatigue
from motivating, reassuring, and
emotionally supporting people.

continues

EXHIBIT 6–6 *continued*

Frequent physical effort lifting and supporting patient (20–400 pounds), lifting and/or pushing equipment (up to 200 pounds), applying traction, resistance, and manipulation (1–200 pounds). Ability to operate a motor vehicle, Three to 4 hours of sitting, standing, walking, pushing/pulling, lifting/carrying up to 300 pounds, repetitive use of both-foot control, repetitive use of both hands, grasping simple/light of both hands to firm/strong grasping of both hands, and fine dexterity of both hands. Job requires continuous standing and walking.

Environment

Somewhat undesirable working conditions. Exposure to body waste, secretions, infectious diseases, cuts, hazardous materials, dust, gas, fumes, walking on uneven ground, physical equipment and machinery, burns, electrical shock from equipment 6–8 hours/day.

EXHIBIT 6–7

Job Description for Senior Occupational Therapist

Job Title	Department
Senior Occupational Therapist	Physical Medicine and Rehabilitation
Reports To	Revised
Manager, Administrative Services	
Physical Medicine and Rehabilitation	

Job Objectives

To supervise OTRs, COTAs, students, volunteers, and aides. Supervision includes orientation, development, and evaluation of personnel and monitoring the provision of quality services. Patient care responsibilities will vary depending upon volume of personnel to be supervised. May serve as student field work coordinator.

EXHIBIT 6–7 *continued*

Job Responsibilities

I. Patient care.

    A. Performs all duties of the staff occupational therapist on a daily basis as described in the staff OT job description and as observed by department director.

II. Remains knowledgeable of and monitors staff compliance with American Occupational Therapy Association (AOTA) professional guidelines, standards, and ethics.

    A. Remains current on professional information and reviews information with OT staff during weekly OT department meetings as documented in meeting minutes.

    B. Reviews OT staff compliance with understanding of professional regulations at least once per year as documented in departmental meeting minutes.

III. Evaluates and monitors job performance of OT staff.

    A. Completes performance appraisals annually.

    B. Reviews job description for modifications on a yearly basis as noted by changes in the job description document.

    C. Follows personnel policy and procedure for disciplinary action as the need arises as noted by written documentation per policy format.

    D. Monitors job performance of supervised employees throughout the year as documented by peer review process and individual employee notes and chart audits.

IV. Provides supervision for the department.

    A. Receives, signs, and submits time sheets with 90 to 100 percent accuracy as noted by communication from department head secretary.

    B. Informs OT staff of their obligation for fulfilling annual health screening requirements on their anniversary date as noted by feedback from the health office.

V. Organizes staff and patient scheduling.

    A. Monitors distribution of outpatients to individual therapists' schedules on a daily basis as noted by inspection of outpatient schedule.

    B. Reviews inpatient schedule daily and changes as necessary as noted in individual therapist's caseload.

continues

EXHIBIT 6–7 *continued*

    C. Acts as "float" therapist during times of need as noted on review of senior OT's daily schedule.

    D. Maintains therapist vacation calendar for the year as documented on department's yearly calendar.

VI. Monitors departmental productivity.

    A. Receives and reviews department labor utilization analysis on a monthly basis and discusses with staff at weekly department meetings as noted in department minutes.

    B. Encourages staff to make inpatient treatment a priority by limiting daily outpatients to five patients per therapist per day as noted on daily department schedule.

    C. Assesses need to identify individual therapist's productivity when an apparent problem is brought to the attention of the senior therapist as noted by documentation in the therapist's file or department minutes.

VII. Facilitates utilization of continuing education allotments.

    A. Encourages staff to attend continuing education courses, seminars, or conferences by posting course information in the department as such information is received.

    B. Counsels employees on courses that may be suitable for their growth and schedules their time off at least once per year as noted by review of their files.

    C. Allocates sufficient funds in the budget for one course per therapist per year as noted in the yearly budget.

    D. Ensures all registrations and payments are 100 percent accurate at course time as noted by receipt of payment.

VIII. Functions as an available reference/interpretive source for other staff members.

    A. Encourages an open-door policy with staff to problem solve on issues of importance (e.g., salaries, staffing, caseload, etc.) as needed as observed by or reported to the Director of Rehabilitation Services.

    B. Maintains open lines of communication with other departments on a daily basis as observed by the Director of Rehabilitation Services or feedback from same.

    C. Presents with an approachable demeanor 90 percent of the time as noted by staff feedback to the Director of Rehabilitation Services.

EXHIBIT 6–7 *continued*

IX. Initiates staff hiring.
    A. Initiates interaction with the human resources department for position recruitment within 10 days of recognized need as observed by Director of Rehabilitation Services.
    B. Schedules interviews with prospective employees with completed paperwork within one week of initial contact as observed by dates logged on resumes.
    C. Completes interviews of prospective employees within one month of initial contact as noted by verification by Director.
    D. Provides orientation to newly hired staff within one month of starting date as noted by signature on the personnel form, completion on job criteria checklist, and completed mandatory inservices.

X. Performs quality assurance (QA)–related tasks.
    A. Attends required quality assurance meetings as scheduled and noted on QA minutes.
    B. Initiates action and follow-up to areas found in neglect as noted by QA meeting minutes and feedback from other involved managers.
    C. Completes studies and reports results quarterly to the department and hospital QA committee.
    D. Interacts interdepartmentally to identify multidisciplinary areas to be monitored annually as noted by study developments and reports.

XI. Maintains a sound fiscal department.
    A. Prepares budget by established deadline as noted by completed items.
    B. Adheres to and compensates for budgetary restrictions and/or allowances as observed by monthly expense reports.

XII. Schedules, presents, and participates in meetings, classes, and presentations in the hospital and/or community.
    A. Attends scheduled and departmental supervisory meetings 75 percent of the time as documented in meeting minutes.
    B. Initiates and organizes staff and ideas for departmental presentations and displays as noted by the Director of Rehabilitation Services.

continues

EXHIBIT 6–7 *continued*

Preparation and Training

Master's degree. Licensed to practice in New York State. Registered in AOTA.

Consequence of Error

Probable errors may be serious involving improper handling or setup of procedures or treatments. Most work not directly verified or checked.

Experience

Three to five years of progressively more responsible work experience required.

Confidential Data

Has full and complete access to patient medical records where utmost integrity is required to safeguard patient, hospital, or employee.

Level of Supervision

Employee and supervisor, in consultation, develop objectives, definition of resources available, projects and deadlines. Five to 20 percent of work is reviewed by first level of supervision.

Directs Work of Others and Number of Employees Supervised

Orients, trains, coaches, schedules, develops, counsels, budgets, measures performance and assists with hiring, promoting, compensating, disciplining, and terminating one employee. Thirty percent of daily time spent in supervision.

Mental/Visual Demand and Physical Effort

Work requires motivating, reassuring, and emotionally supporting diseased or disabled patients. Position requires lifting, pushing, and supporting patients weighing up to 400 pounds. Flow of work frequently produces a high level of mental/visual fatigue.

Environment

Somewhat undesirable working conditions. Exposure to noise, body waste, infection, electrical shock from equipment, and no natural light or ventilation. No element continuously present to the point of being disagreeable.

THE CREDENTIALED PRACTITIONER AS CONSULTANT

Because the contemporary health care organization is frequently involved in new patterns of organization, the credentialed practitioner is sometimes called upon to be an external consultant or independent contractor. Consultants offer advice and counsel and carry out professional activities within the scope of their competence and licensure. Consultative arrangements generally fall into three categories:

- One-time-only arrangements wherein the consultant carries out an in-depth assessment of current practices or assists in development of a major project. For example, an occupational therapist might assist the management team of a long-term care facility with its plan to open an adult day care service. The occupational therapist would typically identify and describe the range of activities for the OT unit's services; calculate and determine the pattern of staffing needs for the unit; and identify equipment and space needs, along with layout considerations.
- Initial survey with implementation. In this instance the consultant and the health care organization's representatives agree that the professional practitioner will remain under contract to implement the initial findings. Using the example given above, the occupational therapist would be given the mandate to contact vendors, compare vendor bids, and, with the organization's approval, select the equipment and oversee its placement.
- Ongoing maintenance of project or program. In this arrangement, the professional practitioner agrees to provide continuous service over some specific, and usually prolonged, period of time. For example, a physical therapist is hired to upgrade the inservice training program at an industrial health clinic. Having developed an overall training plan, based on the facility's needs, the physical therapist commits to a plan to provide the inservice training on a regular basis—for example, one day per month for the upcoming year.

THE INDEPENDENT CONTRACTOR

When the professional practitioner is hired to provide regular, ongoing services for a protracted period of time (as in the third example above), the relationship of the practitioner to the contracting organization may fall into the category of independent contractor. Both parties to such an arrangement need to review pertinent federal and state laws and regulations regarding independent contractor status. Particular attention should be given to the Internal Revenue Code's definitions of independent contractors. The recently enacted HIPAA regulations contain specific provisions concerning privacy and confidentiality requirements for business partners and independent contractors. Professional liability insurance provisions, worker compensation laws, collective bargaining agreements, and similar labor-related mandates need review as to their applicability to the particular arrangements.

GUIDELINES FOR CONTRACTS AND REPORTS

Whether fulfilling the role of consultant or independent contractor, the professional practitioner works under written contract and provides formal reports to the administrative coordinators of the facility. Following are guidelines for the content of contracts and reports.

The Contract

The professional practitioner, working with a properly qualified attorney, would develop a contract specific to the given situation. The contract typically includes at least the elements of a clear statement of parties to the contract, the time period covered, services to be provided, fees and payment schedule, ownership of materials, privacy and confidentiality of patient and business information, and provisions for termination of the contract. An attorney would provide the appropriate level of detail and additional provisions necessary for a sound agreement. Appendix 6–A is a detailed excerpt from a contract between a health information specialist who provides ongoing services to a long-term care facility.

The Written Report

The consultant provides the administrative coordinators with periodic written reports, formal and detailed in their content. Following are guidelines for such reports:

1. Remember that consultant reports are formal business records and, as such, must be retained by both the consultant and the organization for the required retention period for such business records. See the specific state laws and federal tax laws governing the retention period.

2. Remember that consultant reports are subject to inspection and review by licensing and accrediting agencies and by third-party payment auditors. The report, therefore, should be complete, formal, and accurate.

3. Keep the report focused on compliance with required licensure, accreditation, and professional practice standards. Include both positive and negative findings. A useful practice, and one that also motivates the recipients to continue to strive for excellence, is to list the positive findings first, followed by the heading "Areas Needing Improvement."

4. Provide specific recommendations for each topical area needing improvement. For example, suggest the content of an inservice training program on the topic or provide sample forms or procedures.

5. Prioritize the findings in order of importance. To prioritize findings:

    Priority Class One: Address any practice that has potential for direct harm to the patient. An example in health information documentation would be contradictory physician orders concerning medications. This finding would be reported orally to the nursing staff as soon as it is identified by the consultant. The written report, as follow-up, would contain the formal recommendation for corrective practices, with the notation that an oral report was made to the nursing staff in a timely manner.

    Priority Class Two: Address any practice for which the facility received a citation in the last external survey or auditor review, with particular attention to the practices for which a plan of correction was filed with state or federal agencies. Also, address any practice having repeat citations over the past several years, even if the current survey showed full compliance for the immediate year.

    Priority Class Three: Address any practice that is out of compliance with:

    - State licensure requirements. For example, mention record retention practices that do not meet the state's required retention period.
    - Federal conditions of Medicare. For example, cite any failure to update the patient plan of care according to the required time frames.
    - HIPAA regulations. For example, note any failure regarding the disclosure of patient information without appropriate consent.
    - Accrediting standards (if the facility participates in an accreditation program). For example, address the failure to document interdisciplinary progress notes according to suggested standards.
    - Generally accepted principles of professional practice. For example, mention failure to put complete patient identification on each page of the hard copy record or on each data entry for an electronic record.

Appendix 6–B provides an example of a cover letter, a formal report with priority indications, and a project timetable.

EXERCISE: CREATING ORGANIZATIONAL CHARTS

For a work organization and a specific department or function with which you are familiar, create two organizational charts—a master chart for the organization overall, and a supplementary chart depicting the structure and arrangement of the specific department or function. (If you have no familiarity with an actual work organization, invent an organization and department in chart form using the chapter's material for guidance.) Use your charts to answer the following questions:

1. Is the organization more appropriately described as centralized or decentralized? Why?
2. What management position appears to have the broadest span of control in terms of number of direct reporting employees? Why?
3. What is the longest single departmental chain of command in the organization, and how many levels does it consist of?
4. Assuming that dramatic losses of business activity have necessitated reorganizing, revise your original master chart for the organization overall to "flatten" the organization by at least one level in two principal chains of command.

EXERCISE: DEVELOPING A JOB DESCRIPTION

Select a health care profession or occupation and write a job description for it. It will be most helpful to use an occupation in which you have worked or for which you are preparing, subject to one condition: Since you will logically refer to the job description exhibits in the chapter to guide you (Exhibits 6–3 through 6–7), be sure to use an occupation other than those represented by the samples. Following completion of the job description, prepare a condensed description of that job in less than one-half page that could be used for recruiting purposes.

Appendix
6-A

Sample Contract for Health Information Consultant

Note: The following is not intended as legal advice. The consultant should consult an attorney for the development of a specific contract. This sample is for use by an external consultant.

CONSULTANT AGREEMENT FOR HEALTH INFORMATION SERVICES

This agreement is between Robert Alexander, Health Information Consultant, and Care Center Nursing Facility, Anywhere, Vermont. This agreement is entered into as of March 20, 2007. It is governed by the applicable state laws of Vermont. The consultant services of Robert Alexander are retained exclusively for Care Center Nursing Facility, 652 Plain Street, Anywhere, Vermont, a licensed skilled and assisted living facility. Materials developed by the consultant for this facility, including but not limited to policies, procedures, forms, and inservice training manuals, become the property of Care Center Nursing Facility for its exclusive use in the facility as it is currently configured. These materials may not be sold or distributed to other facilities. Consultant retains the right to continue to use similar materials without facility identification.

Independent Contractor

Robert Alexander and Care Center Nursing Facility agree that this relationship is that of independent contractor and not that of an employee or agent. Therefore,

Source: Adapted with permission from Aspen Publishers, Inc. Joan Gratto Liebler, *Medical Records Policies and Guidelines*, 1997, 13: 86: 2–8.

any withholding for tax requirements by any taxing authority, Social Security contribution, or any other purpose will be the responsibility of the consultant. It is further understood that the consultant participates in no fringe benefits or labor union contractual agreements or programs offered by the facility.

Responsibilities

1. Consultant will review the health information services and health care documentation practices of Care Center Nursing Facility in accordance with applicable state and federal laws and regulations, accrediting standards, and generally accepted principles of professional practice. The specific duties are listed below under the heading "Key Activities of Health Information Consultant."
2. Consultant will file written reports according to the following schedule:
   a. quarterly reports at the conclusion of each quarter, within five working days of end of quarter.
   b. one interim report at a mutually agreed-upon time during each quarter. Consultant will make formal, oral reports to the chief executive officer/administrator or designate at the conclusion of each quarter and one interim report at a mutually agreed-upon time during each quarter.
3. Confidentiality: Consultant agrees to hold all information relating to any Care Center Nursing Facility practice confidential and will not disclose such information to anyone but the designated official contacts, or as required by federal or state law or regulation, without specific written consent of the owners of the facility; this consent shall be obtained prior to the use of the information. Strictest compliance with HIPAA and similar patient privacy and confidentiality will be maintained. All files, notes, and related documents shall be returned to the facility at the end of the business relationship between the consultant and the facility.
4. Maintenance of Professional Competence: Consultant agrees to continue to meet the standards of professional credentialing, including continuing education requirements, as set forth by the national professional association for health information practice.

Terms of Payment

Consultant shall present a formal bill for professional services at the conclusion of each quarter, at the time of filing the formal written report. Care Center Nursing Facility agrees to pay the consultant within five working days of receipt of this bill. The agreed-upon fee for service is ($____) per quarter. This is the whole and entire reimbursement; no other costs incurred by the consultant are reimbursed by the facility.

Entire Agreement

This agreement as stated in these terms and signed on the date listed below is the entire agreement; no other written or oral agreement is entered into; this agreement supersedes any other agreement. This agreement may be amended in writing, with acceptance of changes indicated by the dated signatures of the parties.

Termination of Contract

Except for cause, the contract shall remain in effect until one party notifies the other in writing, one month before the desired cessation of contractual relationship.

_____	_____
Administrator	Robert Alexander
Care Center Nursing Facility	Health Information Consultant
Date:	Date:

KEY ACTIVITIES OF HEALTH INFORMATION CONSULTANT

1. Identify applicable laws, regulations, and standards for documentation and systems and determine degree of compliance by this facility with these requirements.
2. Monitor trends in professional practice and impending changes in laws, regulations, and standards for documentation and systems to provide the facility with timely information for planning and budgeting purposes.
3. Develop a policy manual for documentation and systems in health information.
4. Develop detailed procedures for documentation and systems in health information.
5. Develop job descriptions for health information support personnel.
6. Develop forms for data capture and documentation and modify data entry processes to meet computerization specifications.

7. Analyze and review each aspect of the health information system through systematic sampling methods:
   a. patient identification
   b. chart initiation, concurrent review, and final completion
   c. dictation-transcription support
   d. storage and retrieval
   e. release of information
   f. coding and reimbursement support
   g. statistics, registries, and reportable diseases and incidents
   h. quality improvement support studies
8. Assist in budget development, staffing pattern assessment, and space and equipment assessment.
9. Carry out periodic inservice training:
   a. professional staff involved in direct patient care
   b. health information support staff
10. Assist administrative and professional staff committees and review groups through preparation of reports for and attendance at committee and review group meetings.
11. Assist administrative and professional staff in preparation for periodic licensure and accreditation review reports.

Appendix
6–B

Sample Cover Letter and Report

Note: Background information for this fictitious report is as follows:

1. The facility is state licensed for skilled and assisted living care of a long-term nature, for frail elderly patients.
2. Facility is Medicare certified under the applicable Conditions of Participation.
3. No external accrediting agency participation currently in place or planned for the immediate future.
4. General pattern of care:

70 beds	skilled	average length of stay	3.5 years
90 units	assisted living	average length of stay	4 years
100 units	independent living	average length of stay	7 years

   Admissions from independent living to another level of care in this facility is 90 percent.
5. Participant: Medicare-Medicaid programs of reimbursement.
6. Nonprofit, privately owned by church-related organization.
7. Last licensure survey: December of last year.
8. 100 discharges per year, on average, including:
   48 discharged to acute care
   12 deaths (natural causes)
9. There is no full- or part-time credentialed health information practitioner employed by the facility.

COVER LETTER

June 1, 2007
E. B. Bond, Administrator
Care Center Nursing Facility
652 Plain Street
Anywhere, Vermont 01234

Dear Mr. Bond:

Enclosed is the quarterly report reflecting my findings and recommendations for the health information services at your facility. The quarterly bill is also included.

If you have any further questions about the contents of the report, please call me to arrange an additional meeting. I will continue my quarterly visits to implement the recommendations in this report, as we agreed at our May 29 meeting.

Sincerely,

Robert Alexander
Health Information Specialist

Enclosures: Quarterly Report for March, April, and May 2007;
            Quarterly Bill for period ending May 31, 2007

QUARTERLY REPORT—HEALTH INFORMATION SERVICES JUNE 1, 2007

Dates of Site Visits

March 19, 22, and 23	Initial survey
April 3 and 4	Data gathering/fact finding/continued review of systems
April 19	Inservice training—health information support staff
April 26	Inservice training—health information support staff—coding and reimbursement; billing department support staff
May 14	Administrative meeting
May 29	Administrative meeting

Availability Between Visits

I was available to your staff as needed during this period by means of telephone contact.

Persons Interviewed During Site Visits

E. B. Bond, Administrator
C. G. Ellsworth, Director of Nursing
M. C. Comfort, Director of Social Services
D. L. Logan, Coordinator of Health Information Services
P. T. Bari, Director of Finances
Various clerical support staff: Health Information Service and Finance Service

Key Activities

1. Reviewed each aspect of the health information system.
2. Reviewed open and closed records (closed records for past year).
3. Developed policy for concurrent record review, including development of record review form.
4. Held inservice training sessions on confidentiality, release of information, and compliance with HIPAA regulations.
5. Held inservice training session on coding and reimbursement review and compliance.

6. Conducted ethics committee study on compliance with advance directives.
7. Developed policy and procedure for release of information.
8. Developed policy and procedure for processing charts with high-volume content.

Findings and Recommendations—The Overall Health Information Services

Patient Identification System

A complete identification system is in place for patients admitted directly to the skilled level units. A 10 percent sample was carried out to determine errors; no errors found.

Practices Needing Improvement: All patients/residents need numbers/identification on the first occasion of care. The patient identification/numbering system needs expanding to include assisted living and infirmary stays for residential care units.

Recommendation: Adoption of a comprehensive patient identification system, computerized to coordinate with finance service.

Priority Class One: Inadequate information of patient care documents could result in misfiles and other loss of such documentation, with the potential for direct harm to the patient.

Creation and Maintenance of an Official Record for Each Patient

A 40 percent sample of chart creation and availability for each level of care was carried out. All patients had an official medical/health record, created at the time of admission to the unit. Based on this sample study, there is evidence of full compliance with requirements in this area. No misfiles were found; charts were available in designated locations and found on first try.

Recommendation: Continue this excellent practice and level of compliance.

Recommendation: Provide information to the residents of independent living units about their personal health records: content of such records; working with their private care providers to coordinate information exchange.

Concurrent and Discharge Chart Analysis and Completion

A 10 percent sample of records for each level of care was carried out, both for in-house patients (all units of care) and recently discharged patients (the last month's discharges). Review of charts is thorough and timely at discharge, but this is not adequate for the longer stay, in-house records.

Practices Needing Improvement: Timely and thorough review of in-house patients (all units).

Recommendation: Adoption of a comprehensive concurrent chart review process.

Priority Class Two: Past surveys show regular citations relating to lack of timely documentation during inpatient stay. The last plan of correction indicates that a chart review process would be developed, but this has not been carried out to date.

A detailed plan for developing and implementing such a concurrent chart review process has been made available to the health information and nursing staff. It shows in detail:

    a. planning objectives and time line to develop and fully implement by July 1.
    b. detailed time line, displaying each specific activity, with weekly targets for completion of each phase of this process.
    c. schedule of inservice training sessions for personnel involved in implementing this process.

Release of Information Processes

A 20 percent sample of release of information responses was carried out, comparing requests with adequacy of consent for release of information and adequacy of timeliness of response. No problems were noted in the adequacy and timeliness of response.

Practices needing improvement: Family members occasionally signing the consent for release of information, without indication on the chart that the patient is not competent to sign or is unable to sign because of medical frailty. This practice is not consistent with generally accepted legal principles, which guide release of information practices, nor with the licensure requirements that patient rights be safeguarded.

Recommendation: Review and update the policies and procedures regarding release of information; carry out an in-depth inservice training for support personnel involved in release of information. Clarify, through patient care policy team and committee, and legal counsel review, the practices associated with release of information consents when patient is unable to sign for himself or herself.

Priority Class Three: This is needed because the licensure requirements and the conditions of participation for Medicare call for the honoring of patient rights, including release of information consents. The current practice is also at variance with commonly accepted legal principles associated with release of information.

Storage and Retrieval Processes

Charts have been maintained in hard copy since the opening of the facility in 1964. A study was carried out to determine chart usage after discharge. No chart was accessed after two full years following discharge.

Recommendation: Consideration might be given to the appropriate destruction of records that meet record retention schedule for destruction.

Priority Class Three: This is a low priority compared to the more pressing concerns such as chart completion. However, it is common practice to destroy records when the required retention period has been satisfied; this reduces potential for unauthorized access to data and is a more cost-effective use of space. It also reduces fire hazard potential.

Another finding relating to this system concerns the lack of a systematic process for thinning out those charts for long-stay patients. The chart holders are so full that pages are being inadvertently torn, folded, and removed from designated sequence.

Recommendation: For the short term, institute a systematic process for thinning charts into active section (kept at primary location at the nurses' station) and secondary volume, also kept at the nurses' station, but in a specially designated cabinet. A detailed procedure is needed. For the longer-term solution: consideration of a more computerized data collection and patient record is needed.

Priority Class Three: Lack of systematic debriefing process is leading to the inadvertent loss or destruction of documents.

Coding, Registries, and Statistics

A coding audit was carried out; coding accuracy is at an acceptable level. Discussion with billing unit personnel was held; no problems either in timeliness or completeness of coding were noted. A similar review was carried out for the registries and statistics; although there is a slight delay in data entry (about six days), this does not, at this time, seem to be causing difficulty for the administrative and professional staff review teams. External reporting requirements have been met on a timely basis.

Recommendation: Continue the excellent practice of coding and compliance audits. Carry out at least an annual review of statistics and registry input to determine need for the data.

Health Information Documentation

A 40 percent sample of charts was reviewed in detail using the approved chart review form. The following areas of documentation meet the generally accepted levels of documentation:

- physician orders
- interdisciplinary progress notes
- admission and discharge notes and assessments
- ongoing flowcharts of daily and periodic care
- use of psychotropic medications
- restraint-free protocols
- pharmacy review of medications
- occupational and physical therapy notes
- social service summaries
- activities therapy notes

Practices Needing Improvement: The following areas of documentation need improvement:

1. Admission documentation: the transfer documentation was missing in approximately 50 percent of charts reviewed.
2. Admission physical examinations need to be completed within the time frame prescribed by the state regulations. In 15 cases, the physical had not been completed for as long as 12 days after admission.
3. Patient care plans need at least quarterly updates, with particular attention to the long-stay patients. Particularly problematic is the lack of documentation in the care plan regarding the final year of care.
4. Advance directives and health care proxy documents need filing in the chart and a complete notation made on front of chart, face sheet, and order sheet as to the existence of these directives.
5. Notation concerning guardianship: no patient's chart showed such notations, which is unusual given the patient population. This information needs to be gathered at the time of admission and periodically updated.
6. Transfer out to acute care or other health care facilities: 50 percent of the transfers lack the appropriate documentation.

Priority Class Two: Most of these items were noted as deficiencies in the past three annual licensure reviews.

Recommendation: Implement the concurrent chart analysis process; this will foster timely identification and follow-up relating to documentation requirements.

A final comment: the general atmosphere of cooperation among the professional and support staff is noted as a positive attribute of your facility. I look forward to continuing our mutual work toward continual improvement of the health information service.

CHAPTER 7

Improving Performance and Controlling the Critical Cycle

THE CONTINUING SEARCH FOR EXCELLENCE

The search for excellence, striving for perfection, creating a climate of continuous improvement: these and similar mottoes reflect the overall theme of performance improvement initiatives associated with the management functions of quality improvement and controlling. The search for excellence flows from the health care organization's fundamental vision and purpose, the timely and thorough care of the patient. Its values of stewardship and integrity further infuse the organization with energy directed toward continuous quality. This continuing search for excellence has a long and varied history. A review of this history provides managers with a framework within which to consider effective approaches to continuous quality improvement.

Emerging with a vengeance in the late 1980s, *quality* became the most fashionable business term of the 1990s in the way that *excellence* had dominated much of the 1980s. The total quality management (TQM) movement and the earlier excellence movement had somewhat different origins, but so far the results of the quality movement have been much the same as the visible results of the excellence movement, although more widespread. In each instance a basically sound, well-intentioned philosophy has been adopted, promoted, and implemented with extremely mixed results.

Many of the organizations that attempted to adopt dedication to excellence as a guiding philosophy ran into the same problem that has stymied may otherwise effective organizations: how to instill a *philosophy* in people so that it will cause them to behave in the desired manner.

Between the philosophy, which may initially be accepted by a few members of top management, and the actual practice, which involves many employees living out the philosophy, there lies a matter of *process*. There has to be some process available to successfully transfer the philosophy from the few to the many.

A great many people never see past the process and are thus unable to truly adopt the philosophy. They simply go through the motions, appearing to do what they perceive top management wants them to do. Invariably, when a philosophy is proceduralized—that is, when a process is superimposed upon something as ethereal as a concept, idea, or belief—something essential is lost. Those who simply adopt the process as part of the job without buying into the philosophy will not truly reflect the philosophy in their behavior.

When a philosophy of management is overproceduralized, overpromoted, overpublicized, and overpraised, it becomes a fad. It becomes fashionable for its own sake. It was in this manner that *excellence* essentially went down the same path traveled years earlier by *management by objectives* (MBO). We have reason to wonder, therefore, whether the quality movement will prevail or devolve into just another fad, the current "flavor of the month" destined to go the way of MBO, quality circles, excellence, and others.

Quality Control, Quality Assurance, and Quality Management

For years many of the manufacturing and service industries had what was referred to as *quality control.* Quality control ordinarily concentrated on finding defects, rejecting defective products, and providing information with which to alter processes so they would produce fewer defects.

Health care organizations had what they called *quality assurance.* This consisted largely of record scrutiny under which errors consisting of departures from some dictated standard were counted, providing information with which steps would be taken to reduce the frequency of recurrence of the same kinds of errors.

In addition to correcting the processes that produced the errors, both quality control and quality assurance were often responsible for instituting more frequent quality checkpoints so that errors might be caught earlier. The most important similarity between quality control and quality assurance, however, was that both focused primarily on finding errors after the fact. Both were, and yet remain, retrospective processes.

During the 1980s, using philosophical grounding and methods exported from the United States to Japan decades earlier and later brought back as "new, revolutionary management techniques," the emphasis on quality began to shift from catching errors before they go out the door to avoiding errors in the first place. Thus we have the basis of the quality movement embodied today in labels such as *total quality management* (TQM), *continuous quality improvement* (CQI), and *performance improvement initiatives.*

Old Friends in New Clothes?

Many of the tools and techniques included under the performance improvement umbrella should look familiar to some people who have been in the work force for a few years. Many of the "current" tools and techniques have been around for quite awhile, some for decades. They have been resurrected, revitalized (especially through computer technology), and in some instances renamed. For example, a number of TQM-implementation case histories mention the acronym TOPS, standing for *team-oriented problem solving*. As the name suggests, workers who have concerns with various aspects of particular problems approach problem solving as a team, with a common goal and purpose. These problem-solving teams espoused under TQM look, sound, and function the same as *quality circles* promoted during the brief popularity of "Japanese management."

Also essentially renaming quality circles are the other TOPS look-alikes such as *self-directed work teams* and *team-oriented process improvement*. These particular labels are but two of several similar designations that have emerged as representing a significant part of the path to continuous quality improvement.

Quality circles were themselves nothing new when they were so named. In years past, many work organizations utilized what they called *work simplification project teams,* in function and intent essentially identical to quality circles and the problem-solving teams of TQM. Written about in the 1950s and earlier, work simplification teams found their way into hospital methods improvement work as early as 1956.[1]

Even many of the specific tools used by today's performance improvement problem solvers go back 50, 60, 70 years. Industrial engineering techniques already existing for decades scored a number of modest, if not long-lasting, successes when implemented in hospitals from the second half of the 1960s to the mid-1970s—renamed *management engineering,* probably owing to a general aversion in health care to anything perceived as "industrial"—has fallen short of its potential value in health care. Yet there is a return to these practices (process flow, control charts, cause-and-effect diagrams, for instance) as part of today's performance improvement programs.

The Common Driving Force

Regardless of how many previously popular techniques are returned to the spotlight or how many genuinely new features are added, there remains one ingredient that is fully as essential to performance improvement as it has been to any other approach by any other name. That crucial ingredient is top management commitment. This should come as no surprise. Top management commitment to new ideas and approaches has been a prerequisite to complete success for as long as organized enterprise has existed. Without sufficient top management commitment most organized endeavors are destined to, at best, generate results that fall short of intentions, or, at worst, fail altogether and cause harmful results or leave residual damage.

One cannot imagine any rational top manager openly avowing opposition to the principles of quality improvement. Ask any top manager whose organization has espoused performance improvement or TQM initiatives if he or she is truly committed to it—or, for that matter, ask any top manager at all if quality, period, is a personal commitment; surely each will state unwavering commitment. We know that many such endeavors fail because of insufficient top management commitment, but since almost all managers will voice commitment there is but one conclusion to be drawn: top management commitment is a matter of degree, and it is the degree of commitment that is critical.

None of today's total quality programs will work as intended unless top management is actually involved and actively promoting the concept. Superficial commitment at the top results in similarly weak commitment at lower organizational levels. Beware of skyrocket commitment of the top manager who gets all fired up over performance improvement initiatives, distributes information to everyone, creates a steering committee, advisory committee, or other body, chairs the first meeting or two or three—but then starts missing meetings because of "pressing business" and transfers the guiding role to subordinates.

A total quality program also will not work if managers, especially first-line supervisors, will not let go and truly delegate to the employees. This means not simply giving employees the responsibility for doing different tasks or determining more efficient methods; it means also giving them the *authority* to make the decisions to implement their own findings. Further, letting go also means accepting what the employees decide and living with it.

Letting go as just described is difficult for the majority of managers. A great many managers, far more than would be able to see it in themselves, possess a recognizable streak of authoritarianism. Upon reflection, the reasons for a fairly strong presence of residual authoritarianism are understandable. Modern management—true, open participative management—is a phenomenon of the past two or three decades. While the spread of participative management has been steady it has also been gradual; there remain many areas of organized activity in which employees have yet to experience any management style other than straightforward bossism.

Managers learn about management mostly from other managers, and especially from those organizational superiors who, for good or ill, were by virtue of their positions role models for those newer to management. At one time virtually all management everywhere was authoritarian; even now, management that is at least partly authoritarian predominates. Most management role models thus convey at least a modicum of authoritarianism. Subtle proof of the existence of the authoritarian streak can be experienced by the manager who might ponder his or her reaction to being pushed abruptly into a fully participative management situation—the manager may feel that participative management exhibits weakness and that delegating decision-making authority to subordinates is somehow abrogating one's responsibility.

Managers also have trouble letting go and adjusting to a true participative environment because, for the most part, TQM runs contrary to classical organizational theory and our old notions about how a work group is to be managed. Classical theory stresses structure, lines of authority, and the chain of command, and it suggests that as far as each level is concerned someone just above it is in charge. In classical organizational theory, one works *for* the manager; in a true participative environment, one works *with* the manager.

It remains clear, however, that changes in management style and approach may have to occur in order for a quality management program to be successful. In most instances the manager will need to shift from being the boss—from planning, telling, instructing—to being the leader of a team—to counseling, teaching, coaching, and facilitating.

Management's commitment, then, can be seen as a total commitment not only to participative management and employee empowerment but also to intra- and interdepartmental teamwork and improved communication throughout the organization.

Will Total Quality Management Prevail?

The answer is yes; the focus on quality is a mandate flowing from the very purpose of the health care organization. However, its forms and approaches will vary from time to time. Total quality management has every chance of working where previous and perhaps partial efforts undertaken under other names have failed. There is a great deal going on with performance improvement initiatives; activity undertaken in the name of quality improvement has become so widespread that the impression that "everyone is doing it" places considerable pressure on the supposed few who have yet to commit to true quality improvement.

In the health care setting, quality improvement has become the norm. It flows from the organization's overall vision: quality patient care, with emphasis on timely, effective care, given in a climate of safety. The Joint Commission as well as state and federal regulatory bodies mandate performance monitoring and improvement. Examples include the Department of Health and Human Services' Agency for Healthcare Research and Quality; studies focus on such topics as wrong-site surgery. The Centers for Medicare and Medicaid Services have developed a Hospital Consumer Assessment of Healthcare Providers and Systems initiative. Congress passed the Patient Safety and Quality Improvement Act of 2005 ("Patient Safety

Act"). The Institute for Healthcare Improvement launched the "100,000 Lives Campaign" concerning patient safety. The Office of Inspector General has, in its annual work plan, topics relating to quality of healthcare information. The National Committee for Quality Assurance, which manages HEDIS (Health Plan Employer Data and Information Set), has standardized performance measures. Quality, excellence, continuous improvement have become the permanent underlying themes in the health care setting.

Performance Improvement Focus

Performance improvement functions generally fall into one of four categories.

1. Continuous quality improvement, focusing on maintaining the quality of standard operations—for example, the quality of medical transcription; detection of fraudulent line counting; completeness of documentation; spoliation of medical evidence in documentation. These studies are routine and frequent (e.g., monthly).
2. Routine periodic studies, stemming from external requirements as well as internal commitment to excellence—for example, the Joint Commission's quarterly reports or the annual licensure survey.
3. Adoption of a new process or approach, focusing on the "debugging" of such undertakings and eventually moving it into routine practice. Examples include "dry runs" using the tracer methodology of the Joint Commission, following the course of care and services the patient received during the course of hospitalization, including "real time" review involving several departments. Rapid Cycle Improvement strategies may be used in a major project such as a major overhaul of the master patient index, culling out duplicate numbers, and consolidating the related medical record documents. Once the solution has been found to this problem, the topic becomes one of routine focus, as noted above. Another focus of rapid cycle improvement is point-of-care documentation and coding using tablet personal computers or PDAs.
4. Critical areas of interest stemming from internal or external concerns: from time to time, an issue demands intense review. Examples include:
   a. *Patient Safety* While this has been an area of focus of risk management for many years, fresh impetus has been given to this topic, as noted earlier. The Patient Safety Act, the Joint Commission standards, internal malpractice-related reviews, infection control concerns: these all lead to renewed interest in such studies as wrong-site surgery, medication

errors and "read back" requirements, and any of the sentinel events noted by the Joint Commission.

b. *The Revenue Cycle:* Efforts in improving both the timeliness and the accuracy of billing, along with the prevention of fraud, is a multi-department effort including the physicians, the admitting department, the emergency service, the finance office, and health information management. Studies typically include such topics as:

- tracking the time elapsed from the time of clinical events through the final payment of a bill
- analysis of billing rejections
- selection of high priority coding and billing (e.g., a $200,000 inpatient bill versus a $500 clinic visit). All are important, but priority effort devoted to rapid, high-revenue return is sometimes indicated
- comparison of present practices to the planned reviews announced by the Office of Inspector General and its efforts at fraud control

c. *Disaster and Emergency Preparedness:* A major catastrophe (hurricane, tornado, blizzard, fire) brings renewed attention to this aspect of organizational plans. In addition to overall preparedness as reflected in the disaster/emergency plan, topics of study could include:

- aspects of the business continuity plan for patient care and financial records
- compliance with the HIPAA/DHHS guidelines for release of information about the aged and persons with disabilities during a disaster event
- the proper use of the condition modifiers in coding and billing relating to catastrophic or disaster-related events

Managers of each department develop and carry out such studies within their immediate organizational jurisdiction; they also partner with other units in the organization through committees, teams, and special projects to achieve the goals relating to organizational excellence. The management function of controlling is the traditional term associated with these detailed processes.

THE MANAGEMENT FUNCTION OF CONTROLLING

Controlling is the management function in which performance is measured and corrective action is taken to ensure the accomplishment of organizational goals. Performance improvement, continuous quality efforts, total quality management:

these initiatives make up the controlling function. It is an oversight operation in management, although the manager seeks to create a positive climate so that the process of control is accepted as part of routine activity. Controlling is also a forward-looking process in that the manager seeks to anticipate deviation and prevent it.

The manager initiates the control function during the planning phase, when possible deviation is anticipated and policies are developed to help ensure uniformity of practice. During the organizing phase, a manager may consciously introduce the "deadly parallel" arrangement as a control factor.

Two styles of leadership are necessarily blended in this function:

- Close supervision and a tight leadership style reflect an aspect of control. Through rewards and positive sanctions, the manager seeks to motivate workers to conform, thus limiting the amount of control that must be imposed. Finally, the manager develops specific control tools, such as inspections, visible control charts, work counts, special reports, and audits.
- Participative management/leadership style, with wide participation in the quality cycle, is the generally accepted principle in performance improvement initiatives.

Participants

The governing board's commitment to excellence, stated in the vision/mission statement and overall organizational goals, is the starting point for such initiatives. Relying on both external benchmarks and internal assessments, the board takes the lead in continuous quality improvement.

Process improvements and routine quality control initiatives are the purview of the line managers who are involved in day-to-day operations. These managers do not work in isolation; they partner with other stakeholders and super-users. Physician satisfaction surveys as part of the annual strategic plan review is one major area of input. The findings can be used to set priorities and outline strategic initiatives to improve the working environment (e.g., space allocation; renovations) and systems improvements (e.g., upgrading technologies).

Quality improvement teams and committees are yet another common approach: patient care providers and support department managers cooperate in a variety of reviews such as patient safety and risk management, infections control, and medication error prevention. Employee involvement through quality circles is a long-standing feature of performance improvement. These workers, close to the daily routines, provide important insight and feedback to operational managers.

Clients are included in quality improvement initiatives. Patient satisfaction questionnaires are used routinely to capture information about wait times and adequacy of information provided about such delays. Privacy considerations, intake processing procedures, and related aspects of admission are commonly included in such questionnaires.

The Basic Control Process

The control process involves three cyclic phases: establishing standards, measuring performance, and correcting deviation. In the first step, the specific units of measure that delineate acceptable work are determined. Basic standards may be stated as staff hours allowed per activity, speed and time limits, quantity that must be produced, and number of errors or rejects permitted. The second step in the control process, measuring performance, involves comparing the work (i.e., the goods produced or the service provided) against the standard. Employee evaluation is one aspect of this measurement. In manufacturing, inspection of goods is a routine part of this process; studies of client satisfaction are key elements when services are involved. Finally, if necessary, remedial action is taken, including retraining employees, repairing equipment, or changing the quality of the raw materials used in a manufacturing process.

Characteristics of Adequate Controls

Several features are necessary to ensure the adequacy of control processes and tools:

- *Timeliness.* The control device should reflect deviations from the standard promptly, at an early stage, so there is only a small time lag between detection and the beginning of corrective action.
- *Economy.* If possible, control devices should involve routine, normal processes rather than special inspection routines at additional expense. The control devices must be worth their cost.
- *Comprehensiveness.* The controls should be directed at the basic phases of the work rather than later levels or steps in the process; for example, a defective part is best inspected and eliminated before it has been assembled with other parts.
- *Specificity and appropriateness.* The control process should reflect the nature of the activity. Proper laboratory inspection methods, for example, differ from the financial audit and machine inspection processes.

- *Objectivity.* The processes should be grounded in fact, and standards should be known and verifiable.
- *Responsibility.* Controls should reflect the authority-responsibility pattern. As far as possible, the worker and the immediate supervisor should be involved in the monitoring and correction process.
- *Understandability.* Control devices, charts, graphs, and reports that are complicated or cumbersome will not be readily used.

Types of Standards

Standards may be of a physical nature, in terms of both quantity and quality (e.g., the number of charts processed according to the required regulations). Such standards make it easier to develop inspection processes because such information can be recorded relatively simply on visible control charts, work logs, and similar tools. Standards may also be set in terms of cost; a monetary value is attached to an operation or to the delivery of a service (e.g., the cost per square foot per employee, the cost per patient per visit, or the cost per object in a factory). Occasionally, the standard is expressed somewhat intangibly, such as the success of a volunteer drive, competence or loyalty in an employee, or ability in a trainee. Whenever possible, however, a quantifiable factor should be introduced. For example, behavioral objectives could be developed for each level of trainee functioning.

The Intangible Nature of Service

Health care organizations face a special difficulty in that their primary activities are services, which do not always lend themselves to quantifiable measurement. Furthermore, it is difficult to monitor the delivery of a service because of its dynamic nature. Patient privacy is a major consideration. Another dilemma stems from attempts to delineate services in terms of cost; many services must remain available even if the patient census has dropped during a given period. An emergency service must have adequate coverage no matter how many patients come for service at a particular time.

SIX SIGMA STRATEGIES

Six Sigma is an approach to total quality management and continuous performance improvement based on statistical analysis of variations in performance measures. Sigma, the Greek symbol, is used in statistics to measure variation (standard deviation) from the mean. In the Six Sigma approach, process improvement teams seek to minimize variation from the desired norm. The target is six sigma (99.999%) or less of variation from this desired level of performance. The emphasis is on prevention of error, reduction of variation, zero defects, and continuously increasing customer satisfaction. This management strategy, applying proven management principles, was widely used in the 1990s and continues to be implemented. Streamlining processes, reengineering total systems, and focusing on cost reductions while at the same time increasing productivity and quality: these are characteristics of Six Sigma. Measurement and statistical analysis are central. The ongoing analysis focuses on process variation and then rapid response to correct undesirable variations. Projects are run through a process referred to as DMAIC:

D   Define the project goals and customers/clients (both internal and external)
M   Measure the process to determine current performance
A   Analyze and determine root cause(s) of the defect
I   Improve the process by eliminating the defect
C   Control future process performance[2]

Health care organizations have a long history of monitoring performance and seeking continuous improvement. Risk management reviews, infection control monitoring, clinical audit studies, patient safety analysis, coding error rates, reducing accounts receivable delays, filing accuracy studies: all are examples of ongoing quality reviews, suitable for Six Sigma application. Projects relating to compliance measures mandated by licensure and accrediting agencies are yet another set of examples of continuous control and improvement. For example, the quality-of-life indicators associated with long-term care of the frail elderly or the core compliance areas of the Joint Commission provide ideas for topics of study. Coding-Billing-Documentation correlation in the revenue cycle is another suitable focus for studies.

The various control charts presented in this chapter provide working tools for tracking data for such studies. By coupling the Six Sigma approach with the motivational aspect of appreciative inquiry, discussed in Chapter 10, a manager helps foster a climate of success. This culture of celebrating success, giving it tangible expression in results-oriented projects, sets up a chain reaction in the organization, with each part of the system becoming fine-tuned and continuously improved. These approaches to quality reflect the fundamental values of the organization, spelled out in its vision and core values statement. Continuous quality improvement helps reduce cost, prevents error, increases a climate of patient safety and satisfaction, and fosters positive communication among the caregivers and support staff.

BENCHMARKING

Benchmarking is simply comparison of one's own activity or results with the level of activity or results of another department or organization. This involves as a "benchmark" the experience of some other entity, the operating results of which appear to be reasonable or perhaps to represent a desirable target. Benchmarking frequently involves targeting various organizations' best practices and comparing with their results in an effort to improve results in the benchmarking organization. Benchmarks may be derived internally from data obtained from peak performance analysis.

The present-day emphasis on benchmarking activities provides the manager with the impetus to develop standards of practice, deriving them from and comparing them with organizations having characteristics similar to one's own. The ORYX initiative of the Joint Commission provides yet another means of controlling one's performance against externally developed targets.

Sources of Benchmarking Measures

Managers use benchmarking measures developed by external groups, develop measures unique to their organizations, or combine external and internal sources for comparison. Examples of external sources include those taken from federal agencies, national associations, and specialty groups—for example, the core performance measures or the patient safety practices of the Joint Commission; the ECRI (formerly the Emergency Care Research Institute) guidelines for emergency care; and the American Society for Testing and Materials (ASTM) and its standards for medical transcription quality programs. National associations of the various credentialed practitioners offer benchmarking studies appropriate to given fields of practice, such as AHIMA's best practices model. Regional associations (such as a regional hospital group) have benchmarks custom-tailored to the particular characteristics of patient care in the geographic area.

Sample Benchmarking Studies: Health Information Management

These four studies reflect various aspects of benchmarking as found in typical health information management activities. Table 7–1 uses internal benchmarks and reflects issues of interest to medical staff review groups. Table 7–2 relates to personnel management, specifically turnover rate comparisons. Tables 7–3 and 7–4 focus on specific systems within the department: release of information and medical

Table 7–1 Adequacy of Discharge Summary Content

Department of Health Information Management Memorial Hospital

Source of Benchmark: Hospital policy manual and Medical Staff bylaws concerning documentation standards
Participants: Active Medical Staff—Internal Medicine Service
Study Prepared by: Quality Assurance Coordinator, Department of Health Information Management
Time Frame Covered: January, February, March 2007 discharges
Date of Study: April 15, 2007

Elements Noted	January	February	March
Diagnosis and procedures stated in acceptable terminology	92%	90%	96%
Brief summary: reason for admission; chief complaint	94%	94%	91%
Summation of pertinent laboratory and diagnostic studies	80%	82%	87%
Statement of negative findings and special conditions	50%	57%	51%
Summation of treatment rendered and brief justification	94%	95%	95%
Condition at discharge	91%	91%	90%
Instructions to patient or family	82%	84%	82%
Final dispostion	82%	83%	83%

Table 7–2 Turnover Rate—Clerical Workers in Job Grades 3 through 6 in Health Information Department

Department of Health Information Management Memorial Hospital

Source of Benchmark: Areawide turnover rates for hospitals in greater metropolitan area; data developed by hospital council and labor union representing hospital workers in geographic area
Participants: Management Team: Department of Health Information Management assisted by Director of Human Resources
Study Prepared by: Director, Department of Health Information Management
Time Frame Covered: October–December 2006; January–March 2007
Date of Study: April 20, 2007

Turnover Rate Area Rate	October 2006	November 2006	December 2006	January 2007	February 2007	March 2007
			Department Rate			
5%	3%	8%	4%	0	6%	2%

Table 7–3 Medical Transcription Productivity

Department of Health Information Management Memorial Hospital

Source of Benchmark: Consortium of five medical school hospitals in urban area, using productivity standards developed by systems engineers through special contract
Participants: Medical Transcription divisions in each of the five hospitals
Study Prepared by: Medical Transcription Coordinator, Memorial Hospital
Time Frame Covered: March 2007

Work Standard Met	Memorial Hospital	Hospital One	Hospital Two	Hospital Three	Hospital Four
	87%	94%	89%	95%	94%

Note re: Standard

1. 150 lines per hour

2. Based on 70 characters per line using 12 point Courier font

3. Standard brand software

4. Discharge summaries and operative reports

transcription. For the purposes of these studies, the data should be considered fictitious. The examples include both internal benchmark sources as well as external sources.[3]

TOOLS OF CONTROL

Certain tools of control may be combined with the planning process. Management by objectives, the budget, and the Gantt chart are examples of tools used for both planning and controlling. Other techniques may also be used in planning workflow or assessing a proposed change in a plan or procedure. They may also be adapted for specific control use, such as when a flowchart is used to audit the way in which a task is actually being done as compared with the original plan. Some controls are directed at employee performance, such as the principle of requalification whereby the employee is tested periodically to ensure quality standards are met. Specific, quantifiable output measures may be recorded and monitored through a variety of control charts. In addition to these specific tools, the manager exercises control through the assessment and limitation of conflict, through the communication process, and through active monitoring of employees. Specific tools of planning and control are dealt with here.

Table 7–4 Release of Information: Adequacy of Consent

Department of Health Information Management Memorial Hospital

Source of Benchmark: State Legislation—Requirements for ROI consent; Federal Regulation—Requirements for drug and alcohol ROI consent; Hospital Policy Manual—Requirements for adequate consent
Participants: Release of Information Team: Supervisor and day shift ROI specialists
Study Prepared by: Supervisor of ROI unit
Time Frame Covered: May 2007
Date of Study: June 4, 2007

	Week of			
Elements Noted	**May 6**	**May 13**	**May 20**	**May 27**
Name of patient	100%	100%	100%	100%
Addressed to this facility with full title and address	96%	92%	94%	94%
Purpose of release stated	92%	92%	90%	90%
Kind of information to be released specified	78%	78%	81%	76%
Name and title of person to whom information to be released	40%	42%	45%	45%
Signature of patient OR Parent or guardian as applicable	94%	95%	95%	95%
Date signed: current within six months	93%	92%	89%	92%
HIV restrictions applicable? If yes, additional authorization provided to cover HIV-AIDS–related information	96%	96%	97%	97%
Drug/alcohol requirements applicable? If yes, additional authorization provided to cover drug and/or alcohol information	98%	98%	98%	97%

Gantt Chart

A visual control device, the Gantt chart was developed by Henry L. Gantt (1861–1919), one of the pioneers in scientific management. Sometimes referred to as a scheduling and progress chart, it emphasizes the work-time relationships necessary to meet some defined goal. The time needed for each activity is estimated, and a time value is assigned. This information is plotted on the chart. As the work progresses, entries are made to reflect the work completed. The chart focuses on the interrelationships among the phases of work within a given task. The Gantt chart may be used to reflect different aspects of the work:

- machine or equipment scheduling (in this application it is also called a load chart)

- overall production control
- individual worker production

Basic Components of Gantt Charts

Each Gantt chart contains the same basic components regardless of the application. The estimated time allotted for the work is plotted against a time scale that shows the appropriate time frame in days, weeks, or months, as well as calendar dates (Figure 7–1). The calendar legend may be placed at the top or bottom of the chart. As work progresses, items completed are entered and compared to those planned. In using the chart as a visual control tool, the manager uses shading or color coding to enter lines proportional in length to the percentage of work accomplished.

Standard Symbols

Standard symbols are used for plotting the Gantt chart:

1. The "opening angle" is entered under the date an operation is planned to start.
2. The "closing angle" is entered under the date the operation is planned to be completed.
3. A straight line joining the opening and closing angle shows the time span within which the operation is to be done.
4. A heavy line shows work completed. This progress line is usually proportional to the amount of work completed.

Employee	Month: June			Days				
	12	13	14	15	16	17	18	19
M. Higgins	sorting							
S. Morton	sorting							
K. Ollis			filing					
S. Watkins			filing					

FIGURE 7–1 Gantt Progress Chart for Planning and Controlling Filing Backlong: Laboratory Reports

5. A check mark is placed at the date when the progress was posted and is entered on the time scale.

An additional entry may show cumulative work done as time progresses. Codes may be entered to show the reason for being off schedule, such as:

- W: worker unavailable due to illness or personal day
- M: lack of materials
- E: equipment breakdown

In constructing and reading any charts, codes should be used and interpreted consistently (Figure 7–2).

The Flowchart

The manager may use a flowchart to depict the chronological flow of work. A flowchart is a graphic representation of an ordered sequence of events, steps, or procedures that take place in a system. The following are various types of flowcharts:

- *Procedure flowchart:* a graphic depiction of the distribution and subsequent steps in processing work.
- *Program block diagram:* a detailed description of the steps that take place in computer routines. Specific operations and decisions, as well as their sequence in the program, are indicated.

Therapist		Week 1						Week 2					
		M	T	W	Th	F	S-S	M	T	W	Th	F	S-S
A. Clay	AM			acute-2nd							W W Emerg. acute		
	PM												
D. Francis	AM							Acute admiss.					
	PM												
S. Scott	AM	W W						Emerg. acute-2nd					
	PM												
L. Matt	AM			Progress update staff									
	PM												
O. Rank	AM												
	PM												

FIGURE 7–2 Gantt Chart for Evaluating New Admissions

- *Logic diagram:* a graphic representation of the data-processing logic.
- *Two-dimensional flowchart:* a depiction of complex work flow. This type of flowchart allows the procedures analyst to show a number of flows at the same time, such as a procedure that begins with a single action and branches out into several work flows.
- *Systems flowchart:* a display of the information flow throughout all parts of the system. These flowcharts may be task-oriented (i.e., emphasize work performed) or forms-oriented (i.e., depict the flow of documents through the functional structure) (Exhibit 7–1).

Uses of the Flowchart

Flowcharting is associated with computerized data processing because of its emphasis on logical flow, but it is not restricted to program documentation. The flowchart may be used to advantage by any manager who must analyze, plan, and control work flow.

The flowchart may be used for both planning and controlling activities. As a planning tool, it may be used for the following purposes:

1. To develop a procedure. The chart forces the manager to think logically, since it reveals how one aspect of the task is linked to others, which areas of work flow must be made consistent, and where coordination mechanisms are needed.
2. To illustrate and emphasize key points in the written procedure. The flowchart may be used as companion documentation to the written procedure, as it provides an overall picture of the work flow in concise form. Key points in the work flow may be emphasized by color-coding critical decisions or actions.
3. To compare present and proposed procedures. A comparison of a flowchart for a proposed procedure with a flowchart for the existing procedure may show that there are as many, or more, delays in the proposed procedure.

It is less costly to assess the probable outcome of a procedure before it is implemented than to find that the procedure is not workable after it has been implemented.

As a control device, the flowchart may be used for these purposes:

1. To compare the actual work flow with that originally planned. In order to for the charts to remain effective guides to actions, procedures must be updated and the work flow must be monitored for changes that occur imperceptibly. By developing a flowchart of a procedure as it is currently

EXHIBIT 7–1

Processing Written Requests for Release of Information

BEGIN: Receipt of written request

END: Response completed and placed in outgoing mail

DATE: October 15, 2003

PAGE: 1 of 5

Assumptions:

1. These general steps conform to policy on release of information (ROI).
2. Release of information policy contains details about authorization and fee requirements.
3. There are standard form letters to facilitate response.
4. This procedure correlates with storage and retrieval; storage and retrieval personnel obtain the chart, following the designated procedures.
5. No outside copy service is used for ROI.

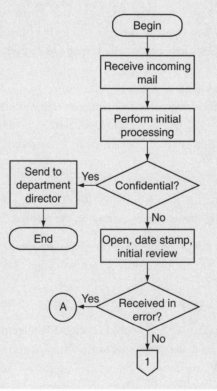

EXHIBIT 7–1 *continued*

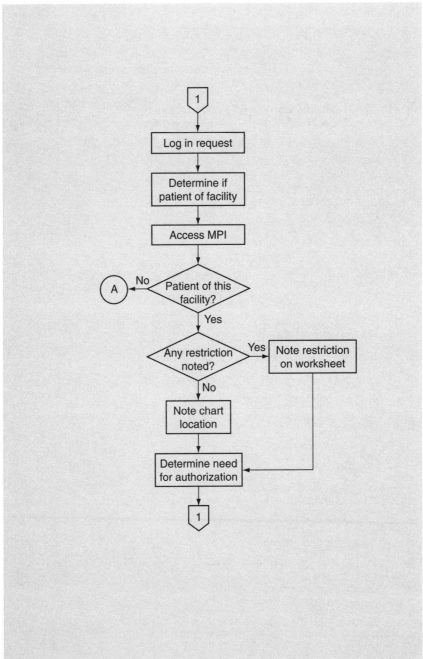

continues

EXHIBIT 7–1 *continued*

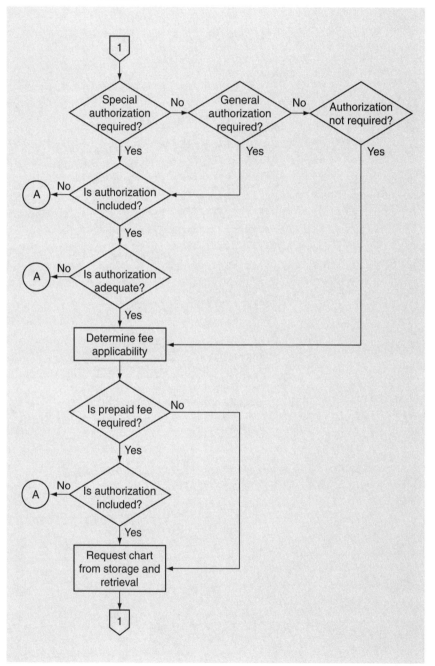

EXHIBIT 7–1 *continued*

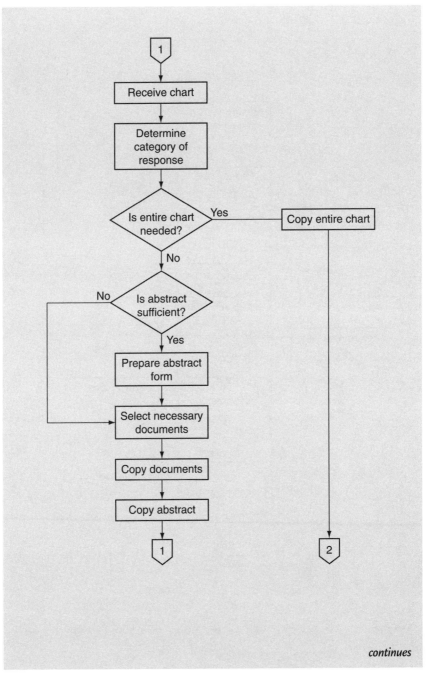

continues

EXHIBIT 7–1 *continued*

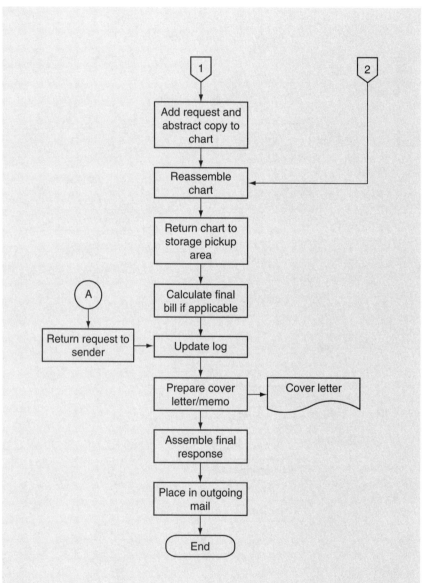

Source: Reprinted from Aspen Publishers, Inc. Joan Gratto Liebler, *Medical Records: Policies and Guidelines*, 1997, 13:46–13:50.

performed and comparing it with the original plan, the manager can see changes that have occurred in the work flow and may then decide whether to change the procedure so that it reflects existing practice or to enforce compliance with the original plan.

2. To audit the work flow. Every loop in a flowchart is a potential delay; the manager can pinpoint areas of delay, investigate the legitimacy of the delays, and determine how to shorten or eliminate them.

Flowchart Symbols

On a flowchart, each distinctive symbol stands for a certain kind of function, such as decision making, processing, or input-output. Symbols provide a shorthand method of describing the processes involved in the work. These symbols, which have become standardized in data processing, are used for flowcharts in connection with both computer programs and with noncomputerized systems analysis. Commonly accepted flowchart symbols are shown in Figure 7–3.

Support Documentation

Sometimes the flowchart is a companion document to a fully written procedure. When the flowchart depicts the overall systems flow or when the procedure has not yet been developed, support documentation is needed to complement the information on the chart. This documentation may be in the form of notes in the body of the flowchart or in the form of a narrative statement. Notes are brief, clarifying statements that supply information in conjunction with a process. They are keyed

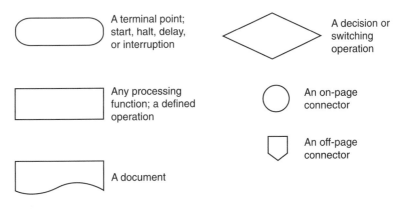

FIGURE 7–3 Flowchart Symbols

to their proper place in the chart by a number or a letter. Notes are placed in side or bottom margins where they will not interfere with the flowchart proper. A narrative statement covers assumptions, questions, and areas that need additional follow-up. A brief summary of the overall setting of the work flow may be included. Any special terms or abbreviations used are defined in this document.

Total Quality Management Display Charts

A manager may use modifications of the total quality management (TQM) charts associated with the Deming approach to management and the TQM movement in general. Exhibits 7–2 through 7–7 provide examples of such charts, including the

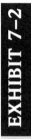

Run Chart

Number of Requests for Charts for Walk-in Patients—
  Weekday Clinics
Time Period: January 1, 2007 to March 31, 2007
Unit of Measure: Individual chart

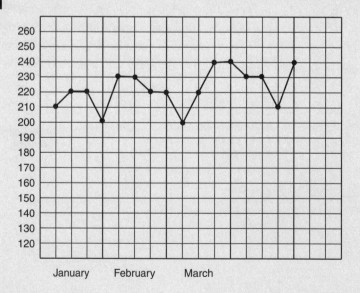

Source: Adapted with permission from Aspen Publishers, Inc. Joan Gratto Liebler, *Medical Records: Policies and Guidelines,* 1997, section 13.

customary chart format and a statement of the primary purpose of each type of chart.

These data display charts are those traditionally associated with total quality management processes. The examples given here reflect application to medical records systems.

Run Chart

Purpose: To identify trends (e.g., number of requests for charts for walk-in patients during first quarter of fiscal year).

Display format: Simple graph.

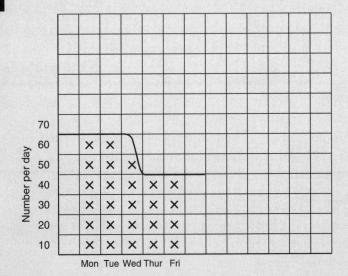

EXHIBIT 7–3

Histogram

Chart Requests for Walk-in Patients—Weekday Clinic According to Day of the Week

Time Period: January 1, 2007 to March 31, 2007

Unit of Measure: Individual chart-average per day of the week

Source: Adapted with permission from Aspen Publishers, Inc. Joan Gratto Liebler, *Medical Records: Policies and Guidelines,* 1997, section 13.

EXHIBIT 7–4

Scattergram

Chart Requests for Walk-in Patients by Clinic Specialty
Time Period: July 2007
Unit of Measure: Individual chart

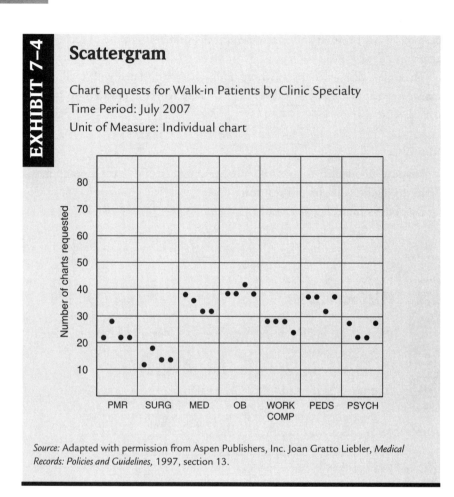

Source: Adapted with permission from Aspen Publishers, Inc. Joan Gratto Liebler, *Medical Records: Policies and Guidelines,* 1997, section 13.

Histogram

Purpose: To measure rate and frequency of occurrences to determine usual, most predictable pattern when averaging is not a reliable indicator.

Display format: Simple graph showing frequency distribution.

Scattergram

Purpose: To show the relationship between two variables or factors (e.g., number of chart requests for walk-in patients by clinic specialty).

Display format: Simple graph.

Cause-Effect Chart ("Fishbone Diagram" or Ishikawa Diagram)

Purpose: Identify major problem and associated cause. Causes are usually clustered by category: people, procedure, equipment, and policy.

EXHIBIT 7-5

Cause-Effect Chart: Charts Unavailable for Appointments—Day Clinics

Time Period: Date current as of August 6, 2007

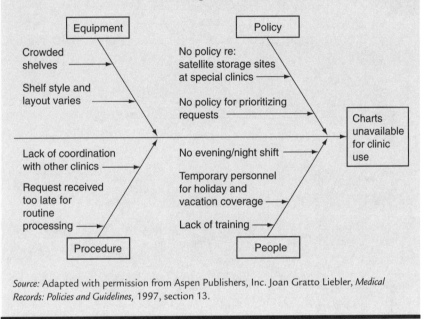

Source: Adapted with permission from Aspen Publishers, Inc. Joan Gratto Liebler, *Medical Records: Policies and Guidelines,* 1997, section 13.

Display format: Cluster diagram of causes, flowing toward the identified problem.

Note: This chart is developed through team effort and it is displayed so that additions may be made as information becomes available.

Statistical Quality Control Chart

Purpose: Ongoing monitoring of variation.

Display format: Graph showing mean, upper control limit, and lower control limit. These charts are usually completed by the worker(s) involved in the daily processing of the work. The manager is typically notified when variation is moving close to the upper or lower control limits. The manager also reviews these charts periodically to isolate problem areas.

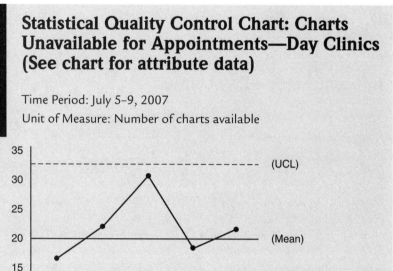

EXHIBIT 7-6

Statistical Quality Control Chart: Charts Unavailable for Appointments—Day Clinics (See chart for attribute data)

Time Period: July 5–9, 2007
Unit of Measure: Number of charts available

Source: Adapted with permission from Aspen Publishers, Inc. Joan Gratto Liebler, *Medical Records: Policies and Guidelines,* 1997, section 13.

Note: LCL=lower control limit; UCL=upper control limit.

Note: Variation occurs as a result of normal, random cause that is expected. It also occurs due to specific events that may be problem indicators. The first step in developing statistical control charts is to determine the average, then set the upper control limit (UCL) and the lower control limit (LCL), usually using three standard deviations as the interval from the mean value.

Pareto Chart

Purpose: To determine priorities by comparing factors; to facilitate sorting the few critical elements from the less urgent.

Display format: Bar graph.

The foregoing and similar graphic displays of data may be incorporated into dashboard reporting systems that provide at-a-glance summaries of findings. They

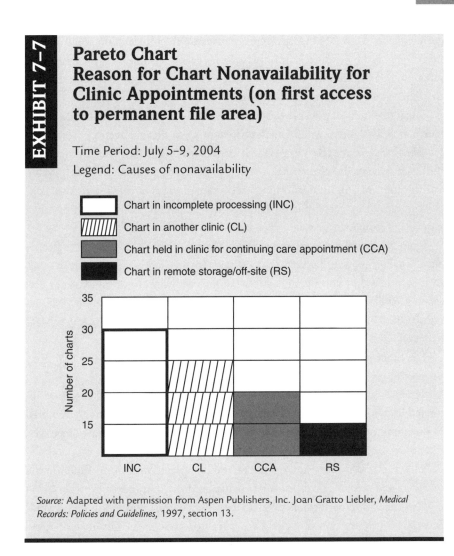

EXHIBIT 7-7

Pareto Chart
Reason for Chart Nonavailability for Clinic Appointments (on first access to permanent file area)

Time Period: July 5–9, 2004
Legend: Causes of nonavailability

☐ Chart in incomplete processing (INC)
▨ Chart in another clinic (CL)
▨ Chart held in clinic for continuing care appointment (CCA)
■ Chart in remote storage/off-site (RS)

Source: Adapted with permission from Aspen Publishers, Inc. Joan Gratto Liebler, *Medical Records: Policies and Guidelines,* 1997, section 13.

are simple, flexible, and informative methods for supplying support to decision makers in the organization.

THE CRITICAL CYCLE

In the opening portion of the chapter it was stated that the control process involves three phases that are cyclic: establishing standards, measuring performance, and correcting deviations. Standards were addressed in the information about benchmarking, and the measurement of performance has consumed a great deal of the remainder of the chapter. As of yet, extremely little has emerged along the way that directly addresses the correction of deviations.

Taken together, all possible means of measuring performance, those discussed herein as well as others, will themselves do nothing to effect correction. Correction requires that someone take some positive steps based on what has been learned from the measurements. In other words, one may possess all possible control information, but this information means nothing unless something is done with it. Also, controlling cannot be accomplished without active directing, which is ultimately a part of all of the management processes.

There are actually *two* cycles involved in controlling. One is the cycle already cited: establishing standards, measuring performance, and correcting deviations. In this cycle we are continually addressing the adequacy of our standards as well as the reliability of our measurements as we continue to correct deviations. Neither standards nor measurements are ever considered carved in stone; these must always be reevaluated as the environment changes.

The other pertinent cycle is the directing-and-controlling cycle, or, as it may be referred to, the cycle of directing, coordinating, and controlling.

Rarely are plans and decisions of any consequence implemented exactly as intended in every respect. Many changes, often moment-to-moment, are required in pursuit of our objectives. In this cycle, progress is evaluated against objectives, intentions, or needs and adjustments—new decisions are made as we go along. Perhaps the terms most descriptive of the complete controlling function are *follow-up* and *action*. The follow-up provides information; this is the observation or measurement of performance. Again, however, all the information in the world is useless without action that translates this into correction. Continually observing how things are going as compared with how they should be going and making new decisions provides new direction to effect corrective action.

Controlling is often the most neglected of the basic management functions, especially in terms of the strength of follow-up on the implementation of decisions. Rarely are all circumstances and all details anticipated in full. Also, for even a routine decision of modest scope it is highly likely that the environment in which it occurs will experience changes between the start and finish of the decision process. Controlling is, quite appropriately, quarterbacking—observing the conditions of the moment and adjusting actions based on current information. It is sometimes simple and sometimes complex, but it is always cyclic.

EXERCISE: THE MULTIPLE-PATH FLOWCHART: THE PURCHASING REQUEST

Utilizing the activity symbols that are presented in the flowchart in Exhibit 7–1, chart the complete processing of a five-part form identified as the Purchasing Request (PR). This is an old form and the subject of considerable complaining throughout the organization concerning its cumbersome nature and its supposedly unnecessarily complicated processing procedure. In the lower levels of the organization and especially among those persons whose job includes the execution of PRs on behalf of their supervisors, it is often cynically declared that the process has been kept deliberately complicated to discourage casual purchases ("You've really got to need something badly to willingly take on this bureaucratic process").

Following a key change in administration and the arrival of a new purchasing executive, you have been assigned to study the Purchasing Request thoroughly and determine whether positive changes can be made. The information-gathering phase of your investigation reveals the following:

- The five-part PR is generated either by or at the request of any supervisor or manager requesting a purchase.
- If it is generated by a supervisor or manager below the level of department head or division director, it must be approved by that higher level. Department heads and division directors and above approve their own PRs.
- The originator places Part 4 of the form in an open file and holds it until the item is received, at which time it goes into a closed file. You have discovered that sometimes Part 5 is filed along with Part 4, and sometimes Part 5 is discarded.
- Parts 1, 2, and 3 go to the purchasing department.
- Purchasing places the order and so notifies the originator.
- Part 1, the original PR, remains in an "on order" file in purchasing and Part 2 is sent to receiving.
- Part 3, for which no current purchasing staff can remember the original purpose, goes into a tray in purchasing. When the tray is filled the accumulated Part 3s are discarded.
- When the purchased item arrives, receiving sends the invoice to purchasing along with another form known as a receiver. Receiving files Part 2 of the completed PR.

- If the content of any invoice is disputed (which has been happening with increasing frequency), accounts payable contacts receiving and requests a copy of its Part 2.
- Your organization is paying a premium to have the PR forms printed by an outside supplier, because a five-part form is one or two parts beyond the capability of your internal print shop.

When you have completed your chart:

1. Determine how you can improve the process for future consideration and chart your recommended process. State whatever reasonable assumptions you may have had to make.
2. In outline fashion, recommend for management's consideration a "Forms Control Procedure" calling for periodic review of the appropriateness of existing forms and specifying a controlled approval process for the introduction of new forms.

EXERCISE: CHOOSING AN ADEQUATE CONTROL MECHANISM: WHAT FITS BEST?

Refer to the chapter section titled "Characteristics of Adequate Controls." For each of the tasks or circumstances described below, recommend a specific kind of control mechanism. Your selected mechanism should provide you with information on which you can base corrective actions as needed. In each case state why you selected that particular mechanism, describe how it satisfies the characteristics of adequate controls, and state whether you believe there are one or two additional mechanisms that might work almost as well as your chosen mechanism.

- Display the status of the accomplishment of routine scheduled preventive maintenance activities by the plant engineering department.
- Track the number of repeat patient chart requests fulfilled beyond a stated two-hour response-time limit.
- Follow the processing of a letter of complaint from its initial receipt to the disposition of the problem.
- Track the timeliness of the clinical laboratory's responses to STAT test requests.

- Track the department's financial operating results as compared with the departmental budget.
- Report on employment turnover throughout the organization by quarter and by year.

EXERCISE: PROMOTING TOTAL QUALITY MANAGEMENT (TQM)

You are a professional employed at a large urban medical center. You have been appointed to serve as a nonmanagerial member of a steering committee established to guide the implementation of TQM throughout the organization. The committee has been through a week of intensive education in TQM/performance improvement principles and has held the first two of an indefinite series of weekly meetings to pave the way for translating the TQM philosophy into practical actions that can be implemented. You are encouraged by what you have learned and experienced during these first few weeks; however, you are also conscious of the organization's past failures with management by objectives (MBO) and quality circles, and you are aware of a fairly widespread tendency to regard such undertakings as dabbling in the latest management "flavor of the month."

Your second steering committee ends late, leaving you only two minutes to get to your next commitment. As you leave the conference room and enter the hospital's main corridor, a colleague, heading toward the same destination as you, falls into step beside you and asks, "What's this total quality management all about? Looks to me like the same stuff that's been pushed at us in different wrappers several times over the years, and it'll probably go the same way. Nowhere. More fancy notebooks and reports that end up collecting dust. Why should we think this will be any less of a waste of time and resources?"

You have less than two minutes available while on the move to provide your colleague with a positive response in a few sentences. Write out your proposed response.

NOTES

1. H. B. Maynard, ed., *Industrial Engineering Handbook,* 2nd ed. (New York: McGraw Hill, 1963), section 10, 183–91.

2. Forrest Breyfogle, James Cupello, and Becki Meadows, *Managing Six Sigma: A Practical Guide to Understanding, Assessing and Implementing the Strategy that Yields Bottom-Line Success* (Indianapolis: John Wiley and Sons, 2000). See also Mikel Harry and Richard Schroeder, *Six Sigma Quality Management* (New York: Random House Audio Publishing Group, 2000).

3. The charts and figures in this chapter are updated versions of those originally published in Joan Gratto Liebler, *Medical Record Policies and Guidelines* (Gaithersburg, Md.: Aspen, 1996–1999).

Budgeting: Controlling the Ultimate Resource

Budget preparation and administration are major duties of the department head. Before dealing with the actual budget calculations, the manager must understand the basic concepts and principles of budgeting. The budget details presented here are treated from the perspective of the department head rather than the accountant, comptroller, or top-level administrator. In addition, this presentation is intended for the inexperienced manager; terms are defined and examples are given in detail to facilitate budget preparation and analysis by an inexperienced user. The first part of the discussion treats basic concepts such as budget periods, types of budgets, uniform code of accounts, approaches to budgeting, and the overall budget process. The second part of the discussion focuses on the details of the budget proper: the capital expenses, personnel budget, supplies, and related expenses.

Sound budgetary procedures are based on six requisites:

1. sound organizational structure so that the responsibility for budget preparation and administration is clear
2. a consistent, defined budget period
3. the development of adequate statistical data
4. a reporting system that reflects the organizational structure
5. a uniform code of accounts so that data are meaningful and consistent
6. a regular audit system so that variances are explained in a timely manner

USES OF THE BUDGET

Budgeting is both a planning and controlling tool. As a plan, the budget is a specific statement of the anticipated results, such as expected revenue to be earned and probable expenses to be incurred, in an operation for a future defined period. This plan is expressed in numerical terms, usually dollars. A statement of objectives in fiscal terms, the budget is a single-use plan that covers a specific period of time; it becomes the basis of future or continuing plans when the incremental approach to budgeting is used whereby the next budget is formulated through the addition of specific increments to the existing budget. It is a statement of what the organization intends to accomplish, not merely a forecast or a guess.

When the budget is properly administered, it becomes a tool of control and accountability in that it reflects the organizational structure, with each unit or department given a specific allocation of funds based on departmental goals and functions. The budget is an essential companion to the delegation of authority; the line manager who has the responsibility for developing the plans for the department or unit must be given the necessary resources to accomplish the approved plans. In turn, this manager accepts responsibility for assigning specific budget amounts to the personnel and material categories and monitoring the use of these resources. Because the budget permits a comparison of planned with actual performance, control is enhanced. The department head is responsible for those costs that are controllable, such as overtime authorization, supplies, and equipment purchases, but not for those that are arbitrarily assigned to the departmental budget, such as fringe benefits calculated as a flat percentage of personnel budget or administrative overhead calculated as a flat percentage of operating costs.

BUDGET PERIODS

A budget specifies the amount to be spent in a predetermined period. This budget period varies according to the purpose of the budget. The capital equipment or improvement budget may be developed for a long period, such as a three-, five-, or ten-year period; the budget for supplies, expenses, and personnel costs may be developed for the immediate fiscal year. Given the various regulatory requirements for long-range planning and budgeting for capital improvements in health care organizations, these organizations commonly have such a combination of long- and short-term budget periods.

The accounting period encompassed by the overall budget framework is the fiscal year. The fiscal year may or may not coincide with the calendar year. In years past many hospitals, especially teaching institutions, used the July through June cycle, which tended to reflect the movement of house staff at the end of the teaching year. In recent years, however, a number of government entities have encouraged—and in some instances have essentially required—the adoption of the calendar year as the fiscal year.

Within the accounting year there are a number of accounting periods. It is common practice to keep track of payroll and certain other expenses on the basis of one, two, or four weeks and to accumulate this information for 13 four-week accounting periods in the year; however, other important financial information is accumulated by calendar month either because it is necessary to do so or because this is clearly the most sensible data collection period.

Because of the inevitable presence in the budget of some information in two- and four-week increments and some in full-month increments, it is usually necessary to manipulate some of the figures by adding in or backing out certain amounts at either end of a period in order to have complete financial information for the period of interest.

Periodic Moving Budget

Another approach to the definition of budget period is the periodic moving budget. In the moving budget, the basic forecast for the year is adjusted as specific periods are completed. As each period is completed, an equal time period is added:

2007	Jan.	Feb.	Mar.	
	Apr.	May	June	
	July	Aug.	Sept.	
	Oct.	Nov.	Dec.	
2008	Jan.	Feb.	Mar.	(Added when the Jan.-Feb.-Mar. 2007 period is completed.)

The cycle of completion and addition may be shorter, as when the July-Aug.-Sept. period is added as soon as the Jan.-Feb.-Mar. period is completed. The periodic moving budget allows the manager to make use of the more up-to-date information that becomes available as each period closes and to thus make a more accurate prediction. In organizations using the 500-day plan or similar long-range plans with periodic (e.g., 200-day moving update) review points, this type of budgeting is the natural process.

Milestone Budgeting

In milestone budgeting, the budget periods are tied to the subsidiary plans or projects. As these milestone events are accomplished, costs can be determined and budget allocations for the next segments of the project can be established. The budget periods are not uniform but depend on the projected time frame for the subsidiary plan. During the implementation of the electronic health record, for example, several milestone events would be noted, with budgeting forecasts associated with each segment. Milestone budgeting usually covers more than one year.

TYPES OF BUDGETS

The budget may be developed to give emphasis to one of several aspects of the overall plan. The revenue and expense budget is the most common type of budget. It reflects anticipated revenues, such as those from sales, payment for services rendered, endowments, grants, and special funds, and it includes expenses, such as costs associated with personnel, capital equipment, or supplies. In the personnel or labor budget, projections are based on the number of personnel hours needed or types and kinds of skills needed rather than on wages and salaries, as in the personnel costs of the revenue and expense budget. A production budget expresses the information in terms of units of production, such as economic quantities to be produced or types and capacities of machines to be utilized.

The fixed budget presumes stable conditions; it is prepared on the basis of the best information available, such as past experience and forecasting. The plans, including cost and expense calculations, are made on the basis of this expected level of activity. The variable budget concept was developed because operating costs and level of activity may fluctuate. For example, a university may calculate its unit budgets according to credit hours generated, but student enrollment may be lower than anticipated; a hospital may use dollars per patient day or average census as its basis, but the daily census in the hospital may drop and remain low. Thus, costs and expenses are established for varying rates. As actual income and operating costs become known, the budget is adjusted. The periodic moving budget is used with variable budgeting, as is the step budget.

The step budget is a form of variable budgeting in which a certain level of activity is assumed and the impact of deviations from this level of activity calculated. If the manager wishes to show several possibilities predicated on various factors, such as level of production or number of clients served, the step budget is used. These other levels may be greater or less than the basic estimate. For example, a step budget showing probable estimates plus pessimistic and optimistic allowances might be developed. The advantage of using the step budget is that it permits, even forces, the manager to examine the actions required in the event of a variation from the estimated revenue and expense. When a step budget is prepared, the fixed costs and revenues—that is, those that are not tied to volume of service, production levels, or other factors related to operational costs—are stated. Then the variable revenues and costs are calculated according to the volume of service, operating costs, anticipated revenues, and similar factors.

The master budget is the central, composite budget for the total organization; all the major activities of the organization are coordinated in this central budget. The department budgets are the working, detailed budgets for each unit; they are highly specific so as to permit identification of each item as well as close coordination and monitoring of revenue and expense. In order to coordinate the several department or unit budgets into a master budget and in order to make budget processes consistent, a uniform code of accounts and specific cost centers must be developed.

The Uniform Code of Accounts

The standard classification of expenditures and other transactions made by an organization is the uniform code of accounts (also referred to as a uniform chart of accounts). Such a uniform code of accounts contains master codes and subdivisions to reflect such information as the specific transaction (e.g., personnel expense, travel expense, capital improvement) and the organizational unit within which the transaction occurred (e.g., purchasing department, dietary department, public relations unit). The delineation of the specific organizational unit facilitates responsibility reporting, as it is possible to relate specific expenditures to the manager in charge of that organizational unit.

The chief financial officer of the organization develops the necessary guidelines for a uniform chart of accounts. These guidelines typically reflect those of national associations such as the Healthcare Financial Management Association (HFMA). These account codes are used in the budget to group line items, such as a purchase requisition or a position authorization request. Account codes for a particular institution might include

200	Furniture
210	Capital Equipment
520	Equipment Rental
530	Equipment Maintenance and Service Contracts
580	Purchased Services (e.g., an outside contract with a coding and abstracting service)
600	Education and Travel
610	Dues and Subscriptions

Budget worksheets are coordinated with these account codes, with specific items listed, line by line, under each account code. *Line item* is a term commonly used to refer to such specifications. For example, the worksheet for budget preparation and, subsequently, the line items of the budget for the category of Dues and Subscriptions reflect the item in detail and the unit with which it is associated.

610.1	Hospital association (regional) dues	$1,000.00
610.2	Professional dues paid for Chief of Service	300.00
610.7	Accrediting agency regulations annual update subscription	150.00
610.8	Attendance at annual meeting of professional association	
	50% cost for Chief of Service	700.00
	25% cost for each staff assistant	350.00
610.9	Inservice workshop for support staff (2-day seminar, in-house)	480.00

The code of accounts varies from one institution to another; the items and costs given here are for illustrative purposes only.

Cost Centers

An activity or group of activities for which costs are specified, such as housekeeping, maintenance and repairs, telephone service, and similar functions, is a cost center. Usually predetermined, cost centers generally parallel the department or service structure of the organization. For example, direct patient care cost centers, with their associated codes, may include

45	Physical Therapy
46	Occupational Therapy
47	Home Care Program
48	Social Services
49	Radiology

Administrative cost centers may include

50	Computer and Information Service
51	Health Information Service
52	Admissions Unit
53	Dietary
54	Laundry and Housekeeping

Additional cost centers reflect costs associated with the overall expense of operation:

1	Employee Health and Welfare Benefits
2	Depreciation: Buildings and Fixtures
3	Depreciation: Equipment
4	Payroll Processing

Responsibility Center

A unit of the organization headed by an individual who has authority over and who accepts responsibility for the unit is a responsibility center. These centers parallel the organizational structure as outlined in the organizational chart. The departments or services are responsibility centers, each with its detailed budget. The cost center codes and responsibility centers normally parallel one another.

APPROACHES TO BUDGETING

The two major approaches to the budgeting process are incremental budgeting and the zero-based system (historically referred to as the planning-programming-budgeting system (PPBS)). In incremental budgeting, the financial database of the past is increased by some given percentage. For example, the personnel portion of the budget may be increased by a flat 5 percent over the last budget period allotment, capital expenses by 7 percent, and supplies by 4 percent. There is some efficiency in this approach, since the projected calculations are relatively straightforward. There is also a danger, however; significant changes, shifting priorities, or pressing needs within some unit of the organization may be overlooked. As with incremental decision making, there is an implicit assumption that the original money and resource allocation was appropriately calculated and distributed among organizational units. Incremental budgets are object-oriented—that is, they are developed in terms of personnel, materials, maintenance, and supplies. Traditional budgeting is control-oriented, while PPBS is planning-oriented.

PPBS was mandated in the Department of Defense in the early 1960s. PPBS, as the name implies, emphasizes the budgeting process in systems terms. The outputs for specific programs are assessed, and resource allocation and funding are related directly to the program goals. It is also referred to as "zero-based" budgeting because past dollar allocations are not the basis of projection.

A major feature of PPBS is its departure from the traditional one-year budget cycle. Funding is projected for the period of time (frequently three or more years) needed to achieve the goals of the program. In the planning phase, the general objectives are stated and refined, the projected schedule of activities is established, and the outputs are specified. These refined objectives are grouped into programs, resulting in a hierarchy within the plans.

The alternate means of achieving the plans are assessed through cost-effectiveness analysis. Units of measure for the outputs are developed (e.g., number of clients to be served, length of hospital stay, geographical area to be covered). Costs and resulting benefits for each approach are calculated, and the best alternative in terms of cost-benefit is selected. In the PPBS approach, managers seek to increase the number of factors that can be used to provide top-level decision makers with sufficient information to make the final resource allocation. An adequate information system is, therefore, required; this is consistent with the classic systems approach, which includes an information feedback cycle.

The PPBS approach has several disadvantages. First, it is a time-consuming process, involving long-range planning, development and comparison of alternatives in terms of cost-effectiveness, and the final budgeting. Second, not all goals can be stated precisely; not all worthy objectives can be quantified in specific measures, with a specific dollar cost attached. Third, there is the presumption that all alternatives are known and attainable. Fourth, in PPBS, the value, the legitimacy, and the actual survival of the program or organization are questioned. This, in turn, reopens conflict and exposes the accumulation of internal and external politics—the power plays, the bargaining, the trade-offs that have developed over time. The concern for program survival may intensify to the point that line managers may seek to withhold negative information, and the feedback cycle may become distorted.

Although the zero-based budgeting approach is probably not used in preparing the routine budget for the ongoing operations of the organization, it is the approach underlying the cost justification for special projects of great magnitude. For example, the managers of a health care facility might commit to a major change in computer applications or support systems. Millions of dollars may be involved in the conversion to the new system. Detailed analysis of the project will typically include cost comparisons of several vendor options, with specifics provided for each. Cost breakouts for such a project are presented by category, such as:

Financial services module:
Application software $700,000
Software maintenance/yearly 150,000
Implementation services 600,000
(one-time cost in year one)

Training
no cost in year one; included in implementation
annual cost for consultant training staff 90,000

Licensing fees—annual 50,000
(subject to review at end of three years)

In both approaches, the budgeted funds are used during the designated period, with any unspent funds turned in at the end of the fiscal year. However, some organizations follow a revenue retention rule to reward efficiency: a department keeps a portion of unspent funds at the end of the year to augment the upcoming year's funds.

THE BUDGETARY PROCESS

Initial Preparation

The budgetary process is cyclic; the feedback obtained during one budget period becomes the basis of budget development for the next period. The budget process usually begins with the setting of overall limits by top management. The specific guidelines for budget preparation reflect the mandatory federal, state, and accrediting requirements as well as union contract provisions and the financial assets of the organization. The timetable and particular forms to be used in budget preparation are issued along with these guidelines.

Development of the unit budget is the specific responsibility of the department manager. In some instances, a department manager may wish to use the "grassroots" approach to budgeting; unit managers or supervisors prepare their budgets and submit them to the department manager for coordination into the overall department budget. The supervisors or unit managers must, of course, be given sufficient information and guidance to carry out this function. An alternate way of involving supervisors and subordinates is to ask for suggestions about equipment needs, special resources, or supplies. In highly normative organizations, such as a university, there may be an advisory or review committee composed of selected employees who make recommendations to line officials regarding budget allocations. In any event, the department head bears the responsibility for final preparation, justification, and control of the budget.

During the budget preparation phase, the manager reviews, challenges, and updates the working assumptions. Trends are noted, priority needs are identified, and initiatives for the upcoming year are stated. Effective managers rely on a continuous process of gathering facts throughout the year. Information includes changes in workload quantity and patterns (e.g., an increase in the number of industrial health-related cases; the opening of a satellite clinic for school health). Equipment and maintenance logs reflect the useful life estimates or depreciation values of all major items, including the cost of maintenance and repair. Delayed maintenance of the physical structures is noted. The department history log (similar in concept to the classic wheel log of a ship's captain) is reviewed; this log shows the ongoing history of departmental changes in systems and in departmental capital improvements (e.g., rewiring or painting) as well as major systems changes (e.g., introduction of off-site storage).

The availability of previously unavailable external resources is identified, as in ensuring the availability of a reliable transcription service for outsourcing this function in health information services. The increased availability of specialists in an area of occupational therapy opens up the possibility of introducing new service in that unit of patient care.

Major trends in the field of professional practice, along with emerging department issues, are noted and appropriate initiatives stated. A department manager's initiatives might include increasing retention through inservice education programs and bonus or incentive plans; developing more specialist coverage; upgrading work stations; introducing new treatment modules; or developing outreach programs in community-based locations.

The Review and Approval Process

Competition, bargaining, and compromise in the allocation of scarce resources (personnel, money, and space) occur in the review and approval phase of the budget process. It is important for the manager to have the necessary facts to support budget requests; control records to demonstrate fluctuations in the workload, staffing needs, equipment usage, and goal attainment are essential sources of such information.

The internal approval process begins with a review of the department's budget by the department head's immediate budget officer. Compliance with guidelines is checked; justifications for requests for exceptions are reviewed. The organization's designated financial officer (usually the comptroller) may assist the chief executive officer in coordinating the department budgets into the master budget for the organization, but the chief executive officer is the final arbiter of resource allocation in many instances.

There is continuing emphasis, both within the organization and from external pressures, on cost containment, and a cost containment committee may be involved in the budget review process. Current voluntary efforts contribute to the routinization of this aspect of budget review. Cost-containment committees vary in structure and mandate, but their tasks typically include advising, investigating, and even participating in the implementation of cost-containment measures. Such a committee should have a questioning attitude as its primary philosophical stance; data are scrutinized and compared in an effort to identify areas where cost can be contained.

The budget hearing or review provides the department manager with an opportunity to make the case for his or her unit. Forthrightness and thorough preparation should characterize the manager's presentation. As the individual closest to the special issues of the particular unit, the manager should use this occasion to brief higher-level managers on critical issues. The manager should indicate a willingness to trade off certain costs so that another department, with a more pressing need, may be accommodated; in turn, the manager should be able to make the argument for why such a trade-off is not possible. A manager might be willing to defer major improvements as well as routine maintenance (such as annual painting of the department) until another year, thus freeing money for use by another department needing new equipment or increased staffing. This deferred maintenance might be tied to planned changes for the coming year, such as implementation of a major upgrade in equipment because of a technological change not yet available this coming budget year but definitely available in two more years (e.g., voice recognition technology). Instead of viewing the budget process as a win-lose proposition, a manager could partner with other department heads to preview mutual needs and trade-offs, thus fostering a win-win approach.

The customary planning approach of overaim or contingency planning is the usual principle followed in budget development. During the budget review, the manager would be prepared to give an optimistic, best-case scenario estimate (e.g., revenue increased; turnover decreased), a worst-case scenario with definite indicators of expenditures that can be reduced or cut should this become necessary at a later time in the budget year, and a middle-ground estimate.

During the review process, the values of open communication and integrity are paramount so that prudent, cost-effective decisions can be mutually agreed upon.

The final approval for the total budget is given by the governing board. In practice, a subcommittee on budget works with the chief executive officer, and final, formal approval is then given by the full governing board, as mandated in the organizational bylaws and/or charter of incorporation.

The budgets of organizations that receive some or all of their funds from state or federal sources may be subject to an external approval process—for example, by the state legislature or the federal Bureau of the Budget. There is a certain predictable drama in the budget process that becomes more evident in the external review process. There is a tacit rule that budgets are padded because budget requests are likely to be cut. The manager attempts to achieve a modicum of flexibility in budget maneuvering through overaim. There is also a necessary aspect of accountability, however. The public more or less demands that federal or state officials take proper care of the public purse. Even as clients (the public) seek greater services, they want cost containment, especially through tax relief. Public officials, then, must in fact dramatize their concern for cost containment, partly by a highly specific review of budget requests and a refusal to approve budgets as submitted.

On the other hand, should an agency request a budget allocation that is the same as, or less than, that of a previous year, it might be seriously questioned whether the agency is doing its job. At best, the manager must recognize the subtle and overt political maneuvers that touch the budget process.

Implementation Phase

The final phase of budgeting is the implementation stage, when the approved budget allocation is spent. During this phase, revenues and expenses are regularly compared—for example, through periodic budget reconciliation. Should revenues fall short of the anticipated amount or should unexpected expenses arise, there may be a budget freeze or certain items may be cut. For example, overtime may be prohibited; personnel vacancies may not be filled, except for emergency situations; supplies or travel money may be eliminated.

There are specific internal procedures that must be followed to activate budgeted funds in the normal course of business. For example, the budget may contain an appropriation for certain supplies, but a companion requisition system must be used to effect the actual purchase of such supplies. When an individual worker is to be hired, a position authorization request may be used to activate that position as approved in the budget. Finally, during the budget year, preparation for the following budget period is made, bringing the manager full circle in the budget process (Exhibit 8–1).

Budget variance review and the periodic audit are discussed later in this chapter.

CAPITAL EXPENSES

An organization owns and operates capital facilities of a permanent or semipermanent nature, such as land, buildings, machinery, and equipment. Capital budget items are those revenues and costs related to the capital facilities. These expenses may be centralized as a single administrative cost for the entire organization, or they may be specified for each budgetary unit. The manager at the departmental level is normally concerned primarily with capital improvements for the department, such as acquisition of additional space, renovation and repairs, special electrical wiring, and painting.

The second capital expense in the departmental budget is major equipment. The equipment budget usually includes fixed equipment that is not subject to removal or transfer and that has a relatively long life. Major equipment that is movable is also included. The distinction between major and minor equipment is usually made on the basis of the cost and life expectancy of the item; major equipment commonly includes any item over a specific cost (e.g., $1,000) that has a life expectancy of more than five years. As with other aspects of budgeting, however, a specific organization may use some other cost or life expectancy factor to define major equipment/capital equipment expense. Major fixed equipment includes the heating fixtures, built-in cabinets or shelves, and appliances; major movable equipment includes file cabinets, patient beds, computer stations, and a variety of treatment modular equipment.

EXHIBIT 8–1 Exhibit 8–1 Annual Budget Plan— Based on Fiscal Year July 1 to June 30

Activity	Current year — Jul	Aug	Sep	Oct	Nov	Dec	Jan	Feb	Mar	Apr	May	Jun	Projected year — Jul	Aug	Sep	Oct	Nov	Dec	Jan	Feb
1. Current budget executed; monthly reconciliation & adjustments made	▬▬▬▬▬▬▬▬▬▬▬ (Jul→Jun)																			
2. CEO & Controller develop forecasts; issue budget guidelines to departments						▮														
3. Dept. heads formulate budgets and submit								▮												
4. CEO & Controller develop master budget									▮											
5. Department revisions made and submitted									▮											
6. CEO & Controller finalize budget										▮										
7. Board of Trustee subcommittee review; further adjustments made and final approval given											▮									
8. TRANSITION: close out current year accounts												▮								
9. New fiscal year budget in effect OR tentative budget in effect, pending full approval and/or further revisions												▬▬▬▬▬▬▬▬ (Jun→Feb)								

When budgeting for major equipment expenses, the manager may calculate the acquisition cost and prorate this cost over the expected life of the equipment. Depreciation costs are a factor in equipment selection. The budget guidelines developed by the chief financial officer's staff includes reference tables for estimating the useful life of major equipment and a formula to calculate composite depreciation rates for each unit of equipment. Vendors for major equipment generally provide depreciation data as part of the support information relating to their products. An item that is more costly to acquire may be less expensive in the long run because of a lower operating cost, long life expectancy, or slower rate of depreciation. This information should be included on the supplemental information forms used to justify equipment selection.

The worksheet for capital expenses includes the account code number from the uniform code of accounts, item description, unit cost, quantity, and total cost (Exhibits 8–2 and 8–3).

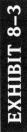

EXHIBIT 8–2

Sample Worksheet for Capital Expenses— Health Information Services

Department: Health Information Services

Fiscal Year: July 1–June 30

Account Code	Account Title: Item Description	Item Quantity	Item Cost	Total
210.6	Secretarial Desk	1	$760.00	$760.00
210.7	Side Chairs	3	150.00	450.00

EXHIBIT 8–3

Sample Worksheet for Capital Expenses— Physical Therapy

Department: Physical Therapy

Fiscal Year: July 1–June 30

Account Code	Account Title: Item Description	Item Quantity	Item Cost	Total
210.3	Parallel Bars—10 foot	1	$2,800.00	$2,800.00
210.4	Shoulder Wheel— Deluxe Heavy Duty	1	620.00	620.00

SUPPLIES AND OTHER EXPENSES

The many consumable items that are needed for the day-to-day work of the department are listed under the category of supplies. It may be tempting at first to group all these items under "Miscellaneous," but the clear delineation and listing of such items in the appropriate budget category alerts the manager to the magnitude of these costs and facilitates control. Items considered consumable supplies typically include routine items such as pens, pencils, notepads, letterhead stationery, staples, scissors, rubber bands, and paper clips. Such detailed calculations for these kinds of supplies may seem tedious, but the dollar value of these items is, in fact, significant. The stockpiling of unnecessary quantities takes up space, invites petty theft, and may lead to excess inventories of items that become outdated (e.g., forms, specialty supplies for equipment no longer in use). Commonsense practices of regular inventory control and good recordkeeping by an office manager provides a department head with both the planning and control appropriate to a seemingly incidental cost. Postage is included in this category unless it is absorbed as a central administrative line item.

A given department may have special consumable supplies that are essential to its operation. The direct patient care units incur expenses related to medical and surgical supplies. The clinical laboratory has a major expense in reagents. A health information department has as a major expense the color-coded, preprinted folders used for patient records. Special forms approved and mandated for medical record documentation (e.g., the fact sheet/identification sheet used in the admission unit, the preoperative anesthesia report form used in the surgical unit, the laboratory requisition/report form for laboratory studies) may be charged to each department as they are requisitioned and used. An alternative practice is to charge the health information department or central forms design unit with the cost of all preprinted forms. When the emphasis in the budgeting process is on control, however, it is preferable to charge the unit using such supplies so that administrative control may be fixed.

Special expenses commonly incurred at the department level include the lease and rental of equipment, the purchase of technical reference books and periodicals, training and education costs, and travel and meeting expenses. Contractual services for a special activity (such as transcription, statistical abstracting, and special laboratory studies) are included under the expense category.

The worksheet for budget requests for consumable supplies and expenses typically includes the required account number from the organization's uniform code of accounts, the item description, the item cost, and the total requested (Exhibits 8–4 and 8–5).

EXHIBIT 8–4

Sample Worksheet for Supplies and Other Expenses—Health Information Services

Department: Health Information Services

Fiscal Year: July 1–June 30

Account Code	Account Title: Item Description	Item Quantity	Item Cost	Total
610.2	Annual Professional Dues Paid for Department Head	—	$135.00	$135.00
610.7	Accrediting Agency Regulations Annual Update Subscription	1	90.00	90.00
610.4	Drug Usage Manual, Current Edition	4	28.00	112.00

EXHIBIT 8–5

Sample Worksheet for Supplies and Other Expenses—Physical Therapy

Department: Physical Therapy

Fiscal Year: July 1–June 30

Account Code	Account Title: Item Description	Item Quantity	Item Cost	Total
322.2	Ultrasound Gel	2	$20.00	$ 40.00
322.3	T.E.N.S. Pads	10	13.50	135.00
600.4	Four-Day Education Seminar	—	$140/day	$560.00

Notice that the budget worksheets reflect the totals for each line item. The manager retains the detailed calculations in a working file for reference during budget presentation and then for use during budget implementation. These working files contain levels of detail about specifications such as brand names, software details, discounts, and usual vendors. Examples of such detail include the following working file notations:

Books, Subscriptions, and Training Materials	$600.00
Audio Seminars for Training	300.00
Coding Update for Emergency Department Services	161.00

DRG FY 2007 Update	161.00
Hospital Outpatient Reporting Module	161.00
Non-physician Practitioner Services: Coding and Reporting	161.00

Obtain from AHIMA as authoritative source; also use discount by purchasing four at one time. The first three references are needed for coding and reimbursement update for the coming year; these three will need annual replacement. The fourth module is suitable for use over two or three years.

Maintenance and Repair

Cost allocations are made under this category to reflect both routine maintenance and occasional repairs. Two approaches to these arrangements are:

- The fee-for-service plan: payment is made for time and materials per service. The price may vary, usually by way of an increase, but this method may be cost-effective for equipment that is new and still under warranty. Newer equipment generally needs few if any repairs early in the life of the item.
- The service agreement: a contract, with fixed cost, is made with a service company. This agreement typically includes preventive maintenance as well as rapid on-call service. For departments having a mix of new and older equipment, such plans are cost-effective.

A mix of the two approaches is a third possibility. Cost comparisons of these approaches would provide the manager with a basis for decisions in this matter.

Specialty References and Licensure Software

A required line item is associated with the legal requirement to pay licensure fees for software packages. Specialty software is needed in most departments; the associated licensing fees are generally charged to the department. This is a line item that must be calculated in detail and may not be cut even when other expenditures must be reallocated. The budget justification document is the licensure software agreement, which specifies this obligation to pay a periodic fee for usage.

Specialty references (books, periodicals, and software) constitute another consideration for resource allocation. Certain references change from year to year, reflecting external agency requirements and practices. Examples include the latest interpretations of coding and reimbursement guidelines, accrediting standards, prescription drug references and compendia, and guidelines on certain aspects of clinical practice. This line item may total more than $2,000 but the cost savings are readily identifiable: these references are needed for the proper processing of mandated reimbursement practices. As with software licensure agreements, some of these costs cannot be omitted or reduced. These items are, of course, differentiated from other journal subscriptions, software, or references that, while highly desirable and convenient, are not absolutely necessary and could be cut should a financial emergency occur.

Staff Development

This set of line items reflects costs associated with staff development, including travel and training opportunities and material. Costs associated with travel are among the most vulnerable of line items. The manager should have a well-developed rationale for such expenditures; these costs should be linked to specific departmental and organizational goals, with their related projects. For example, attendance by the manager at a national meeting of a professional association provides the manager with opportunities to preview systems and equipment on a scale not available locally. Such a meeting may also provide critical updates concerning new mandates, as well as methods of complying with existing requirements such as accreditation, risk management, or reimbursement requirements. Specialty-oriented tutorials may be available at such events, providing the manager with updated skills that he or she can then teach to department staff. For example, a hospital may be planning to increase its observation unit capacity; the health information services must therefore be up to date in the coding and billing strategies under outpatient prospective payment. Attendance at a training session at a national meeting would pay dividends because of the resulting upgrade in coding and billing quality.

In developing travel budget estimates, the general policies of the organization are followed; for example, travel should be conducted by the most cost-effective means, with lodging and per diem limits specified.

As part of recruitment and retention of specialty staff, managers (with appropriate approval) sometimes offer a guaranteed amount of time and money for such travel. When such agreements have been entered into, that part of the travel cost is a given and may not be cut.

Examples of cost calculation associated with training, along with ideas for cost justification, are included in Chapter 11.

THE PERSONNEL BUDGET

The cost of personnel is typically the largest category of expense, accounting for as much as 85 percent of the total budget in many cases. Personnel costs include the wage and salary calculation for each position and for each worker, including anticipated raises (e.g., cost of living increases, merit increases) and adjustments resulting from a change in status (e.g., from probationary employee to full-time, permanent employee). The department manager normally calculates these costs; special justification for an increase in the number of positions or for adjustments to individual salaries or wages is also included.

Also calculated and justified by the department manager are those costs associated with vacation relief, overtime pay, temporary or seasonal help, and sign-on bonuses. Specific support information may be required for these budget requests, such as a calculation of the personnel hours required to give proper departmental coverage and a calculation of the hours not available to the organization because of vacation time and holidays. If there is a high employee turnover rate or a distinct pattern of absenteeism, historical information, such as the average time lost over the past year or several years as a result of these circumstances, may be cited as support information.

In calculating the costs for personnel needs, the manager deals with impersonal costs, that is, those associated with the position, regardless of the incumbent; such costs include the wage or salary range for the position and the number of full-time equivalent positions. In addition, there are other costs that are associated with the incumbent and change with the holder of the position; these costs include those associated with the number of hours scheduled for work each week, the number of years in the job category, the eligibility for merit increases, and the anniversary date for a scheduled increase in pay. The following factors must be considered in any budget calculation:

1. *Minimum Wage.* Federal and state laws mandate a base pay rate for certain jobs. Some categories of temporary help may be exempt from this wage; the manager must seek the guidance of the human resource specialist for details of this provision.

2. *Union Contract Stipulations.* Each class of job and each incumbent must be reviewed in light of contractual mandates for basic wage as well as mandatory increases. Where there is more than one contract in effect, the provisions of each contract must be reviewed and applied as appropriate. Wage and salary increases on a straight percentage basis may be mandated. In some cases, the contract may state that either a given percentage or a flat

dollar amount, whichever gives the greater increase, is to be awarded. A hiring rate may be indicated for employees on "new-hire" status; a related job rate may be indicated, with the employee moving to the job rate at the end of the probationary period (Table 8–1).

3. *Organizational Wage and Salary Scale.* Except for the specific provisions of union contracts, the organizational wage and salary scale applies. Positions are listed by job category or class, and the individual employee's rate is calculated from this scale. Increases may be in terms of a percentage or in terms of step increases dependent on the number of years in the position.

4. *Cost of Living Increase.* The organizational guidelines and/or contract provisions establish cost of living increases. Frequently, this amount is given as a flat percentage increase added to the base rate of pay, although it may be given as a flat dollar amount added to the base rate of pay.

5. *Area Wage and Salary Considerations.* Periodically, benchmark data are made available within a geographic region. Such data are generally developed by a chamber of commerce group, regional health care organizations, or labor unions, to reflect the market-basket costs of the region. Similar to overall cost of living calculations reflecting nationwide factors, these area wage and salary surveys drive the costs associated with hiring and retention of workers. These data are usually refined to reflect several variables: size and complexity of the health care organization; profit versus nonprofit enterprises; years on the job; specialty training and credentialing.

6. *Merit Raise or Bonus Pay.* These costs may be shown as an overall amount given to the department as a whole. The manager may not be able to assign dollar amounts to an individual worker at the beginning of a year, since the merit award may not be given until some time period has passed and the worker has earned the increase. Specific guidelines are given to the manager concerning the calculation of merit or bonus pay as part of the base rate of pay or as a one-time increase that does not become part of the employee's base rate of pay.

Table 8–1 Sample Salary Structure (Clerical)

Pay Grade	Hiring Rate (weekly)	Job Rate (90 calendar days)
B	$280	$300
C	$300	$316
D	$310	$342

7. *Special Adjustments.* From time to time, a special adjustment may be made to the wage or salary structure. An organization that is adjusting its wage and salary structure to satisfy Equal Employment Opportunity Commission (EEOC) mandates may grant a one-time adjustment to a class of workers or an individual (e.g., women and/or minority workers) to bring their rate of pay in line with other workers' pay scales. When long-term employees' rates of pay "shrink" as compared with those of incoming workers, a special one-time adjustment may be made to keep the comparative wages of new versus long-term employees equitable.

The budget worksheet and/or budget display sheet generally includes the following items, which progress logically from the factual information based on the present salary of the incumbents to the projected salary through the coming budget period.

1. Position code or grade code, obtained from the master position code sheet for the department and organization.
2. Position description: abbreviated job title or category.
3. Budgeted full-time equivalents (FTEs): the number of personnel hours per position divided by the hours per full-time workweek. Example (based on a 40-hour workweek):

   Worker A   40 hours
   Worker B   27 hours
   Worker C   20 hours
   Worker D   13 hours
           Total 100 hours = 2.5 FTEs

4. Employee number, usually assigned by personnel division or payroll division for identification of payroll costs and employee records.
5. Employee name: name of incumbent. If position is vacant, this information is noted.
6. Actual FTEs: number of employed workers and number of vacancies (see Exhibit 8–6 for an example of calculating FTEs in the health information department budget process).
7. Current rate of pay: hourly rate, biweekly rate, or job rate. The hourly rate is calculated by dividing the total salary by the number of work hours per budget period; the biweekly rate, by dividing the total salary by 26. The job rate is usually specified in the wage scale, especially as given in a union contract.

EXHIBIT 8-6

Calculating FTEs for Health Information Services

To calculate the number of employee hours needed to process the work in a given function, the manager first establishes the basic definition of a full-time equivalent position. This calculation is based on the usual workweek as defined by the facility:

one FTE = 40 hours/week
40 hours/week × 52 weeks = 2,080 hours/year

The hours needed may be concentrated in one full-time position or distributed between two or more part-time workers to total 2,080 hours/year. The latter method provides flexibility.

The second part of the staffing calculation consists of estimating the volume of work to be done.

Work standard: 24 minutes to process one chart
Volume per day: 30 charts needing DRG assignment
30 charts × 24 minutes = 720 minutes needed
One FTE - 480 minutes per work day

$$480)\overline{720.0} = 1.5$$

Needed: 1.5 FTE to process 30 discharge charts per day

8. Projected annual base salary, calculated by multiplying the rate by the appropriate unit of time. This projected salary is specific to the incumbent. Should the incumbent separate from the organization with the replacement worker hired at entry-level pay, the annual base salary would be lower.

9. Incumbent's anniversary date, used to calculate cost of living or other raise associated with date of employment.

10. Projected annual increase because of cost of living increase, merit or bonus pay, or special adjustments.

11. Projected total salary: present salary plus projected annual increase.

Example:

Grade Code	4
Position Title	Compliance Specialist
Shift	Full-time, day
Incumbent	M. Caretto
Current Biweekly Pay	$1,412
Projected Annual Base	$36,700
Anniversary Date	12-20-07
Projected Annual Increase	$1,800
Projected Total Salary	$38,500
Hours Per Pay Period (biweekly)	80

DIRECT AND INDIRECT EXPENSES

A department budget also reflects costs under the categories of direct and indirect expenses. Direct expenses typically include salaries, services and contracts, dues and subscriptions, and equipment. Indirect expenses are charged to the departmental budget on a formula basis or some process of assessment. These indirect costs are associated with the organization as a whole and are prorated per department. Examples of indirect costs and their units of assessment are shown in Table 8–2.

Table 8–2   Indirect Expenses Charged to Health Information Services

Item	Amount	Basis of Calculation
Fringe benefits/health and welfare	$156,000	Percentage of salaries
Equipment depreciation	30,000	Depreciation schedule
Telephone costs (equipment)	8,000	Number of telephones
Maintenance and repairs	2,300	Number of work orders
Physical plant operation (e.g., heat, A/C)	42,000	Number of square feet
Building depreciation	6,000	Number of square feet

BUDGET JUSTIFICATION

As mentioned earlier, support or explanatory documentation may be required for budget requests. If a particular type of equipment is requested, the manager is expected to explain why that particular model or brand is needed. The reasons may include compatibility with existing equipment, guaranteed service contracts, availability, or durability. Projected patient usage is another element of support data; the acquisition of a particular item may enhance patient care because of its safety features or it may attract more patients to the facility.

Sometimes the facility may need an item simply to remain competitive and thereby retain a given patient population. The budget justification may take the form of a cost comparison, such as that between rental/long-term lease of equipment and outright purchase plus maintenance costs. For a health information department, a cost comparison between an in-house word processing/transcription unit and a contractual service might be included.

The Budget Cut

When financial exigencies warrant a budget adjustment, either in the form of a partial reduction in a line item or category or the elimination of an entire expenditure, the manager uses the budget justification details to guide this process. Certain items cannot be cut (e.g., software licensure agreements, sign-on bonuses promised to specific employees). The manager looks to those categories of planned overage to determine what items to reduce or cut. For example, desired staff training programs may be best accomplished by sending workers off-site, but adequate programs could be developed by the management staff and offered at substantial savings.

Similarly, bulk purchases (for example, three years' worth of file folders) could be cut back to one year at a time. The discount for the bulk purchase rate might be lost, but in a tight budget situation of a given year, this more limited expenditure might be necessary to meet the "bottom line." Another option might be available from wage and salary lines: a manager could delay hiring a replacement when a vacancy occurs. The wage and fringe benefit amount could be used to pay for a temporary/contractual worker. By delaying the hire of the new full-time worker until the next fiscal year, the pay increase is also saved. Alternatively, the manager could fill the position immediately, but at an entry-level pay grade.

Cost Comparison

Budget justification also includes cost comparison. One example would be that of comparing costs of in-house or commercial storage of patient records. A sample worksheet for this type of cost comparison is shown in Exhibit 8–7. This type of information would also be the basis for Requests for Proposals (RFPs) when the selection process is implemented.

BUDGET VARIANCES

During the fiscal year, the manager receives periodic reports showing budgeted amounts versus amounts spent. This report may categorize such information under the headings of "over budget" or "under budget" for the period and for the year. The manager uses this information as a monitoring and control device. A particular unit's budget may include money for overtime that is assigned arbitrarily to budget quarters. A periodic report may show that the manager was over budget in that category for the quarter but not for the year. Such a report is an internal warning system that alerts the manager to that line item. Filed with higher-level management, the variance report reflects the manager's awareness of the expenditure for the quarter and its relationship to the yearly amount as a whole. Should there be some unexpected cause for utilizing these overtime funds, such as high absenteeism because of employee illness or injury, this information is noted in the variance report.

Under-budget indicators require similar explanations as part of the control process in budgeting. Explanations for under-budget items are not required in every instance, but particular attention must be given to large sums that have not been spent because of delay factors in the outside environment. For example, the purchase of a large, expensive piece of equipment may be included in the budget for the fiscal year. If it is not available until the next fiscal year, the delay could throw a carefully planned budget out of balance; that is, funds are not expended in one year, and no funds are allotted for this purchase in the upcoming budget. The manager should anticipate such a situation and make arrangements for the transfer of funds in a timely way.

Direct patient care service budgets include projections of care to be rendered. Actual revenue generated per patient visit is compared with projected revenue. The explanations—over- or under-projections of care to be rendered—are made by the budget officer for the service. If patient care services are below those projected, plans for increasing services may be included with the explanation.

Example of Variance Analysis

Exhibit 8–8 displays a year-to-date summary of expenditures. The fiscal year in this sample runs from July through June. This report reflects year-to-date costs as

EXHIBIT 8–7

Worksheet for Comparison of Storage Options

Factors	In-House Hard Copy	Commercial Storage Hard Copy
Personnel		
• labor costs		
• training		
Equipment and supplies		
• camera		
• processing equipment		
• supplies		
Physical space		
• for equipment		
• for processing		
• for temporary holding		
• for permanent holding		
Availability of data/records		
• during processing		
• after processing		
• access time		
—STAT/emergency		
—readmission		
—administrative use		
• additional cost for special access		
Custom features		
• not allowed		
• done at additional cost		
Project completion time		
Confidentiality		
• during processing		
• after processing		
Bonded/insured		
HIPAA compliant		
Authentication certificate provided		
Certificate of destruction		
Quality controls		
Volume discounts		
Total cost per year of retention		

EXHIBIT 8–8

Summary of Expenditures, Year-to-Date

Cost Center 234

Object Code	Supplies	Budgeted	Actual	Over/under
021	Printed forms, stationery, office supplies: Vendors	51,999.00	50,000.00	1,999.00
026	Books	400.00	304.80	95.00
027	Journals and magazine subscriptions	620.00	754.00	(134.00–)
028	General stores, supplies—internal	2,400.00	1,987.00	413.00
035	Parking	-0-	30.00	(30.00–)
044	Travel	1,700.00	1,483.00	217.00
051	Film rental	-0-	42.00	(42.00–)
	Supplies—subtotal	57,119.00	54,600.80	2,518.00
Object Code	**Services**			
122	Contractual temps	850.00	600.00	250.00
131	Equipment rental	2,000.00	1,811.00	189.00
134	Outside contractual service	5,000.00	3,750.00	1,250.00
136	Equipment repair contracts	380.00	31.60	348.40
138	Computer license agreement	12,000.00	9,000.00	3,000.00
	Services—subtotal	20,230.00	13,192.60	5,037.40

posted through April 30, the close of the third quarter. The department manager reviews these figures to:

1. Verify accuracy of posting (making sure costs are posted and none are omitted due to error). The department daily ledgers are compared to this official listing prepared by the finance office.
2. Review specific object codes where the actual costs exceed the approved budgeted amounts. An item may be over budget for the period but not for the year. The manager would note these and prepare explanations.

3. Review specific object codes where actual costs are below the approved budgeted amounts. If the allotted money is not going to be spent in the approved category, the manager may seek approval to use these funds for some other need. Particular attention is given to an under-budget category in which a major expense has been, or soon will be, incurred but which has not yet been posted. Object code 138, Computer License Agreement, reflects a major cost yet to be posted—namely, the fourth-quarter payment.

THE GENERAL AUDIT

Through the related processes of posting entries to the proper line items, monitoring variances and explaining their causes, and tracking each item from its budgeted approval entry through its actual expenditure, the manager has developed an audit trail. The required forms, documentation, and approvals for actual expenditures all dovetail with these practices to provide sound control over the financial resources. The department manager will usually carry out periodic partial audits during the fiscal year, and both internal and external auditors will carry out a full audit at least once during the year.

Examples of such audit practices include the prevention of "ghost employees" or "ghost patients"—every employee will be clearly identified as to job title, hours worked (payroll data), and paycheck issued and processed. In some organizations, all employees must sign in person for paychecks on a random or regular basis to prevent such potential fraud. The audit trail of a given patient is easily tracked: the master patient index provides name and other identifying information; a complete and accurate patient care document should match this; names of care providers are matched against provider rosters; billing records are matched against the documentation of the care.

Similarly, expenses relating to purchases of equipment can be tracked by noting the purchase requisition, the installation date, the actual location of the equipment at the time of the audit, and the appropriate entries in the equipment inventory.

The Audit Committee

Such a committee is formed to assist the board of trustees in fulfilling its oversight responsibilities. This committee monitors the integrity of the organization's financial statements and its compliance with legal and regulatory requirements (e.g., the Centers for Medicare and Medicaid payment/fraud controls) and works with independent outside auditors. The committee also reviews and monitors compliance with ethical codes for senior financial officers, chief executive officers, and department managers. The organizational values of integrity and stewardship are promoted through such ongoing activities, closing the loop from plan through execution, with each step properly documented.

EXERCISE: ADJUSTING THE BUDGET

Review the information presented below in the Sample Operating Budget—Department of Physical Therapy and adjust this budget according to the following:

- You have just learned that inpatient charges will probably be 3 percent higher than projected and that outpatient charges are expected to increase by 8 percent, and that your research grant support will be reduced by half.
- The continuing education conference projected to net $3,200 has been canceled.
- Salary expenses will likely be 2 percent higher than originally anticipated.
- You are required to show a projected net profit of at least 50 percent of total revenue. If your revised budget generates less than this level of net profit or surplus, indicate where you can probably cut expenses to meet the target and explain why the expenses you have chosen to cut are your best choices.

SAMPLE OPERATING BUDGET— DEPARTMENT OF PHYSICAL THERAPY

(July 1, 2007, through June 30, 2008)

I. Revenue and Income

A. Inpatient Charges	$550,000
B. Outpatient Charges	310,000
C. Research Grant Support	29,000
D. Continuing Education Conference	3,200
E. Supplies and Equipment Sales	11,500
Total Revenue	$903,700

II. Expenses

Direct Expenses

A. Salaries	$260,000
B. Consultant	2,500

C. Honorarium	1,500
D. Minor Equipment	6,000
E. Equipment Rental	2,000
F. Travel	2,500
G. Telephone	5,000
H. Supplies	6,000
I. Postage	350
J. Copy Machine Rental	11,000
K. Advertisement	1,500
L. Dues	800
M. Books	350
N. Equipment Maintenance and Service Contracts	2,000
Total Direct Expenses	$301,500
Indirect Expenses	
A. Employee Benefits (23%)	$59,800
B. Administration	23,000
C. Equipment Depreciation	7,200
D. Physical Plant Operation	39,000
E. Maintenance and Repairs	2,000
F. Building Depreciation	6,000
G. Laundry/Linen	2,500
H. Housekeeping	4,900
Total Indirect Expenses	$144,400
Total Expenses	$445,900
Net Profit or Loss	$457,800

EXERCISE: BELT-TIGHTENING—MORE BUDGET ADJUSTMENTS

Answer the following questions using the Health Information Department Budget furnished below, specifically the data included in Table 8–3:

1. What would be the dollar impact if the 5 percent increase planned for January 1 were reduced to 3.5 percent and postponed until April 1?
2. As an alternate cost-saving strategy, determine the annual savings if all hourly staff were reduced from 40 to 37.5 hours as their standard workweek.

Consider the top three staff—director, compliance specialist, and registries coordinator—as salaried and thus unaffected by the workweek change.

3. Determine the total dollar impact if both of the foregoing strategies were implemented together. Remember that the pay increase affects everyone, but the 37.5-hour week affects just hourly staff.

SAMPLE HEALTH INFORMATION DEPARTMENT BUDGET

This budget is based on the following premises:

1. Fiscal year: July 1 through June 30
2. Workweek: 40 hours/week; 2,080 hours/year per FTE
3. Cost of living increase: 5 percent of current base rate (see Table 8–3 for detailed cost of living calculations by position title)
4. Effective date of cost of living increase: January 1
5. Overtime rate: time and a half, based on current base for employee
6. Holiday pay: regular base rate (for employees who work on a scheduled holiday: double time, calculated on current base for each employee)
7. Temporary agency rate: average rate is $13/hr. for clerical worker, no fringe benefits given
8. Sick pay: calculated on each employee's current base
9. Fringe benefits: 29 percent of total wages and salaries for the department; 29 percent for each individual employee
10. Wage and salary calculations are displayed to show these details:

Factor	Example
Current annual base	$58,000
July–December of current calendar year—total earnings	29,000
January 1 cost of living increase (5%)	2,900
New annual base effective January 1	60,900
January–June of coming calendar year—total earnings	30,450
Total needed for full 12-month period of the fiscal year	29,000
	+ 30,450
	59,450

Table 8–3 Wages and Salaries by Position Title

	Current Base	July Through December	January 1 5% Increase	New Base	January Through June	Total For Fiscal Year
Director	75,000	37,500	3,750	78,750	39,375	76,875
Compliance Specialist	42,000	21,000	2,100	44,100	22,050	43,050
Registries Coordinator	42,000	21,000	2,100	44,100	22,050	43,050
Coder	32,000	16,000	1,600	33,600	16,800	32,800
Coder	30,000	15,000	1,500	31,500	15,750	30,750
Billing Compliance Specialist	29,120	14,560	1,456	30,576	15,288	29,848
Release of Information Specialist	25,000	12,500	1,250	26,250	13,125	25,625
Secretary	20,800	10,400	1,040	21,840	10,920	21,320
Medical Transcriptionist	27,040	13,520	1,352	28,392	14,196	27,716
Medical Transcriptionist	26,000	13,000	1,300	27,300	13,650	26,650
Medical Transcriptionist	22,000	11,000	1,100	23,100	11,550	22,550
Release of Information Clerk	18,100	9,050	905	19,005	9,505	18,555
Registries Specialist	25,000	12,500	1,250	26,250	13,125	25,625
Medical Record Specialist II	19,400	9,700	970	20,370	10,185	19,885
Medical Record Specialist I	17,000	8,500	850	17,850	8,925	17,425

Note: These figures are examples only. Actual rates will vary geographically and over time.

Health Information Department Budget

Personnel Costs

Object Code		
01	Wages and Salaries	$461,724.00
02	Fringe Benefits	133,900.00
03	Vacation Relief Coverage	2,000.00
04	Sign-on Bonuses	10,000.00
	Subtotal A	$607,624.00

Equipment

Object Code

	10 office chairs (6 at $128 each)	$768.00
	Automatic paper shredder	429.00
	Stepstools (3 at $59 each)	177.00
	Multi-terminal word-processing system	74,000.00
	Subtotal B	$75,374.00

Supplies

Object Code

021	Printed Forms, Stationery, Office Supplies: Vendors	$51,999.00
026	Books	1,000.00
027	Journals and Magazine Subscriptions	1,620.00
028	General Stores Supplies—Internal	3,400.00
035	Parking	-0-
044	Travel	1,700.00
051	Film Rental	-0-
	Subtotal C	$59,719

Services

Object Code

122	Contractual Temporaries	1,850.00
131	Equipment Rental	2,000.00
134	Outside Contractual Service	5,000.00
136	Equipment Repair Contracts	2,000.00
138	Computer License Agreement	32,000.00
	Subtotal D	$42,850.00

Cost Transfers

Object Code

150	Telephone	$3,840.00
151	Work Orders	-0-
152	Postage	360.00
153	Photocopy/Print Shop	200.00
154	TV-VCR Rental	-0-
158	Dietary	560.00
	Subtotal E	$4,960.00

Summary

Personnel Costs	$607,624.00
Equipment	75,374.00
Supplies	59,719.00
Services	42,850.00
Cost Transfers	4,960.00
Total	$790,527.00

Committees and Teams

CHAPTER OBJECTIVES

- Provide a generalized definition of a committee.
- Differentiate among committees, standing as well as ad hoc, and plural executives and task forces.
- Describe the generally accepted purposes and uses of committees.
- Enumerate the advantages as well as the limitations and disadvantages of committees.
- Provide guidelines for ensuring committee effectiveness.
- Identify the role and functions of the committee chairperson.
- Provide guidance for creating and preserving documentation of a committee's formal proceedings.
- Examine the modern management phenomenon of the employee team (in a number of possible forms) as a special case of the committee.

Committees have become a fact of life in modern organizations. The democratic tradition in American society, the committee system's history of success in organizations, and the legal and accrediting authority mandates for such activity contribute to the widespread use of committees in health care organizations. Committee participation is an expected part of the daily routine of the chief of service, department head, or manager. The committee structure complements the overall organizational structure, because it can be used to overcome problems stemming from specialization and departmentation. The weakness of specialization is the potential loss of broad organizational vision on the part of the individual manager; however, coordination of action and assessment of the overall organizational impact of a decision may be facilitated when a committee brings together a number of specialists for organized deliberation.

Health care organizations need committees to help consolidate the dual authority tracks within the medical authority structure and the administrative/support structure. The joint conference committee, consisting of representatives from the medical staff, the board of trustees, and the administration, is commonly used for this purpose. Functions of health care organizations typically monitored and assessed by committees include pharmacy and therapeutics, infection control, patient care evaluation, surgical case review, medical records, quality assurance, and utilization review. Table 9–1 summarizes typical committee participation by various health care professionals.

THE NATURE OF COMMITTEES

A committee may be defined as a group of persons in an organization who function collectively on an organized basis to perform some administrative activity. A committee is more than an informal group that meets to discuss an issue and share ideas, even if such a group meets regularly. The manager who informally calls together a team of subordinates or other managers to talk over an idea or problem is not dealing with a committee. The emphasis in the committee concept is the creation of a structure that has an organized basis for its activity and interaction and that is

Table 9–1 Examples of Committee Participation

Department Head	Utilization Review	Clinical Documentation	Risk Management	Quality Assurance
Occupational Therapy	*	*	X	X
Physical Therapy	*	*	X	X
Medical Technology		*	X	X
Dietary	*	X	X	X
Health Records	*	X	X	X
Nursing	X	X	X	X
Social Service	X	X	*	X

* = rotating membership with other department heads; X = permanent ex officio membership.

accountable for its function. The predominant characteristic of the committee is group deliberation on a recurring basis done in the context of a specific grant of authority.

Committees may be temporary or permanent. The temporary, or ad hoc, committee is created to deal with one issue, such as the implementation of the problem-oriented medical record or cost-containment compliance, and its work is limited to that issue. If the problem assigned to an ad hoc committee becomes a recurring one, it may be handled by an existing committee, it may be referred to an existing department, or a new standing committee may be created to deal with it.

Standing committees, which are relatively permanent, focus on recurring matters. The individual members change, but the committee is continuing with respect to the number of members, the distribution of representatives, and its basic charge. Typical standing committees in health care organizations include those responsible for dealing with credentials, infection control, patient care policies, medical records, and quality assurance. A department may have specific standing committees, such as departmental quality assurance, safety control, or professional development committees.

A committee may have either line or staff authority. If the committee has authority to bind subordinates who are responsible to it, it is part of the line unit structure. For example, a governing board may have an executive committee that gives directives to the chief executive officer of the institution and thus exercises line authority. A grievance committee, whose decision is binding because of a policy or union contract, exercises line authority in producing its determinations; managers are not free to act contrary to such decisions. If, on the other hand, the committee has an advisory relationship to line managers, it is a staff unit.

In actual practice, the distinction between line and staff authority of a committee is sometimes blurred. A credentials committee of the medical staff may have limited line authority in that, except for unusual cases, the next levels of authority are bound by the recommendations it makes. A union contract governing faculty at a medical school or university may require that a faculty committee review each case of promotion and tenure and make a recommendation to the line officer, the dean, who in turn must add a recommendation, with the final decision made by the board of trustees. Participation in the decision process by several layers in the hierarchy is mandatory in such cases. In that sense, the credentials committee of the medical staff, as well as the promotion and tenure committee of a college, may be viewed as a line committee with limited but explicit input into decisions concerning professional colleagues. Their decisions are not final, but their recommendations are well protected by custom and, in some cases, by law.

The Plural Executive

Although most committees are nonmanagerial in nature, there is a structural variation in which a committee is created that has line authority and undertakes some or all of the traditional functions of a manager. These committees are created as a result of policy decisions. A familiar example in the health care setting is the executive board of a national professional association. Established through the bylaws of the organization, the executive board typically consists of the elected officers and has the authority to act on behalf of the membership in prescribed areas. The board of trustees in a hospital is also a plural executive, although it is almost universal practice to appoint a chief executive officer and assign management functions to that officer.

The plural executive may be established by law, as in federal regulatory agencies (e.g., the Federal Communications Commission and the Securities and Exchange Commission). The law creating such agencies stipulates that there be a regulatory board (usually) of 5 to 11 members who have line authority as a board. The board varies greatly in the amount of power held and authority exercised. Although the board has formal authority, the center of true power in the organization may shift from the executive board to the appointed chief executive officer, who reports to the executive board.

The individual officeholders who constitute the plural executive must rely greatly on an appointed officer, such as the executive director, and on the staff chosen by that officer. While the executive officer is in a continuing position, the plural executive group may meet infrequently, and its membership may change as frequently as every year. Furthermore, the members of the plural executive unit tend to remain less visible, as they give directives to the executive, who issues these under the office's title. This common practice often obscures the authority constellation proper to the plural executive and may even reduce it to one of symbolic rather than actual authority and power.

The Task Force

A temporary organizational unit, the task force is created to carry out a specific project or assignment and present its findings to some person or committee that has line authority. It has as its focus highly specific work that requires technical expertise. The task force analyzes the question, completes the research, and makes its recommendations, which may take the form of a complete plan of action. Unlike committees, which remain in existence until specifically dissolved, the task force automatically ceases functioning when its assigned task is completed.

Members of a task force are chosen on the basis of technical competence and specialized training to form a composite, interdisciplinary team. They are not selected to represent a special group interest, and not every department or organizational unit is represented. A task force rarely, if ever, has line authority. Its findings sometimes are referred to a committee that deliberates issues of a basic policy nature; the work of the task force complements that of committees by providing technical research and preparing background information. The group may be created as a result of committee deliberations; for example, the executive committee or the board of trustees of a health care institution may wish to expand its services or to develop an entirely new physical complex. These technical problems could be referred to a task force for study; when the work of the task force is done, the executive committee or board takes appropriate action.

A task force sometimes is created for its symbolic value—a common political use. The various presidential commissions of the past decades are examples of the use of task forces to call attention to an important issue (e.g., civil rights, space technology, and care of the aged). In order to provide an arena that is relatively free from vested interests and particular biases, a task force rather than an administrative agency or department personnel may be assigned the responsibility of studying an issue.

THE PURPOSES AND USES OF COMMITTEES

Committees are created to fulfill various specific needs. The following purposes and uses of committees include the advantages that accrue to an organization as a result of effective committee structure development.

To Gain the Advantage of Group Deliberation

Many management problems are so complex that their impact on the organization as a whole is best assessed through group deliberation and decision making. Decisions may have a long-range effect, and no single manager has the knowledge necessary to see all the ramifications of a problem. In a committee structure, no one manager bears the burden of a decision that will have far-reaching consequences. Probing of the facts and their implications is likely to be more thorough if the knowledge, experience, and judgment of several individuals are brought to bear on the problem in a coordinated manner. The stimulation of shared thinking may lead to a better decision than could be reached by an individual. Finally, group deliberations may be mandatory in some organizations because of the stipulations in a union contract, an accrediting agency, or a regulatory body.

To Offset Decentralization and Consolidate Authority

In the process of organizing, each manager is given only a portion of the organization's authority. Normally, each manager receives sufficient authority to carry out the responsibilities of the branch or unit of the organization over which that individual has charge. When the organizational structure is consolidated, efforts are made to avoid splintered authority. Yet, because of the limits placed on the manager's authority, not every problem a manager faces can be solved, nor every plan implemented. It is necessary to consolidate organizational authority through specific coordinating efforts, and committees provide an additional organizational structure that can be used for this purpose.

The creation of a special purpose committee to deal with a project or problem involving several units of an institution is an acceptable means of augmenting the normal organizational structure. If the problem is a recurring one, the structure itself should be adjusted to consolidate authority in a formal manner. For nonrecurring special problems, however, special-purpose committees are appropriate.

Coordination among units in a highly decentralized organization may be fostered through committees. The focus under these circumstances is on the need for consistency of action and coordination of detailed plans among several units, which are often separated geographically. The statewide health coordinating committee in health care planning is an example of a committee created specifically for the purpose of coordinating activity among units with wide geographical distribution and multiple categories of membership.

To Counterbalance Authority

The check-and-balance system in an organization is subject to many pressures. When individuals in decentralized locations surrender authority to higher levels in the hierarchy, there is an attendant desire to monitor those higher levels. For example, in order to avoid a concentration of power in an executive director, a professional organization or a union with nationwide membership may create an executive committee with power to finalize all decisions, to approve the budget and authorize payments over a stated amount, and to act as sole decision-making body in many areas.

In a situation in which there has been significant fraud or deception or extreme authoritarianism, an officer may be retained temporarily to avoid a public scandal that would have negative effects for the organization. To limit the actions of such an individual during the transition period, the authority of the office is stripped away and placed in a special group that acts as a line committee in place of the official, who retains only the title and selected symbols of office. This committee functions until the officer is safely removed in a politically acceptable manner and a successor is chosen. The committee structure can be costly in economic terms, but an organization may be willing to pay the price to offset concentrated power and to obtain a diffused authority pattern in certain circumstances.

To Provide Representation of Interest Groups

Occasionally, certain groups have a vested interest in an organization and seek representation in its decision-making arenas, including committee participation. Wanting to protect the value of their degrees, alumni of a college seek positions on the board of trustees or on advisory committees to specific programs. Community members concerned with both long- and short-range plans of a health care organization seek input into patient care policies and community health programs through committee participation.

The organization, in turn, is interested in obtaining the support of specific groups and extends to them an opportunity to participate in its deliberations, often through the committee structure. A college may seek alumni representation to consolidate financial support from that group. A hospital or health center may seek community representatives for its advisory committee so that it can better determine local sentiment, assess probable responses to changes in the pattern of services offered, gain tangible financial support, and create goodwill toward the institution.

To Protect Due Process

In disciplinary matters, an organization may seek to reflect the larger societal value of due process, even when there is no legal or contractual requirement to do so. An increase in litigation has added an almost legal flavor to processes in which an individual's performance is evaluated. A committee of the individual's peers, even if the peer group does not have line authority, may be constituted to make a recommendation to the line officer or governing board. Examples of this approach include the promotion and tenure committee of a university, the ethics committee of a professional association, or the credentials committee of a medical staff. A union contract may specify the composition and function of a grievance committee to ensure that it includes line workers as well as management officials.

To Promote Coordination and Cooperation

When individuals affected by a decision have participated in making that decision, they are more likely to accept it and abide by it. Participants in group deliberations develop a fuller understanding of each unit's role. The communication process is facilitated, since the managers affected by the decision have had an opportunity to present their positions, the constraints under which their departments function, and their special needs, as well as to express disagreements. All members can evaluate the overall plan, review their own functions, and become familiar with the tasks assigned to other units that depend on their unit's output or, in turn, constrain the work assigned to their unit. In its final decision or recommendation, the committee states the assignments for each unit, and these are known to all. This is especially valuable when the success of the work depends on the full understanding and acceptance of the decision and plan of execution.

To Avoid Action

A manager who wishes to avoid or postpone an action indefinitely may create a committee to study the question or may refer it to a panel that has a long agenda and sends its findings to yet another committee for action. If members are selected carefully or if the assignment to an existing committee is made strategically, action will be slow. The issue may die for lack of interest or may become moot because of a decision made in some other arena or because of the departure from the organization of the individuals concerned. Although this intentional delaying tactic can be misused by a manager, it may also be a positive strategy; for example, delay through committee deliberation may be a form of "buying" time for issues to become less emotionally charged.

To Train Members

Committee participation may be used as part of the executive training process. Exposure to multiple facets of a decision, the defense of various positions, and the development of insight into the problems and considerations of other managers' decisions are part of this training experience. The potential manager is assessed by other members of the executive team during this interaction, and appropriate coaching and counseling may be given to the management trainee.

LIMITATIONS AND DISADVANTAGES OF COMMITTEES

Humorous and disparaging comments sometimes reflect the limitations and disadvantages of committee use: "A camel is a horse that was designed by a committee," or "There are no great individuals in this organization, only great committees."

Committee interaction, with its emphasis on deliberation and group participation, is slow. The committee structure, therefore, is not the proper arena for making decisions that must be made quickly. The time consumed, including the hours spent in formal meetings, is also costly. In highly decentralized organizations or professional associations, travel and lodging costs alone may run well into the thousands of dollars for a meeting of only a few members. The cost of an individual member's attendance (separate from travel and related costs) is calculated by establishing an average hourly rate per member and multiplying the meeting time by this rate. For example, an executive committee in which ten department heads participate meets a minimum of two hours once a week. Their salaries are calculated and an hourly rate obtained. At an average of $50 per hour per member, a typical meeting of such a group costs at least $1,250, not including preparation, follow-up time, or the cost of staff support and services. The results of committee action should offset the costs in time, money, and overall effort.

Because of time pressures, committee deliberations may be cut short, thus removing the major advantages of the committee structure (i.e., group participation and presentation of multiple viewpoints). The committee may be indecisive because there is insufficient time to deliberate, or the discussion may become vague and tangential, leading to adjournment without action. Members' lack of preparation prevents full discussion of issues. Being present and on time is only part of a committee member's responsibility; member preparation is a critical factor.

There are several pitfalls to be avoided in regard to preparation. Material may be prepared and distributed in a timely manner, but the committee members may fail to brief themselves prior to the meeting. A member of a subcommittee may fail to carry out an assignment that is critical for the panel's further action. Staff aides or the chairperson may be late in preparing items so that committee members arrive to find large quantities of critical material at their places and are expected to reach decisions without the time to develop an informed opinion.

Absenteeism or tardiness may obstruct the committee's work. If a quorum is required, absence or lateness (or early departure) of several members may upset the critical balance. When the discussion of an agenda item is dependent on a particular member's presence, this part of the meeting must be delayed or postponed if that member is absent or late. Furthermore, time spent waiting for members to arrive to provide a quorum or to discuss a particular agenda item generates cost with no offsetting productivity.

Obstructionist behavior in committee meetings can limit debate. On the one hand, a member who continually declines to give an opinion and who continually votes "abstain" muddies the outcome. The committee may be seen as lacking in decisiveness, and its recommendations may be set aside more easily. On the other hand, an individual or a few members may try to dominate the committee. When unanimity or at least major consensus is required, such members may refuse to give in or may insist on their own suggestions for compromise. The committee, in order to act, must accept this dominance by a few. A ready solution to this problem is the encouragement of minority reports. Some open discussion of group dynamics may also foster solutions to this type of roadblock.

Even with much goodwill and a high degree of commitment on the part of members, certain aspects of committee dynamics tend to limit the group's effectiveness. In seeking common ground for agreement and in dealing with small group pressures to be polite and maintain mutual respect, diluted decisions or compromise to the point of the least common denominator may characterize committee decisions.

Furthermore, a committee never can take the place of individual managers who accept specific responsibilities and exhibit leadership. Managers must accept the responsibility for certain decisions, even when they are unpopular. It may be especially important to have a specific individual held responsible for decisions in conflict situations. The proverbial buck stops at the highest level of officers, and one manager must be the first among equals when it is a decision in that manager's area of jurisdiction.

ENHANCEMENT OF COMMITTEE EFFECTIVENESS

Committees, in spite of their limitations, are valuable for organizational deliberations. Their effectiveness may be enhanced by

- viewing committee activity as important and legitimate
- providing the necessary logistical support

- assigning clear-cut responsibilities and specific functions to the committee
- considering committee size, composition, and selection of members carefully
- selecting the committee chairperson carefully
- maintaining adequate documentation and follow-up activity
- creating task forces as an alternative to the proliferation of committees
- ensuring that members are sensitive to group dynamics and organizational conflict

Legitimization of Committee Activity

The top management of an organization must create a climate in which the work of committee members is valued. The evaluation system for merit raises and promotions should include the assessment of individuals' work on committee assignments. Committee membership should be viewed positively by members rather than merely tolerated as a duty. Job descriptions should include committee assignment as a necessary component of the work. When staffing patterns are established, work hours should be allotted for essential committee participation. Committee structure should be streamlined so that action is purposeful and members can see the results of their work. Training specifically for effective committee involvement should be part of the overall training program for members rather than left to chance.

Logistical Support

All necessary staff assistance should be given to the committee chairperson and members. Staff assistants may prepare specific material, devise research questions, gather necessary support data, and carry out follow-up activities. Clerical support should be provided for recording and transcribing minutes and related documents. Adequate space should be made available for meetings. Top management may enhance committee workings by requiring that committee meetings be scheduled regularly and that membership be drawn from several organizational components. Setting aside a certain block of time for interdepartmental meetings and proscribing intradepartmental sessions during that period facilitates the coordination of schedules. If it is deemed preferable, committee meetings may be scheduled for longer periods of time at less frequent intervals.

Scope, Function, and Authority

When a committee is created, its purpose and function, as well as its scope of activity, must be presented clearly. Will its purpose be merely to deliberate? Will it deliberate and make a recommendation, or will its decision be a binding one? What subjects will it consider? For example, will the medical care evaluation committee concern itself only with assessments of the topics of quality assurance that are mandated by outside review agencies, or will it expand its function to organization-wide quality assurance and education? Will utilization review remain a separate function? Will the health information committee focus only on the records of inpatients or on the records of all patients who receive care in the institution regardless of patient category (e.g., inpatient, outpatient, group practice)?

The scope of the committee's work is shaped by its authority. If the credentials committee of the medical staff only makes recommendations to the governing board, while the board retains final authority to make staff appointments, this should be stated in the bylaws creating the panel and setting forth its mandates. The committee's accountability also needs delineation. To whom does it make its reports? How frequently? Is coordination required with certain administrative components or with other committees?

Committee Size and Composition

No absolute figure can be given as the optimum size of a committee. Since open, free deliberation is a major reason for a committee, the size of the group should be small enough to permit discussion. On the other hand, it should be large enough to represent various interests. The organization's bylaws and charter may stipulate required committee composition, which, in turn, will affect a committee's size. Some hospital policies, for example, state that all chiefs of service are members of the executive committee; therefore, the size of the committee is determined by the organization's department structure.

The need for a quorum to undertake official committee action presents special problems if members' schedules simply do not allow them to attend meetings on a predictable basis. Committee size may be increased in order to ensure a quorum so that business may be conducted.

Committee composition is one of the most important factors in the success of a group's work. Whether they volunteer, are appointed, or are elected, members should possess certain personal qualities; they should be able to

- express themselves in a group
- keep to the point
- discuss issues in a practical rather than theoretical way
- give information that advances the thinking of the group about the topic rather than about themselves
- assess a topic in an orderly yet flexible way

- suppress the natural desire to speak for the sake of being heard or of saying what they think the leader or some powerful member wants to hear

The members also should have sufficient authority to commit the unit or group that they represent to the course of action adopted by the committee. If an individual is appointed to a committee to represent a busy executive, that person should have the power to cast a vote that binds the executive who deputized the member. Deputizing is not without its hazards, but they may be avoided by careful review and discussion between the executive and the representative before the meeting.

Generally, committee members should be of approximately equal rank and status in the organization in order to permit the free exchange of ideas. The presence of ex officio members, who may be viewed as more powerful than the elected members, may deter free discussion. Individuals who attend meetings as staff assistants should respect the limits placed on their participation. There should be a clear understanding that the duties of secretary of the committee are those of the individual appointed or elected from within the group; other persons present to carry out the clerical aspects of secretarial work, such as taking down the raw proceedings from which minutes will be extracted, should not be asked to participate in the discussion and should not volunteer information or opinions as they are not official members. If a parliamentarian who is not a member of the committee attends the meetings, this individual should confine any interaction with the committee to points of parliamentary procedure and should withhold all opinions, agreements, and disagreements concerning the issues under discussion. A group that appoints or elects a committee should have confidence that only those individuals duly appointed or elected will make decisions and recommendations on its behalf.

While diverse points of view should be represented in deliberations, not every participant must be a full-time committee member. Individuals can be invited to attend a meeting or a portion of one in order to answer questions from the committee, share information, or present a point of view. Like staff assistants, individuals who attend meetings as guests should respect the limits of their participation.

In summary, committee size and composition are matters of individual organizational determination. Committees should be large enough to represent various interest groups and ensure adequate group deliberation, but small enough to ensure that the deliberation will be effective.

Periodic Review of Committee Purpose and Function

There is an occasionally encountered phenomenon experienced by some committees, primarily standing committees, although even ad hoc committees are not totally immune. That phenomenon is the tendency of some committees to remain in place, meeting regularly and cranking out meeting minutes, when the essential reasons for their existence have either changed or vanished.

Some have likened a committee to a physical structure that, once built, tends to remain in place in its original form even though it becomes empty or perhaps is just partially occupied. On the other hand, some, specifically C. Northcote Parkinson in *Parkinson's Law*, compare a committee to a plant that "takes root and grows, flowers, wilts, and dies, scattering the seed from which other committees will bloom in their turn."[1] In other words, committees are often seen as self-perpetuating or even self-propagating, regardless of whether the reasons for their formation have vanished or changed.

Any committee should be subjected to periodic review of its purpose and function. This purpose and function might be referred to as a "mission," perhaps a "charter," maybe simply a "charge," or some other label to describe the reason for its existence. Certainly some standing committees will not often require such review; consider, for example, the executive committee or the finance committee of an institution's board of directors, which will likely remain in place as long as the organization's basic mission remains unchanged. But even those supposedly stable committees might benefit from periodic review; for example, certain conditions in the environment or perhaps in the organization itself might suggest some appropriate change in committee membership or composition.

The review of a committee's purpose and function should not be left solely to the committee itself. Depending on how some committee members feel about membership on the committee, members could conceivably vote to continue a useless committee or to disband a committee that has valid reasons to continue. Some committee members, and certainly the committee's current chairperson, can legitimately be involved in the review. These people, being closest to committee activity, will be in a position to provide information to others involved in the review. It is most appropriate that the review be led by persons placed at the level of management to which the committee reports. A committee of the board of directors would be evaluated by the full board; a medical staff committee would be evaluated by the medical staff leadership; an institution's safety committee would be evaluated by a member or two of administration, including the executive to whom the committee answers; and so on.

Some of the principal questions to be addressed by those evaluating a committee's purpose and function are:

- Has the mission, charter, or charge of the committee changed somewhat, significantly, or not at all?

- What would appear to be the net effect on the organization if this committee were eliminated?
- If this committee is to be retained, what changes, if any, should be made to its mission, charter, or charge?
- If this committee is to be retained, should the frequency of meetings be altered in any way?
- Can the functions of this committee be constructively combined with the functions of another committee?
- What changes, if any, should be made in committee structure and composition?
- Should there be any changes made to the committee's reporting requirements?

It is true that many committees tend to take on a life of their own. It is also true that many in management feel they are "committeed to death" and could make good use of the time that could be freed if they had fewer meetings to attend. It follows, therefore, that regular, systematic review of committee purpose and function—at least once per year for the majority of committees—can help weed out ineffective or unneeded committees. In brief, periodically make each and every committee justify its continued existence.

THE COMMITTEE CHAIRPERSON

Selection and Duties

The position of chairperson of a committee may be filled in several ways. One is direct appointment by the individual with the mandate and the authority to do so. The bylaws of an organization may direct the president of the medical staff to appoint a committee chairperson. The manager of a department may be the chairperson of a related committee as a matter of course, the director of the utilization review program may be the appointed chairperson of the utilization review committee, and the individual who holds the line position responsible for safety will probably automatically become the chairperson of the safety committee.

Managers may appoint themselves chairpersons of committees that they constitute and over which they wish to exercise control, or they may offset powerful members by appointing as chairperson an individual sympathetic to their position. Selection of committee chairpersons may or may not be left to the group's membership. In committees where members are elected from the panel as a whole and where there is an accepted egalitarianism in the group, this is a common practice. The group conveys the idea that all those selected for membership have equal ability and that equal confidence is placed in all of them. Conversely, the group could also convey the idea that the committee is not very important so it does not matter who is chairperson. A group that elects the members of a committee may select the chairperson as a separate action by a special vote or may direct that the individual who receives the highest number of votes automatically assumes the chairpersonship.

Occasionally, the office is simply rotated among members of the committee in order to avoid a power struggle. When a specific activity of a standing committee requires extensive and recurring follow-up work and staff assistance is limited, the work of the chairperson is divided by rotation; since the burden of staff support must be shared by the chairperson's department or unit, this approach spreads the support work over several organizational units. When the committee's work is viewed as mere compliance with bureaucratic red tape and the work is not valued by its members nor by the group as a whole, the position of chairperson is sometimes downplayed by this rotation process. Finally, individual members may volunteer to accept the assignment as chairperson because of a sense of duty, because of a desire to advance themselves or protect some potentially threatened interest, or because the committee deals with an issue within their field of expertise.

An able, well-qualified individual sometimes refuses to accept the position of chairperson because it would limit his or her ability to participate in deliberations. Eligibility factors sometimes determine the choice of a chairperson. Prerequisites might include prior membership on the committee, tenure as a faculty member, ten years of service as a full-time employee, or a certain technical or professional degree.

A committee chairperson's duties include arranging for logistical support, chairing meetings, and monitoring follow-up assignments. The logistical duties include

- coordinating the schedules of committee members
- correlating committee activities with the work of related committees or departments
- checking for compliance with mandated deadlines and actions
- obtaining meeting space
- issuing meeting notices as to time, date, place, and agenda
- coordinating and distributing support information before meetings
- preparing the agenda, including sequencing items according to priority

Chairing the Meeting

The chairperson sets the tone of meetings, controls the agenda to a major extent, guides deliberation on the issues, and provides or denies opportunities for committee members to express themselves. The degree of formality or informality is indicated not only by the manner in which the chairperson conducts the business of the meeting but also by an explicit statement. At the outset, the chairperson makes known the rules of debate, for example, whether there will be general discussion followed by a formal vote and whether strict adherence to parliamentary procedures will be required throughout the meeting.

It is the duty of the chairperson to conduct the meeting efficiently by starting the session on time, following the agenda, and providing sufficient time for deliberation. Subtle leadership skills must be brought to bear as the chairperson referees the members' deliberations. The process of group deliberation and participation must be protected and promoted. The chairperson must artfully provide time for individuals to be heard, which is far more than merely letting each person have a turn to speak. Group cohesion must be fostered even when there are differences of opinion.

The agenda is usually prepared by the chairperson. It is intended to guide the proceedings, but the chairperson may take an item out of sequence if the course of discussion creates a natural opening for the deliberation of related agenda items. The chairperson keeps the meeting flowing by moving from one agenda item to another at appropriate times, calling the group's attention to work accomplished and work yet to be done.

The chairperson must seek to prevent polarization, overhasty decisions, or the eruption of blatant conflict. It is the chairperson's duty to prevent the group from moving into discussion of unrelated topics or returning to issues that have already been settled. The chairperson periodically integrates the discussion by summarizing major points, calling for motions, and appointing subcommittees or individuals to carry out special assignments.

To summarize the primary duties of the chairperson, in chairing a meeting this individual should:

- Except in the face of highly unusual circumstances, always begin the meeting at the stated time, and do not repeat information for late arrivals.
- State the purpose of the meeting at the start and determine that everyone knows why they are present.
- Ensure that someone (a "recorder") is assigned to record the proceedings for the purpose of minutes and assignments, and that someone (a "scribe") will

capture (via flip chart, etc.) points and ideas that arise for discussion. (At a small meeting these two activities could probably be handled by a single person.)

- Encourage discussion. Ask direct questions, especially of participants who otherwise tend to remain silent. Consciously attempt to secure everyone's participation.
- Remain in control of the proceedings. Do not lecture or dominate, do not tell others what to say, do not argue with participants, and do not try to be funny.
- Remain in control of the group itself. Do not permit tangential digressions, and do not allow monopolizers or ego-trippers to take over or to intimidate less vocal participants.
- End with some specific plan. Allow no one to depart without full understanding of the decisions made, actions to be taken, individuals responsible for implementation, and when things will be done. Every meeting must end with a statement of who will do what by when.
- Follow up after the meeting to ensure, as necessary, that what was decided and assigned has been accomplished.

Follow-up Activity

The final duty of the chairperson is follow-up. The chairperson participates in the preparation of minutes either directly by formulating them or indirectly by reviewing and approving them as prepared by the committee secretary. Periodic reports must be made to administrative officials. In addition, the chairperson must write letters to invite special guests, consult technical staff, hold informal sessions with members between meetings, and attend subcommittee meetings or those of related committees; all these duties fall within the category of follow-up.

The chairperson must periodically review the work of the committee. Is this work satisfactory given the committee's basic charge? Is the committee fulfilling its designated function? The minutes of several recent months may be examined and specific follow-up inquiries made to individuals and subcommittees concerning the progress of work assigned; agenda items that were set aside or those not discussed for lack of time should be brought to the committee's attention again. All unfinished business should be monitored. Exhibit 9–1 is a form a committee chairperson may use to facilitate this follow-up. Exhibit 9–2 provides an example of a tabulated form for recording minutes.

EXHIBIT 9–1	Follow-up of Committee Action

Committee _____

Year _____

Agenda Item/ Topic	Meeting Date Deliberated	Description	Responsibility Assigned to	Next Action Due	Date Action Completed
Outpatient Clinic Records	May 15	1. Develop chart review list.	Health Information Specialist	July 20	
Suspension of Privileges for Admitting Patients	June 11	1. Review legal aspects of procedure for suspending physician privileges.	Chief of Medical Staff	July 20	
		2. Update procedures in light of legal aspects.	Chief of Medical Staff	October 17	

COMMITTEE MEMBER ORIENTATION

Members often come to committees with varying degrees of knowledge about committee purpose, function, and procedures. In most instances, therefore, some orientation to a new committee assignment is recommended. This may amount to little or nothing for a professional appointed to a committee involving a specific function. For example, a nurse functioning as a quality assurance specialist may need very little orientation to membership on the institution's quality assurance committee. On the other hand, someone appointed to a committee that cuts across a number of functional lines may require more orientation and familiarization.

EXHIBIT 9–2

Excerpts from Utilization Review Committee Minutes

Date _____

Client #	Start of Care	Discharge Date	Findings and Remarks
512-02	10/25/06	current	RN, PT, OT: Good records; progress documented by all disciplines. RN evaluation had excellent needs assessment and nursing plan. PT evidenced ongoing teaching and good carryover. OT documentation not always legible, but patient progress in ADL was obvious to reviewer. Team cooperation evident throughout record.
513-07	12/20/05	current	RN; Aide; ST; OT; PT: No list of medications. Two nursing supervision notes missing; doctors' orders not current. Nursing supervision is evident but aide notes are incomplete. Communication among all disciplines is weak. Why no social service referral? Recommend review of case with all disciplines; needs discharge plan.

For example, an individual from the admitting department who is appointed to the institution's safety committee may require more extensive orientation.

To cite some examples of committee member orientation:

- In a particular small hospital, a new member of the safety committee meets with the committee chairperson one on one for about an hour before the new member's initial meeting.
- In a midsize not-for-profit human services agency, a newly appointed member of the finance committee of the board receives a two-hour orientation over lunch with the agency's chief executive officer, finance director, and finance committee chairperson.

- In a midsize hospital a new member of the board of directors receives a half-day orientation with the hospital's CEO and the executive committee of the board.

Before ever agreeing to committee service, one who is invited to serve should be fully advised of the purpose and function of the committee, the time commitment necessary, and the meeting schedule. Once this information has been conveyed and an individual's agreement to serve is secured, the committee chairperson can proceed with arrangements for a customized orientation depending on the needs of the individual. It should, of course, go without saying that a significant part of this orientation should involve answering the questions of the new member.

MINUTES AND PROCEEDINGS

Sound practice requires that an organization maintain official documentation of business transacted. Minutes serve as the permanent factual record of committee proceedings. An explicit statement in bylaws or policies may state that the minutes shall be maintained, including a record of attendance; that they shall reflect the transactions, conclusions, and recommendations of each meeting adequately; and that they shall be kept in a permanent file. Some other time frame for retention that reflects the legal and statutory requirements for the organization may be stated. Committee manuals should contain such information.

Properly formulated, minutes summarize business transacted, including matters that require follow-up action, matters on which there is substantial agreement or disagreement, and issues that remain open for committee deliberation. Minutes are sometimes transmitted to individuals who are not currently members, as determined by the policies on distribution and by legal and accrediting requirements. The historical record provided in the minutes gives new members an overall sense of committee activity. A surveyor checking for compliance with utilization review requirements may request the minutes of the utilization review committee over the past year. Representatives of the Joint Commission may call for minutes and proceedings of the medical staff committees to help in determining whether the staff is fulfilling its medico-administrative responsibilities.

In legal proceedings, the admissibility of committee minutes and proceedings as evidence rest on the premise that these records were made in the normal course of business at the time of the actions or events, or within a reasonable time thereafter. Thus, minutes of the official business of the organization's committees must be prepared, reviewed, and distributed in a timely manner (i.e., close to the time of the actual proceedings). They are reviewed formally at the next meeting to obtain general agreement that their content reflects the business transacted. Should a lawsuit be instituted regarding the possible negligence, malpractice, denial of privileges, or discipline of a practitioner, the minutes of such proceedings might, in some instances, be admissible as legal evidence; the laws on this point vary from state to state.

It could be argued that minutes do not reflect all the business transacted by the committee. The counterargument is a question: Why not? The effort spent on proper documentation in the normal course of business is a legitimate use of organizational time and staff. It has also been argued that minutes could be altered to reflect business that, in fact, was not transacted, but this is true of any form of documentation. Review of minutes by all members is one way to safeguard accuracy. Managers can only go forward guided by their own ethical code as well as by the organizational and societal presumption that the work was carried out "in good faith."

Preparation of Minutes

Minutes are prepared in two stages. First, either the proceedings are transcribed in their entirety by clerical staff or a summary of key points is compiled by a staff assistant. Then, the official secretary to the committee (if there is such an officer) or the committee chairperson formulates the official minutes from the transcript or summary. If there is no clerical assistant or staff aide, the chairperson (or member-secretary) uses self-compiled notes to formulate the minutes. Any required approval is obtained, and the minutes are sent out according to a prescribed distribution list. The distribution process may be simplified by developing a standing list of the names and titles of members, administrative officers to whom certain minutes are sent because of their organizational jurisdiction, and/or the chairpersons of related committees. The chairperson then needs only to check the names of those who are to receive a particular set of minutes. It is useful to include the statement "Standard Distribution" and also to list any additional individuals to whom minutes were sent as a point of information. The inclusion of a list of support material or enclosures makes the minutes more complete.

Exhibit 9–3 illustrates a format that makes it possible to scan the pages of a volume of minutes and focus on specific topics. The topic key should be placed in the right-hand margin; if the left-hand margin is used for the topic key, it may be placed too deeply in a bound or semi-bound margin for ready reference. Inclusion of the dates on which there was previous discussion gives the user an easy means of reference to related information. This format generates an index of committee

EXHIBIT 9–3

Sample Format for Minutes

The committee directed its attention to new guidelines concerning the content of discharge summaries. A random sample of discharge summaries dictated during recent months was compared with the guidelines to determine areas of noncompliance and areas of strength.

DISCHARGE SUMMARIES
2/23/07
9/23/06

topics, and members have the benefit of ready reference to past deliberations of a related nature.

Content of Minutes

Minutes are more than a mere listing of committee actions in chronological order. The topics discussed are normally grouped, a process facilitated by adherence to a formal agenda. In relatively informal meetings, however, the discussion may be diffuse and less focused on discrete topics than is a discussion in a meeting conducted under strict parliamentary procedure.

The minutes should reflect what is done, not what is said. Adequate minutes as a matter of course contain such information as

- the name of the committee
- the date, time, and place of the meeting
- whether it is a regular or special meeting
- the names of members present (specify ex officio if appropriate)
- the names of members absent (include a notation of excused absence if appropriate)
- the names of guests, including title or department as an additional indicator of reason for attending

The opening paragraph of the minutes, which is relatively standardized, normally includes

- the name of the presiding officer
- the establishment of quorum, if this is done routinely or at the request of a member

- a routine review of the minutes of the previous meeting, noting whether they were reviewed as read or only as distributed and whether any corrections were made

The proceedings are summarized. The names of those who made formal motions are given, but the names of those who seconded the motions need not be recorded. All main motions, whether adopted or rejected, are included.

The bulk of the business may be reflected in general discussion only. There are five basic dispositions of agenda items, and each should be listed with its disposition:

1. Item is discussed and a formal motion is made; formal wording of motion is given. Votes for and against, as well as abstentions, are recorded. Notation is made whether motion is adopted or rejected.
2. Item is discussed and there is general consensus. No formal motion is made. Summary statement of general discussion is entered with notation that there was general agreement with action taken.
3. Item is discussed and tabled informally or set aside for discussion at another time because members need more information. Reasons for setting it aside may be stated; indeed, it is useful to give this information for later reference.
4. Item is discussed, with subsequent formal motion to table it permanently.
5. Item is not discussed. This is not stated directly; item is simply carried as old business.

A precaution is in order relative to numbers 3, 4, and 5 above, concerning items that are "tabled informally," "set aside for discussion at another time," "tabled permanently," or "simply carried as old business." These particular actions—representing largely more inaction than action—are often taken for truly legitimate reasons. Perhaps study is required, more information is needed, or the people most appropriate to a particular item are not present. Often, however, items of business that represent thorny, emotional, or generally controversial issues are repeatedly put off via one or another of the means cited. Certain items of business seem to be put off, then brought up again only to be put off again, and so on.

Some unresolved and recurring agenda items can languish without action forever, such that they simply accumulate and nothing happens to them except postponement after postponement. It is suggested that any accumulation of such agenda items be reassessed regularly, with the intention, if possible, of either moving them onto an active schedule—for example, "To be addressed at the February meeting"—or dropping them altogether. Often committee participants and other decision makers behave as though they believe that an issue ignored long enough might just go away of its own accord. It is true that occasionally some issues, even those involving seemingly difficult or insoluble problems, simply vanish. However, according to Murphy (of the oft-cited Murphy's Law), left unto themselves, matters ordinarily proceed from bad to worse.

Whether a particular issue is thorny or controversial or not, whether the issue in question seems to defy rational solution, it falls to every committee member to be aware that postponing a problem is in fact deciding not to decide. There may often be completely valid reasons for doing so, but there can be a price associated with deciding not to decide. The exercise of this "no-decision option" is itself a decision, and frequently it turns out to be the decision of the greatest potential consequences. Therefore, recurring or unresolved agenda items should not be allowed to coast in open-ended fashion for a prolonged period of time. Either place them on a reasonable track toward resolution, or get rid of them altogether.

A useful practice for providing background information for new members of a committee or for review of past committee action is to include a rationale statement for each motion that is made. Although this is not required, such a statement provides a succinct summary of the underlying reasons for an action:

> It was moved and seconded that chart review will be carried out by health information department personnel for all patients in the long-term care/rehabilitation unit whose length of stay exceeds 14 days. This review will be made on a weekly basis for each patient.
>
> Rationale: Because of the extended length of stay for this category of patients (an average of 47 days in this facility), the detection and subsequent correction of medical record documentation deficiencies should be carried out during the patients' stay.

Both the positive and negative discussion of each topic may be summarized. If there is a specific follow-up action to be taken and a committee member is assigned this task, the name of the individual should be included in the minutes. If a subcommittee is created, the names of its members are given. In the minutes of a formal meeting, points of order and appeals, whether sustained or lost, are noted.

At the conclusion of the minutes, the name of the individual who compiled them is given. The legend "minutes compiled by" may be used instead of the somewhat archaic phrase "respectfully submitted." If minutes are approved or reviewed by the chairperson before distribution, this is stated. The minutes should be signed by the person who compiled them (e.g., the committee secretary) and the person who approved them for distribution. If the committee does not have an official secretary, the chairperson's name and signature are entered.

EXHIBIT 9-4

Documentation Review: Geriatric Clients in Home Care

Focus of review: documentation of risk assessment for falls in the home

Number of client records reviewed for proper documentation:	40
Standard of Compliance	100%
Actual Compliance	88%

Elements of documentation to be noted:
  Age 75 or older
  Cardiovascular medication
  Psychotropic medication
  Use of four or more medications
  Cognitive impairment
  Decrease in hip strength
  Poor balance when walking
  Prior falls in the home
  Chronic pain/pain status
  Environmental factors (e.g., rugs; stair rails)
  Compliance by client with safety instructions
  Compliance by family/caretakers with safety instructions

Minutes and proceedings reflecting patient care often are summarized in tabular form. Exhibit 9–4 is an example reflecting client safety assessments in home care.

WHERE DO TEAMS FIT IN?

In these days of expanding employee involvement it is increasingly likely for problem solving to be approached through the use of employee teams. Teams have been at the forefront of the implementation of total quality management (TQM) programs, as they were in previous undertakings under various other names (for example, quality circles, in which an individual "circle" was neither more nor less than an employee problem-solving team).

Today's team essentially fits within the broader definition of committee dealt with in this chapter. There are, however, some points of difference between teams and the more traditional forms of committees. Like other committees, a team may be "standing," with a continuing life beyond its initial concern, such as a departmental team that exists to continually scrutinize the department's procedures. By contrast, a team may also exist temporarily to address a specific problem or situation.

Generally, a team is ordinarily seen as less formal or less structured than a committee. We often see committees as existing by virtue of some higher authority, such as the committees of the medical staff or the board of directors, or at least as deliberative bodies established by higher management. By comparison, teams, although perhaps standing in the sense of having open-ended assignments, are generally perceived as nonpermanent.

The term *committee* is more likely to be associated with more formal processes such as parliamentary procedure and the requirement for thorough minutes of proceedings. Also, when compared with the word *team*, committee is more likely to be associated with voting, which may or may not be a feature of a given team's activities.

Therefore, given the foregoing few points of variation, a team may be referred to as a committee. There is, however, one unique dimension of an employee team that deserves special attention, and that is the questionable legality of some teams relative to their missions.

AS EMPLOYEE INVOLVEMENT INCREASES

Participative management and employee involvement have been talked about for several decades and have been practiced in an increasing number of work organizations since the human relations approach to management began to make inroads into the authoritarian management of the past. Thanks to TQM and other initiatives, more and more is being done with the involvement of employees by way of teams.

There are, however, areas of employee involvement in which teams are seen as intruding on the territory of labor unions. There is constant risk that any given employee team could be adjudged an illegal labor organization under the National Labor Relations Act (NLRA). Many projects that employee teams might tend to become involved in could be considered as infringing on the rights of collective bargaining organizations.

The essence of legal challenges and National Labor Relations Board (NLRB) rulings has been that an employee team that discusses and makes recommendations concerning wages, benefits, and other terms and conditions of employment is essentially an employer-dominated labor organization. An organization behaving as such, ruled the NLRB, was functioning in capacities reserved for legally constituted collective bargaining organizations and was therefore acting in a manner that infringed upon employees' rights to be represented by a union.[2]

EMPLOYEE TEAMS AND THEIR FUTURE

Avoiding "Committee Paralysis"

A number of the legal problems that teams have experienced since the early 1990s have caused some employers to shy away from teams that include rank-and-file employees. The value of including employees in problem solving is undeniable; in most situations nobody knows a job better than the person who does it every day. Surely it makes sense to account for employees' needs and desires in making changes within the organization. Rather than paralyze employee teams because of legal risk, it makes more sense to look for ways in which we may make the fullest possible use of employee input while avoiding legal entanglements.

The active use of employee participation and input, largely via teams or committees, actually lies at or near the heart of every total quality initiative. If management believes what is said to employees about the value of their input, about empowerment, and about individuals "owning" their jobs, then management had better make maximum use of participative processes—including teams.

Occasional Shortcomings of Teams

Some team members, especially managers serving on teams with nonmanagers or others of perceived lesser rank, are unwilling to set aside position and power for the sake of the team. Also, unequal levels of knowledge and ability among team members can lead some to dominate and others to become overwhelmed or lost in the crowd.

Some extremely important and highly disruptive effects on teams lie in reward and compensation systems that continue to focus on individual effort rather than on team performance. This has been a frequently encountered barrier to successful total quality implementations as organizations have tried to alter how they do business without changing the systems by which they do business. Indeed, some reward systems support individual performance to such an extent that they can discourage teamwork.

Performance appraisals that do not account for team performance also present barriers. An organization's performance appraisal process is usually one major business support system that has to change dramatically for successful total quality implementation. Also, it is necessary to change employees' concept of evaluation from a focus on the individual to emphasis on the team.

Whether for total quality management or any other undertaking that involves committees or teams, lack of top management commitment to the process is a sure means of undermining effectiveness. It should go without saying that top management that fails to "walk the talk" will be perceived as insincere.

Some problems with teams are inherent in the labels used to describe these bodies, labels such as self-directed, autonomous, and the like. These names are misleading in that they convey the belief that these groups are independent and free to act as they choose. No effective teams in business really provide their own total direction. Each team should be directed by its specific charge or mission or assignment and by the goals of the organization. As such, all teams should actually be interdependent with other organizational elements. Effective teams require clear direction, comprehensive guidelines, and open, nonthreatening leadership.

What to Avoid in Using Employee Teams

It is possible to empower teams that include rank-and-file employees and utilize them to maximum effect by observing a few simple limitations:

1. Never allow an employee team to deal with terms and conditions of employment, such as wages, hours, benefits, grievances, and such. Even consideration of working conditions in general should be avoided. As a member of management who might be part of a team, do not deal with other team members, and specifically nonmanagers, concerning terms and conditions of employment. If a team's activities take it from a legitimate topic into the realm of terms and conditions of employment, its direction should be altered.

2. Do not solicit from teams complaints, grievances, or suggestions about terms and conditions of employment. If such issues arise on their own, refer them to the proper points in the organization.

3. Do not let team meetings degenerate into gripe sessions in which members simply complain about aspects of their employment.

4. Do not mandate employee participation, ask employees to represent other employees, or sanction employee elections to choose representatives.

5. Do not allow an employee team or committee to exist and function without a clear, understandable mission or charge and without fully and plainly delineated limits on its authority and responsibility.

Proper Focus of Effective Employee Teams

Short of actually establishing teams or committees to wrestle with certain issues, a number of steps can be taken to encourage employee participation. It is possible, and frequently desirable, to consider bringing together loosely defined groups of managers and employees simply to brainstorm ideas, gather information, and help define problems, as long as no proposals are offered or recommendations made. It is also proper to assemble an employee group to share information and observations with management, again, as long as no proposals or recommendations are made.

Beyond one-time or limited informal gatherings and in the realm of actual teams or committees, use the following points of focus:

1. When establishing a team or committee, identify it up front as not intended as an employees' channel to management. Have a clear mission or charge in place before soliciting team membership, and have the team's functions and limits identified before any team activity begins.

2. Keep the team focused on productivity or quality improvements only. This requires clear guidelines and plenty of continued vigilance. It is difficult to talk about quality, efficiency, productivity, and such without conditions of employment becoming involved, so be constantly aware of the potential need to redefine the team's boundaries periodically.

3. Staff teams with volunteers, or use rotating membership selected by some means that is not management dominated.

4. If a team is empowered to make a final management decision, that is, the team decides in place of management, not just recommends to management, it can be seen as acting as management. This is acceptable. In fact, it has been suggested that the ultimate protection against being ruled an illegal labor organization exists when the team can make final decisions in its own right. "The only true safe harbor is vesting the [committee] with the responsibility of making final management decisions."[3]

5. If an issue is sufficiently narrowly defined that all persons affected by it can be included in a single group, a "committee of the whole" including everyone is usually legally safe. In such an instance nobody can be seen as "representing" anyone else.[4]

6. For standing committees or long-lived teams, maintain a majority membership of managers. A committee or team composed of a majority of managers stands less chance of being adjudged illegal under the NLRA.[5] Such teams do present a significant drawback, however; a team composed mostly of managers is far less likely to be seen as a legitimate vehicle for employee participation.

7. Rather than always creating teams or committees that tend to develop a continuing existence, consider establishing specific problem-solving or work-improvement ad hoc groups, each with a specific, well-defined charge and a specific problem to solve, and disband each group after its goal has been attained. Such ad hoc groups can much more safely consist of a majority of nonmanagers than can permanent teams or committees. For teams composed largely of rank-and-file employees, however, it is legally safest to have management representatives serve as observers or facilitators, without the power to vote on proposals or dominate or control the group.

For collaborative group problem solving and participative decision making in general, it is always appropriate to bring into the group those people who have the skills needed for dealing with the group's charge. It is necessary, however, to recognize that those persons who have skills pertinent to the problem at hand will likely have greater influence on group decisions.

Recognize also that teams or committees become unwieldy as they increase in size. Small groups are generally better; active participation in tasks seems to decrease with increases in group size. In fact, team participants tend to rate small groups as more satisfactory, positive, and effective than larger groups.[6]

Employee participation may well be the key to continuing increases in quality, efficiency, and productivity. Employee participation is essential. As noted earlier, nobody knows the inner workings of a job better than the person who does it day in and day out. Also, there are few if any problems the solutions to which are not enhanced by multiple viewpoints and inputs. A team brings to the problem the power of the group. To cite a highly pertinent quotation from an anonymous source: "I use not only all the brains I have, but all I can borrow."

EXERCISE: COMMITTEE STRUCTURES

In no more than 100 words, describe the structure and size of a health care organization that has a board of directors and a formal committee structure. This description would most appropriately be of a hospital or nursing home, preferably one with which you are familiar, but it can be imaginary if you have no direct familiarity.

For your chosen organization, you are to design a complete two-part committee structure. This will consist of naming (1) the committees you would expect to exist under the auspices of the board of directors, and (2) the administrative committees you would expect to exist. For each committee you name, provide a one- or two-sentence description of the committee's mission, and indicate the approximate number of committee members and any primary expertise that might be required on the committee. (To accomplish this it may be necessary to perform some research into health care organization committee practices.)

CASE: THE EMPLOYEE-RETENTION COMMITTEE MEETING

Background

General Hospital has an administrative committee known as the Employee Retention Committee. This group's role is to address issues having a bearing on turnover, with a stated goal of reducing undesirable turnover and thus enhancing retention. The committee consists of the following personnel:

- Dave Andrews, an administrative assistant who inherited chairmanship of this committee upon entering his position with the hospital. He called the present meeting about 10 days earlier, having notified two of the others by telephone and two in person.
- Harriet Roberts, the hospital's employment manager.
- John Dawson, a staff nurse in the intensive care unit.
- Alice Morey, director of food service.
- Arthur Wilson, staff physical therapist.

The meeting was scheduled for 1:00 P.M. in Andrews' office. Andrews returned from lunch at 1:08 to find Roberts and Wilson already there. At 1:12 Dawson entered and Andrews said, "I'd like to get started, but where's Alice?"

Somebody responded, "Don't know."

Andrews dialed a number and received no answer. He then dialed the call center and asked for a page. A moment later a call came in.

Turning from the telephone, Andrews said to the rest of the group, "She forgot. She'll be here in a minute."

"Dave, I wish you had a larger office or a better place to meet," said Dawson. "I don't know how we're going to fit another person in here."

"I know it's small," Andrews answered, "but both conference rooms are in use and I couldn't find another place. Say, holler out to Susan and tell her to find another chair—we'll need it."

Wilson said, "Dave, can you open your window a little? It's already stuffy in here."

Dave opened the window a few inches. Just then Alice Morey arrived, squeezing into the office with the extra chair that had just been located. It was 1:18 P.M.

Andrews said, "I guess we can get started now." He shuffled through a stack of papers and said, "I've got a copy, if I can—oh, here it is—of a recent turnover survey done by the human resource directors in the region." He looked at Roberts and said, "I assume you have this?"

"Yes, there's a copy in my office. But I didn't know I needed to bring it."

Andrews said, "Well, I think that from this we can assume—"

Dawson interrupted, "Dave, wouldn't it be better if we could all see it? Then you could go through it point by point."

Andrews said, "I guess you're right. I have just this copy." He turned toward the door and called out as he waved the document, "Susan, I need four copies of this. Right now, please."

Turning back to his pile of papers Dave said to the group, "The last time we got together there were a number of things we decided to look for. I don't remember just what we assigned to whom, but I've got it here somewhere." For a half-minute or so he leafed through the papers before him, then he turned to his desk and began to leaf through folders in the file drawer.

While Dave was looking, Morey turned to Roberts and said, "Say, what have you been doing about finding that new dietician we need? You've been dragging your feet on the employment requisition for three weeks and Elaine is leaving in another week and we still haven't had any candidates to interview."

Roberts responded. Her sharp tone sparked a defensive reaction and a lively discussion ensued.

Andrews located the paper he was seeking and Susan returned with the requested copies. Andrews distributed the copies and fixed his attention on Morey and Roberts as he waited for an opening in their discussion. At 1:32 the group returned to the subject of employee turnover.

"Now, about this regional survey," Andrews began.

Wilson said, "What about the survey? I thought you wanted to start with the things we agreed to do the last time we met."

"Who cares," said Roberts, "let's just get started."

Dawson looked at his watch and said, "Let's get started and finished. I have an ICU staff meeting at 2:00."

The meeting settled down to a discussion of the regional survey and the preliminary information each person had gathered since the previous meeting. At exactly two minutes before 2:00 Dawson excused himself to attend his staff meeting. At 2:08 Morey was called over the paging system; she left the meeting and did not return.

At 2:12 Andrews said he felt they had tentatively decided on their next step but required some input from the two parties who had already left. He then started to excuse the other two with the suggestion that they get together again after two weeks, but his telephone rang and he answered it himself, his usual practice, and talked some four or five minutes before returning his attention to the two remaining in his office. He said, "I guess that's it for now. I'll set a time for the next meeting and let you know."

When the last of the participants left, Andrews called Susan to remove the extra chair. As she did so he reflected gloomily on how difficult it was to get anything substantive out of a committee in this organization.

Instructions

1. Perform a detailed critique of the Employee Retention Committee meeting. List the occurrences or omissions that you believe indicate faulty committee practice, and state why you believe so and what should have been done differently.

2. Comment on the composition and membership of the Employee Retention Committee, and indicate how you would structure and position such a committee and how you would thoroughly describe its mission, purpose, or charge.

NOTES

1. C. Northcote Parkinson, *Parkinson's Law* (Boston: Houghton Mifflin, 1957; reprint, New York: Ballantine Books, 1971), p. 50.
2. Employee Representation Committees at Electromation Are Illegal: NLRB. Management Policies and Personnel Law, BRP Publications, Inc. (January 15, 1993), 1–2.
3. J. R. Redeker and D. P. O'Meara, "Safe Methods of Employee Participation," *HR Magazine* 38, no. 4 (April 1993): 101–4.
4. Ibid., 102.
5. Ibid., 104.
6. L. Blake, "Reduce Employees' Resistance to Change," *Personnel Journal* 71, no. 9 (September 1992): 27–76.

CHAPTER **10**

Adaptation, Motivation, and Conflict Management

CHAPTER OBJECTIVES

- Address the necessity for properly integrating each individual employee into the organization and describe the common techniques of integration.
- Identify the patterns of behavior through which workers express their attitudes toward the organization.
- Introduce the theories that address present-day employee motivation and provide the manager with insight into motivating employees.
- Develop an understanding of the origins of conflict, especially in the organizational setting, and describe how to address conflict constructively.
- Briefly examine the role of the collective bargaining agreement (union contract) in the avoidance and control of conflict.

ADAPTATION AND MOTIVATION

In order to get work done efficiently and effectively, managers must motivate workers and assist in their adaptation to organizational demands. Individuals must fit into the organizational framework. There is a close tie between motivation and adaptation activities and the controlling function of the manager. The worker who fits into the organization and who values an assigned role is likely to be motivated more easily. In turn, the need to control activity through disciplinary action is reduced.

Adaptation to Organizational Life

Two specific factors that result from organizational structure may be cited to illustrate the need for an explicit management process to help integrate the individual into the organization:

1. the need to offset the effect of decentralization
2. the need to coordinate the many individual functions that result from departmentation and specialization

Overall goals and policies are made at the highest level of the hierarchy, but the work is carried out at every level. Occasionally, conflicting directives are issued from the central authority.

Additionally, the number of individuals who enter the organization and the different manner in which these individuals react to the complexities of organizational life must be taken into consideration. These individuals not only have different values, different personalities, and different life experiences, but they also belong to many other organizations, some of which may have values that compete and even conflict with the values embodied in the workplace. Some of the patterns of accommodation to organizational life may be functional for the organization but dysfunctional for the individual. Potential conflict must be offset, and the personality mixes of workers and clients must be melded into smooth interpersonal relationships.

Techniques for Fostering Integration

Events and conditions should be anticipated as fully as possible, and the courses of action to be taken for designated categories of events and conditions should be described. Authorization of the course of action applicable to any category may be permissive; it may spell out several series of steps among which the employee shall choose. In order to prevent undesirable actions from arising, penalties should be established for those who commit them. The policy manual, the procedure manual, the employee handbook, the medical staff bylaws, and the licensure laws for the various health professionals are all routine management tools for guiding behavior and fostering integration.

Work Rules

Rule formation generally has been accepted as a management prerogative in the control function. Work rules are related to motivational processes because they contribute to a stable organizational environment. They serve several functions in an organization:

- They create order and discipline so that the behavior of workers is goal-oriented.
- They help unify the organization by channeling and limiting behavior.
- They give members confidence that the behavior of other members will be predictable and uniform.
- They make behavior routine so that managers are free to give attention to nonroutine problems.
- They prevent harm, discomfort, and annoyance to clients.
- They help ensure compliance with legislation that affects the institution as a whole.

The organization has a positive duty to protect both clients and workers with regard to health, sanitation, and safety. In addition, it must seek to prevent behavior that has the potential of alienating or offending clients. Because they deal with patients and their families in stressful situations, health care organizations have specific obligations in this area.

Sanctions

Both positive and negative sanctions can be used to induce compliance. Bonus pay, merit increases, and special time off with pay are positive sanctions; demotion, suspension, and written reprimands are negative sanctions. An essential element in any system of sanctions is the development of adequate feedback mechanisms and correction where needed. Employee evaluation and training processes can provide feedback and correction on a routine basis.

Selection

Kaufman stressed that the recruitment and selection process can be used to influence the degree to which employees tend to conform and become integrated into the workplace.[1] The more selective an organization is, the more effective the involvement of the members tends to be. Their commitment to organizational values is deeper, and they need fewer external controls.

In recruiting members, the highly selective organization should try to appeal to an audience composed of individuals who are well disposed toward the values of the organization—even at this preselection stage. Recruitment information may indicate implicitly or explicitly the need to conform.

Training

Kaufman also noted that highly structured orientation training can ensure the technical readiness of new employees and increase the likelihood they will conform.[2] For example, their technical skills can be modified so that they perform the work according to the specific procedures unique to the organization. Orientation programs have been developed in hospitals in order to familiarize professionally trained individuals (e.g., technologists) with particular routines. Businesses use the rotating management internship to foster integration of newly graduated management majors.

Identification with the Organization

The process of developing in employees a strong sense of identification with the organization is enhanced by the internal transfer and promotion process, which can also add to their ability to adjust and broaden themselves.[3] The development of a sense of identification is good for the organization, but it can also be good for each individual. Any continuity, any structure possessed by the person's work life is provided by the organization. The organization becomes, as it were, a major source of personal identity, and through the promotion process a stable career path can be developed.

The Work Group

An employee's particular mindset is continually reinforced by his or her work group. Through the work group, the individual is assimilated into the organization—or is perhaps prevented from being properly assimilated. In addition to the formal prescriptions regarding work activities, informal patterns of behavior arise among members of the group. The individual learns the unwritten rules as well as interpretations of the written rules. The informal organization of the work group also satisfies an essential human need—the need to belong. Nonconformity with group norms could lead to expulsion from the group, which would eliminate a vital source of information and communication as well as an arena in which to air conflicts that stem from the formal organizational role demands.

PATTERNS OF ACCOMMODATION

Individuals adjust to highly organized settings in a variety of ways. Presthus suggested that the bureaucratic situation evokes three types of accommodation: (1) upward mobility, (2) indifference, and (3) ambivalence.[4]

Upward Mobility

An individual who identifies deeply with the organization and derives strength from his or her involvement is upwardly mobile. This strong identification not only evokes a sense of loyalty and affirmation but also provides a constant point of reference. Presthus noted that because the upwardly mobile employee accepts the organization's demand for complete conformity, he or she can overlook the contradictions between the routine operations of the organization and its official myths.

Indifference

Unlike the upwardly mobile employee, an employee who is indifferent refuses to compete for organizational rewards. Although alienated by the structural conditions of big organizations, the indifferent employee has come to terms with the work environment. Presthus noted the use of general psychological withdrawal as a means of reducing conflict. In particular, the individual redirects interest toward off-the-job satisfactions. Work is not the individual's whole life, and his or her off-the-job activities are rarely job-related. Presthus noted that indifferent employees are often the most satisfied members of the organization, since their aspirations are based on a realistic appraisal of opportunities.

Ambivalence

The employee who neither rejects the promise of power nor plays the games required to get power in the organization demonstrates ambivalence. This individual has high aspirations, but lacks the interpersonal skills of the upwardly mobile. The ambivalent employee does not honor the status system and tends to have difficulty with superiors, who are aware that their relationship with the employee is based on formal authority, not on esteem. The ambivalent employee is often a specialist caught between the world of specialized skills and the organizational hierarchy. He or she is usually sensitive to change and can be a catalytic agent in bringing about change.

THEORIES OF MOTIVATION

On one hand, the manager seeks to develop a work force that fits the organization; on the other hand, the manager must remain aware of the basic needs of the workers. The art of motivating is built on this recognition of human need. Motivation is the degree of readiness or the desire within an individual to pursue some goal. The function of motivating or actuating is essentially a matter of leading the workers to understand and accept the organizational goals and to contribute effectively to meeting these goals. In motivating or actuating, the manager seeks to increase the zone of acceptance within the individual and to create an organizational environment that enhances the individual's will to work. As self-motivation increases, the need for coercive controls and punishment decreases.

Bases of Motivation

Needs are the internal, felt wants of an individual (they are also referred to as drives and desires). Incentives are external factors that an individual perceives as possible satisfiers of felt needs. A review of management history reveals shifting emphases in the understanding of motivation.

Maslow's Hierarchy of Needs

Maslow's theory of motivation is predicated on the premise that every action is motivated by an unsatisfied need. Purposeful behavior is motivated by a multiplicity of interests and motivators and therefore varies with circumstances and with individuals. Once a need has been satisfied, another level of need must be appealed to in order to motivate workers, for a satisfied need is no longer a motivator. Maslow's hierarchy of needs consists of the following scale:[5]

1. physiological needs
2. safety and security needs
3. the need to belong and to engage in social activity
4. the need for esteem and status
5. the need for self-fulfillment

Herzberg's Two-Factor Theory

Herzberg approached the theory of motivation by identifying two factors or elements that are operative in motivation: satisfiers and dissatisfiers. There are, according to Herzberg, many factors in organizational life that satisfy or dissatisfy, including company policy, supervisors, working conditions, and interpersonal relationships among work group members. If these are perceived as negative or lacking, they are dissatisfiers. If they are present and perceived as "good," they are satisfiers; they are not motivators, however. Herzberg identifies the following as examples of motivators: opportunity for advancement and promotion, greater responsibility, and opportunity for growth and interesting work. His concept of motivators tends to parallel Maslow's concept of higher-level needs—those of esteem and status and self-fulfillment.[6]

Relationship of Maslow to Herzberg

If you know the motives (needs) of individuals you want to influence (according to Maslow), then you should be able to determine what goals (Herzberg) you should provide in the environment to motivate those individuals. Hersey and Blanchard postulate that this is possible because it has been found that money and benefits tend to satisfy needs at the physiological and security levels; interpersonal relations and supervision are examples of factors that satisfy social needs; and increased responsibility, challenging work, and growth and development are motivators at the esteem and self-actualization levels.[7]

McGregor's Theory X and Theory Y

McGregor set forth a series of assumptions that compare the traditional view of workers (Theory X) with his own view of industrial behavior (Theory Y). The manager who holds Theory X believes that employees have an inherent dislike for work and assumes that they have little ambition, will avoid work if possible, and want security above all else. In contrast, the manager who holds Theory Y assumes that work is as natural as play or rest; that the average worker, under the right conditions, seeks to accept responsibility; and that workers will exercise self-direction and self-control in the service of objectives to which they are committed.[8]

Theory Z

Developed primarily by Japanese managers in the late 1960s and 1970s, Theory Z is a contemporary approach to management and motivation that focuses on increased productivity and job satisfaction among workers. The cultural climate in which this pattern of management developed, that of Japan, emphasizes close linkage of work and the worker's life. The term *Theory Z* was coined by William Ouchi, who describes in detail the elements of this motivational approach.[9]

PRACTICAL STRATEGIES FOR EMPLOYEE MOTIVATION

Motivation may be described as the drive, impetus, or initiative that causes an individual to direct his or her behavior toward satisfaction of some personal need, using "need" in the broader sense of the word to describe something one pursues because its attainment represents fulfillments of a sort. Considering motivation in this light, we might question whether it is possible for anyone to "motivate" another human being to do anything or pursue anything.

It is in fact not strictly possible to motivate another person. The best that can be done is to create the circumstances under which an individual can become self-motivated. It is much like the old saying, "You can lead a horse to water but you can't make him drink." You can create what would seem to be ideal conditions and structure seemingly perfect circumstances, but these alone provide no guarantee of successful employee motivation because there is no way of making someone respond appropriately if the person does not care to respond. Most people in work organizations are subject to the same overall collection of needs, but the mix of needs—that is, the differing emphasis on the various needs that drive an individual—may vary greatly from person to person. In brief, what "motivates" one person may have little or no effect on another. This necessitates generalizing to some extent and recognizing that any particular motivational strategy may work with some people and fail to work with others who are similarly situated.

In dealing with technical, professional, and managerial employees, it is probably relatively safe to assume that the motivation of many of these kinds of workers can be best understood using Herzberg's two-factor theory described earlier, the two kinds of factors being motivators and dissatisfiers.

Motivators

The true motivating forces, or at least the strongest of the genuine motivating forces, are to be found in the work itself and are all describable as opportunities. The genuine sources of motivation are the opportunity to:

- accomplish or achieve, and be recognized for doing so
- acquire new knowledge
- do work that is both challenging and interesting
- do work that is meaningful, that makes a societal contribution
- assume responsibility
- be involved in determining how the work is done

The foregoing opportunities are likely to include the primary motivators for a great many employees, providing these employees are at least nominally satisfied with the environmental factors surrounding their employment, the potential dissatisfiers.

Dissatisfiers

The potential dissatisfiers are the environmental factors that exist in all aspects of an employee's relationship to the organization. These generally do not motivate, but they can easily lead to employee dissatisfaction if they are not maintained at a level acceptable to the employee. These potential dissatisfiers can be grouped in five categories:

1. *Salary administration,* or the perceived overall fairness of salaries and benefits
2. Potential for *promotion and growth,* and the extent to which this is or is not present
3. *Personnel policies,* or how each employee is treated both as an individual and relative to other employees
4. *Working conditions* and the extent to which they promote well-being relative to what is expected
5. *Communication* in all of its forms, including knowledge of the organization's plans and prospects, regular feedback on performance, individual confidentiality, and higher management's responsiveness to employee questions and concerns

Motivational Strategies

The first four of the five dissatisfiers listed above have much to do with the overall organization and are perhaps mostly beyond the control or direct influence of the department manager. The final one on the list, communication, depends in part on the organization's policies and practices but is also considerably dependent on the individual manager's behavior. Any specific motivational strategy must take into account the relative strength of potential dissatisfiers, so it might be said that an initial—and continuing—motivational strategy is the maintenance of the environmental factors so as to minimize their potential effects as dissatisfiers. Other active motivational strategies that might be utilized include:

- *Performance appraisal.* Making full use of the organization's performance appraisal process, preferably including self-appraisal participation and faithfully including appraisal interviews, serves a number of communication needs and can also provide recognition for work well done (only very rarely is it not possible to convey something positive in an appraisal). However, the formal appraisal done annually or perhaps semiannually is not enough; the manager should dispense praise when earned and in general maintain an ongoing communicating relationship with each employee.

- *Job rotation, job enrichment, job enlargement.* These strategies generally involve expanding or enlarging jobs or rotating duties. Such actions provide employees with the opportunity to gain new knowledge and can serve to inject increased interest and challenge into the work.

- *Delegation.* Related to the foregoing strategy concerning job expansion, proper delegation well administered can provide employees with added interest and challenge, the chance to acquire new knowledge, and the opportunity to take on increased responsibility.

- *Awards and honors.* Employee awards and honors programs provide visible recognition that can go a long way in satisfying some employees' needs for recognition and appreciation. Such programs often include "Employee of the Month" and "Employee of the Year" selections.

- *Career ladders and parallel-path progression systems.* Such systems provide the opportunity for capable individuals to advance themselves professionally without necessarily seeking entry into management, satisfying a continuing need for learning, growth, status, and recognition.

- *Incentives and bonuses.* While it may be argued that in and of itself money is not a particularly strong motivator, it nevertheless looms important for some. Often the monetary value of an incentive or bonus does not count nearly as strongly as the act of achievement. For some employees we can truthfully say that the money becomes primarily the "score" in the quest for accomplishment.

- *Employee participation.* Allowing employees to participate in establishing or revising methods, procedures, and processes is potentially one of the strongest individual motivators. In addition to involving the employee in determining how the work is done, doing so provides increased responsibility, adds interest and challenge, and promotes the acquisition of new knowledge.

APPRECIATIVE INQUIRY

Appreciative Inquiry (AI) is an approach to organizational change and development that begins with examination of what is working well and appreciation, through active recognition and expression, of the best of the individual and the group or organization's experience. Developed in the mid-1980s by Dr. David Cooperrider, Suresh Srivastva, and their colleagues at Case Western Reserve University, AI has been applied to a variety of organizational settings, including large federal agencies such as the Department of Health and Human Services, business ventures, and professional associations.[10]

The AI Process

When a manager uses the AI approach, the focus is on the values and mission of the organization, and the positive experiences of the individual members of the organization. In the health care setting, this can be broadened to include client or patient groups as well as the professional, technical, and support staffs. The operative assumption is the understanding that something, even many things, are working well. These positive experiences are explicitly recalled and actively noted as successes. Using these positive accomplishments, the group then builds on them to envision improvements. A set of goal statements is developed, or updated, based on the newly energized vision of the organization's efforts. By way of example, consider the difference in these two methods of dealing with patient safety, risk management, and incident reporting and review. In a more traditional approach, the emphasis is on the number, causes, and characteristics of the problems relating to patient safety—for example, number of falls, medication errors, or misdiagnoses. In an AI approach, the emphasis is on the goal of making this organization the most safe environment for patients, staff, and visitors. The review process would still include specific data such as those noted above. However, the data would be cast in the context of all the care that is given without mishap. Specific problem areas will usually decrease simply as a result of positive efforts at improvement of safety practices.

Motivational Aspects

AI is a planning process that, by its nature, includes motivation through positive reinforcement of the good. The process diffuses potential conflict because the best results of both individuals and departments or divisions are emphasized. Cooperation and enthusiasm for participation is enhanced. Managers have many opportunities in their ongoing work to apply AI. Consider, for example, the usual concerns associated with preparation for outside surveys and reviews, such as accreditation or licensure inspections. The preparation of the survey report necessarily involves fact gathering. Instead of using the mindset that there are many vague problems that will come to light, the management team could start with reaffirming its best practices, noting these, and then isolate those areas needing improvement. Note, by way of example, the consultant report in Chapter 6; the areas of compliance, which represent the majority of the day-to-day practices, are clearly listed, then the areas needing improvement are given. Another situation of potential concern and conflict is associated with periodic labor union contract negations. Typically, each party brings to the table its list of concerns and demands. Using an AI approach, however, the starting point would be a reflection on those areas of management–labor relations and those provisions of the contract that have enhanced the accomplishment of the organization's mission.

When an organization as a whole, or a group within an organization, has experienced much change and yet another major change must be absorbed, AI can be used to coalesce the positive energy needed to carry on. For example, the recent implementation of the HIPAA regulations involved major changes that affected budgeting, vendor selection, collection, processing, and releasing patient care information. In taking on this challenge, the health information manager and the professional association as a whole recalled its long-standing commitment to privacy and confidentiality with the concomitant successes in these areas. These managers were easily motivated to take leadership roles in implementing these new requirements regarding confidentiality and security of patient care information.

Using the AI approach, a manager carries out an employee performance review using as a starting point the employee's assessment of the work and his or her contribution to the department's mission. The manager would invite the employee to identify all the areas where he or she is performing well and then discuss those areas where performance could be improved.

Using the framework of AI, a manager continually seeks to utilize opportunities to express public appreciation for all that is going well. The customary declaration of a week highlighting one or another department is an example of this practice. The nomination of employees as "Employee of the Month" or similar recognition events reflect an AI attitude. The celebration of milestones in a professional organization's life cycle is yet another opportunity to reflect on past accomplishments, leading to emphasis on future endeavors.

CONFLICT

Conflict is an inevitable component of cooperative action, and the effects of conflict are felt by all participants in organizational life. Indeed, in a sense organizational life largely consists of carefully orchestrated conflict, so much so that one of the classic functions of a manager is to ensure coordination, which includes promoting cooperation and minimizing conflict.

Dictionary definitions of conflict use terms such as *variance, incompatibility, disagreement, inner divergence,* and *disturbance.* Conflict is basically a state of external and internal tension that results when two or more demands are made on an individual, group, or organization.

The Study of Conflict

The manager and health care practitioner must understand the phenomenon of conflict within organizations so that they can make it acceptable, predictable, and therefore manageable. Conflict must be accepted as an inevitable part of all group effort. The causes of conflict are located primarily in the organizational structure, with its system of authority, roles, and specialization. The clash of personal styles of interaction can be analyzed so as to deal more effectively with such clashes.

Conflict can be accepted as an element of change, a positive catalyst for continual challenge to the organization. Aggression may be accepted and channeled to foster survival. If conflict is not channeled and controlled, it may have negative effects that impede the growth of both the individual and the organization.

In certain situations, conflict may clarify relationships, effect change, and define organizational territories or jurisdictions. When there has been an integrative solution, resulting from open review of all points of view, agreement is strengthened and morale heightened. Conflict tends to energize an organization, forcing it to keep alert, to plan and anticipate change, and to serve clients in more effective ways.

ORGANIZATIONAL CONFLICT

Managers can assess organizational conflicts by using a theoretical model, since it frees them from the bias created by their own immediate involvement in the conflict. By analyzing conflict in a relatively objective manner, a manager can deal with it more positively and more easily. The following is a basic model for such an analysis:

1. The basic conflict
   a. overt level
   b. the hidden agenda
   c. the source of conflict

EXHIBIT 10–1

Conflict Model with Example

The Basic Conflict

Overt issue	Habitual lateness and/or absenteeism of employee
Hidden agenda	Growing employee resistance to managerial authority
Sources	Human need vs. organizational need
	Organizational structure

Participants

Immediate	Unit supervisor and employee
Secondary	Chief of service, personnel director
Audience	Other employees with similar problems with work schedule, other managers with similar employee disciplinary problems, and higher levels of management who monitor organizational climate

Arena	Grievance procedure
Rules	Work rules re: attendance, procedures for filing grievances
Strategy	Limitation of conflict to unit members

2. The participants
   a. immediate and primary participants
   b. secondary participants
   c. the audience
3. The provision of an arena
4. The development of rules
5. Strategies for dealing with organizational conflict

Exhibit 10–1 is an example of the use of this model.

The Basic Conflict

Overt Level

As a starting point, the manager analyzing a conflict describes the obvious problem. This process of naming the conflict elements provides focus and clarifies the issues that are at stake. Examples include:

- habitual lateness by an employee
- delays in transport of patients from inpatient services to physical therapy or occupational therapy services
- lack of clarity about job responsibilities
- delays in treating patients, causing patients to wait unduly for their appointments

The Hidden Agenda

While the overt issue may be the true and only substance of the conflict, there is sometimes another area of conflict that constitutes a hidden agenda. This hidden agenda may be the true conflict, or it may be an adjunct issue. The process of naming the conflict and describing its elements helps bring to light any hidden agenda that may exist.

Conflict issues are buried for several reasons. They may be too explosive to deal with openly, or subconscious protective mechanisms may prevent a threatening subject from surfacing until the individual in question has a safe structure and the necessary support to deal with it. Within an institution, the climate may not be appropriate for accepting conflict, or organizational resources may be insufficient to deal with it.

The subtleties of intraorganizational power struggles cause certain aspects of conflict to remain hidden. Individuals may choose to obscure the real issue as a means of testing their strength, of determining points of opposition before plunging ahead with an issue, or of checking the intensity of opposition. Periodic sparring over issues that never seem to be resolved is a clue to the existence of a hidden agenda. For example, the hospital budget issue of billing a medical group practice for certain administrative services may surface each year for temporary resolution. The root of the problem is not the allocation of money; it is the creation of a new institutional structure. As a consequence, organizational control of outpatient services is at stake.

The Sources of Conflict

The definition of a conflict should indicate its primary sources: competition for resources, authority relationships, extraorganizational pressures, and so on. As discussed earlier, organizational conflicts are ultimately due to the individuals who participate in organizational activities.

The Nature of the Organization. Organizations with multiple goals face competing and sometimes mutually exclusive demands for available resources. A hospital, for example, must safeguard against malpractice claims through active risk control management, yet it must also contain costs. The rules, regulations, and requirements imposed by the many controllers of the organization identified in the clientele network may be a source of conflict. Shifting client demand and changes in the degree of client participation in the organization lead to conflict when an increase in the allocation of resources for one group is a loss for another. The authority structure is another clue to potential conflict; members of coercive organizations are more frequently in conflict with the organization than are members of normative institutions.

The Organizational Climate. An emphasis on competition as a means of enhancing productivity, as in the use of the "deadly parallel" organizational structure or the use of a reward system that emphasizes competition among individuals or departments, may cause conflict. The intentional overlap and blurred jurisdiction of units can produce continual jockeying for organizational territory. Competition for scarce resources may be sharp, with resulting conflict, coalitions, and compromises. The subtleties of an institution's power struggles, the shifting balance of power (e.g., a growing union movement), and the need to demonstrate power constitute another facet of organizational climate. Denial of conflict is a potential source of trouble, since it removes a safe outlet for the resolution of conflict before it becomes a serious problem.

The Organizational Structure. The complex authority structure in health care organizations (i.e., a dual track of authority coupled with an increasing professionalism among the many specialized workers) creates situations of potential conflict. Professional practitioners, such as nurses, physical therapists, clinical psychologists, and social workers, are trained to assess patient needs and to take actions within the scope of licensure or certification; however, their ability to make decisions is limited by the hierarchical organizational structure. This problem is compounded when the individual practitioner has a legal duty to act or refrain from acting that is directly opposite to the hierarchical system, such as when a nurse refrains from giving a medication that would be harmful to the patient even when the physician has (inadvertently) ordered such a dosage.

Physicians, in holding staff appointments, find themselves required to shift regularly from their roles as independent practitioners when functioning outside the health care facility to more limited roles as members of the organizational hierarchy. This regular role shift may also be required of the physical therapist, nurse practitioner, or occupational therapist who functions as an independent agent in private practice and at the same time participates in the patient care process as a staff member of a health care institution.

Conflict may also arise from specialization within the organizational structure when individuals attempt to carry out their assigned activities. For example, the social worker might seek to place a patient in a long-term care facility, but the utilization review coordinator must impose strict guidelines in terms of days of care allotted under certain payment contracts. The health information manager must develop a system of record control, although many users of records find it more practical to retain records in restricted areas of their own. The purchasing agent must comply with certain regulations on deadlines, budget restrictions, and auditing procedures in spite of individual needs. Specialization within the complexities of bureaucratization leads to frustration, misunderstanding, and conflict.

Superior–subordinate relationships constitute another area of potential conflict. The organizational chart is, in fact, a suppression chart that specifies which positions have authority over and literally suppress other individual jobs or units. The legitimacy of a leader's claim to office is continually assessed. The power, prestige, and rewards built into the hierarchical system all represent gain for some and related loss for others. The erosion of traditional territory associated with line management results from activities clearly intended to remove some authority from line managers. These activities include client or worker involvement in decision making.

The process of management by objectives, in which the workers are directly involved in setting and assessing objectives, commands much attention for its motivational value; streamlined processes, such as central number assignments or patient bed assignments, have much merit as systems improvements; a central pool of patient aides, assistants, and transporters is an alternative to assignment by department. Yet each of these processes erodes the distinct territory of one or several managers, whose ability to make decisions is affected by such changes. Increased specialization in some technical areas leads to a more frequent use of functional specialists. Although the line manager retains authority, the specialist must be included in the planning and decision-making process; the line manager is no longer the sole agent.

Unions may invade managerial territory in several areas relating to personnel management and direct work assignment. In the collective bargaining process, the nature of the work, who will do it, and how much will be done may be issues. Union gains may be management losses.

Individual versus Organizational Needs. Human needs and values must be welded into the organizational framework. A large number of clients and workers enter the organization, and they have different values, experience, motives, and expectations. The degree to which each individual internalizes the values of the organization and accepts a primary identity derived from the institution varies greatly. Individuals who do not participate directly in the accomplishment of organizational goals or in the institutional authority structure tend to identify less with the organization and view its demands less favorably than those who participate more fully in direct, goal-oriented activities.

Solutions to Previous Conflicts. New problems may arise from solutions to previous conflicts. The use of compromise as a strategy in dealing with conflict tends to leave all participants somewhat dissatisfied. At the next opportunity, one or more participants may seek to reopen the issue in order to regain what was lost, particularly if the loss was acute. The loser may build up resources and enter into an active state of aggression when such resources have been accumulated, such as a nation defeated after a war (e.g., Germany after World War I). When there is a consistent denial pattern, the conflict may "go underground" for a time, then emerge again with greater force. Again, managers should realistically examine the negative consequences of conflict resolutions in order to minimize their recurrence.

The Participants

The immediate participants in the conflict can be identified readily as the individuals or groups caught in the open exchange. The secondary participants are the individuals called in to take an active role, such as persons at the next level of the hierarchy. A manager may consult with a senior official to whom the individual involved in the conflict reports or with a staff adviser, such as a labor relations specialist. A unit manager may be required in some instances to refer conflict to the next level for resolution, as in some grievance procedures. In the case of a unionized employee, a representative of the union, such as a shop steward, may be involved. A "neutral" may be called in by both parties in a labor dispute (e.g., a mediator or an arbitrator). Occasionally, a manager may consult informally with certain "marginal" individuals, such as those in the department or organization who have an overlapping role set, a supervisor whose domain spans several activities, a client who is also on an advisory committee, or another department head who has faced similar situations. Because they link groups, these individuals are sought out in order to test a potential solution or to obtain information and even advice.

A third category of participants may be classified as the audience. This category may include the following:

- *The Clients.* If the conflict is overt and severe, the organization may turn to other organizations for the necessary services in order to avoid the conflict. Uncertainty may cause tension within this group, however, and clients may become active participants. A client group alienated from the institution may develop its own system to meet its needs.

- *The Public at Large.* This group may seek action through recourse to some government agency, and an agency's intervention into the conflict may take the form of additional regulation of the organization. The conflict may be brought into the public arena; for example, a labor dispute may be taken to court. The net effect of intervention by some agent on behalf of the public at large is the opening or broadening of the conflict, which removes it from the immediate control of the original parties to the dispute.

- *A Potential Rival or Enemy.* While one group and its opponents are absorbed in conflict, a third group whose energies are not drained by conflict may seek to expand its services and attract the clients of the groups locked in the dispute.

- *Individuals or Groups with Similar Complaints.* Some observers may seek to press a similar claim if "the right side" wins. In the case of employee unrest, a labor organizer may consider more active unionization attempts. Independent practitioners who seek greater autonomy in the practice of health care may monitor changes in organizational bylaws or state licensure regulations and find gains made by one individual or group of practitioners the catalyst needed to obtain similar gains. In malpractice cases, jury awards are monitored and publicized. As the basis for a certain kind of claim is expanded through a trend in court decisions, more individuals may advance their cases. Without extensive publicity of the benchmark cases, this basis of claim might not have arisen. A worker who sees another worker win a concession from the manager about some work rule will more readily press a similar claim.

- *The Opportunist.* Some individual or group may seek to enter the conflict as champion or savior. Such action may be undertaken by individuals seeking to raise themselves to leadership positions.

In many cases, members of the audience not only cheer and jeer but also become active participants, thus expanding the conflict in terms of the number of individuals or groups who must be satisfied in any solution.

Conflict should be resolved at as low an organizational level as possible. The facts are better known by the immediate participants, who are able to communicate directly. Also, because the number of participants is limited, agreement on a solution may be more easily obtained. Top levels of management should be involved only rarely in conflicts within the organization, because their involvement might give undue weight to the problem, establish precedent, and force the setting of policy that escalates resolutions to a higher level. The resources of top management should generally be reserved for critical issues.

The Provision of an Arena

The development of a safe, predictable, and accessible arena tends to create a sense of security and to keep the problems from becoming diffuse. The aggrieved know where to turn and what to do in order to seek redress. The provision of an acceptable arena is also efficient. The individuals involved give their attention to it in a highly structured manner, and it establishes clear boundaries to the conflict. It is legitimate to bring issues of conflict to this place, through this structure, at these designated times. The court system and legislative debate are such arenas in the larger society. In organizations, arenas include the structured grievance process for employees (Exhibit 10–2), the appeals process for the professional staff member seeking staff appointment, or the complaint department for customers. Committees in which multiple input is invited are also common arenas for the resolution of conflict.

The Development of Rules

Rules serve to limit the energy expended on the conflict process. The provision of rules has a face-saving and legitimizing effect; it is permissible to disagree, equal time is guaranteed, and each point of view is aired. The rules also provide a basis for the intervention of a referee or neutral. The rules may be developed to allow a cooling-off period so that the issues can be put in perspective. The time frame given by the rules reduces uneasiness, since participants are assured of a legitimate opportunity to present the issues. Conflict remains under control.

Strategies for Dealing with Organizational Conflict

Two strategies for dealing with conflict are opposite in nature: limitation and purposeful expansion. The limitation of conflict as a strategy was developed by E. E. Schattschneider, who noted the contagiousness of conflict. An organization runs the risk of losing control as conflict is widened, and it is unlikely that both

EXHIBIT 10–2

Excerpts from Grievance Procedure

Any grievance that may arise between the parties concerning the application, meaning, or interpretation of this Agreement shall be resolved in the following manner:

Step 1: An employee having a grievance and his Union delegate shall discuss it with his immediate supervisor within five (5) working days after it arose or should have been made known to the employee. The Hospital shall give its response through the supervisor to the employee and to this Union delegate within five (5) working days after the presentation of the grievance. In the event no appeal is taken to the next step (Step 2) the decision rendered in this step shall be final.

Step 2: If the grievance is not settled in Step 1, the grievance may, within five (5) working days after the answer in Step 1, be presented in Step 2. When grievances are presented in Step 2, they shall be reduced to writing on grievance forms provided by the Hospital (which shall then be assigned a number by the Personnel Services at the Union's request), signed by the grievant and his or her Union representative, and presented to the Department Head and the Department of Personnel Services. A grievance so presented in Step 2 shall be answered in writing within five (5) working days after its presentation.

sides will be reinforced equally. Conflict is best kept private, limited, and therefore controllable.[11]

An underlying purpose of the intentional expansion of conflict is to demonstrate its immediate effect on the clients or the public, who in turn will bring pressure on the opposing party to end the dispute. The immediate involvement of the client group is sought in the hope that it will act as a catalytic factor, forcing quick resolution. For example, a teachers' union may go on strike at the beginning of a school year, a coal miners' union may strike during the winter, and traffic officers may conduct a slowdown or job action during the height of the Fourth of July traffic to the shore.

The routinization of conflict is a third strategy. Another aspect of this strategy may be seen in the symbolic value of the short strike that is a kind of catharsis, an annual or biennial event. Other strategies include concepts noted in other discussions, for example, co-optation, strategic leniency, preformed decisions, and the selection of individuals who fit the organization.

In addition to such conscious strategies, a manager should make use of the general principles of sound organization. When used properly, these principles bring about stability and reduce conflict. Known policies and rules, sufficient orientation and training of members, proper authority-responsibility designations, and clear chains of command and communication: these practices foster cooperation and mutual expectation, with the attendant reduction of undue conflict. Finally, awareness of "burnout" and programs to prevent it can contribute to the reduction of conflict and enhance motivation. Such programs are discussed in the next chapter.

THE LABOR UNION AND THE COLLECTIVE BARGAINING AGREEMENT

Since the National Labor Relations Act was amended in 1975 to remove the exemption of not-for-profit hospitals, workers in health care organizations have been permitted by federal law to organize into labor unions. The specific exemption of not-for-profit hospitals had been in place since 1947, so between 1947 and 1975 the only active union organizing that occurred in not-for-profit institutions was that made possible by the labor relations laws of a few of the states.

The typical collective bargaining agreement reflects management and the union's efforts to contain and control conflict and provide a framework for the resolution of disagreement. Appendix 10–A contains a typical collective bargaining agreement. The entire agreement is included to provide the complete context of the formal relationship between employer and union; however, with specific reference to conflict both actual and potential, attention is called to the following articles:

- Articles Six and Seven, in which the contracting parties agree to the limitation of conflict during the life of the agreement;
- Articles Fourteen and Fifteen, which provide for the orderly resolution of disciplinary actions and complaints by employees against management;
- Articles Eight through Twenty, which address the specifics of working conditions, hours of work, benefits of employment, and other employment-related matters in a manner intended to provide clear guidelines for practice and thus to avoid conflict or minimize the chances of conflict occurring.

Although some members of the health care organization, especially managers and professionals, may find a collective bargaining agreement restrictive because of the apparent limitations it places on actions of various kinds, the overall clarity of the provisions in a well-written contract, plus the fact of its having been negotiated by management and workers together so that both sides "own" the agreement, can sometimes foster positive organizational relationships. When the occasional conflict does occur, the provisions of the contract can guide its resolution.

CASE: A MATTER OF MOTIVATION: THE DELAYED PROMOTION

Background

With considerable advance notice the director of health information management (HIM) resigned to take a similar position in a hospital in another state. Within the department it was commonly assumed that you, the assistant director, would be appointed director; however, a month after the former director's departure the department was still running without a director. Day-to-day operations had apparently been left in your hands ("apparently," because nothing had been said to you), but the hospital's chief operating officer had begun to make some of the administrative decisions affecting the department.

After another month had passed you learned "through the grapevine" that the hospital had interviewed several candidates for the position of director of health information management. Nobody had been hired.

During the next few weeks you tried several times to discuss your uncertain status with the chief operating officer. Each time you tried you were told simply to "keep doing what you're now doing."

Four months after the previous director's departure you were promoted to director of HIM. The first instruction you received from the chief operating officer was to abolish the position of assistant director.

Instructions

1. Thoroughly analyze and describe the likely state of your ability to "motivate" yourself in your new position. In the process, comment to whatever extent you feel necessary on your level of confidence in the relative stability of your position and how this might affect your performance.

2. Describe the most likely motivational state of your HIM staff at the time you assumed the director's position, and explain in detail why this state probably exists.

CASE: CHARTING A COURSE FOR CONFLICT RESOLUTION: "IT'S A POLICY"

Background

The setting is an 82-bed hospital located in a small city. One day an employee of the maintenance department asked the supervisor, George Mann, for an hour or two off to take care of some personal business. Mann agreed, and asked the employee to stop at the garden equipment dealership and buy several small lawn-mower parts the department required.

While transacting business at a local bank the employee was seen by Sally Carter, the supervisor of both human resources and payroll, who was in the bank on hospital business. Carter asked the employee what he was doing there and was told the visit was personal.

Upon returning to the hospital, Sally Carter examined the employee's time card. The employee had not punched out to indicate when he had left the hospital. Carter noted the time the employee returned, and after the normal working day she marked the card to indicate an absence of two hours on personal business. Carter advised the chief executive officer (CEO), Jane Arnold, of what she had done, citing a long-standing policy (in their dusty, and some would say infrequently used, policy manual) requiring an employee to punch out when leaving the premises on personal business. The CEO agreed with Sally Carter's action.

Carter advised Mann of the action and stated that the employee would not be paid for the two hours he was gone.

Mann was angry. He said he had told the employee not to punch out because he had asked him to pick up some parts on his trip; however, Mann conceded that the employee's personal business was probably the greater part of the trip. Carter replied that Mann had no business doing what he had done and that it was his—Mann's—poor management that had caused the employee to suffer.

Mann appealed to the CEO to reopen the matter based on his claim that there was an important side to the story that she had not yet heard. Jane Arnold agreed to hear both managers state their position.

Instructions

1. In either paragraph form or as a list of points, develop the argument you would be advancing if you were in George Mann's position.

2. In similar fashion, thoroughly develop the argument you would advance if you were in Sally Carter's position.

3. Assuming the position of CEO, Jane Arnold, render a decision. Document your decision in whatever detail may be necessary, complete with explanation of why you decided in this fashion.

4. Based on the foregoing, outline whatever steps—policy changes, guidelines, payroll requirements, or whatever—you believe should be considered to minimize the chances of similar conflict in the future.

NOTES

1. H. Kaufman, *The Forest Ranger: A Study in Administrative Behavior* (Baltimore: Johns Hopkins University Press, 1967), 128.
2. Ibid., 170.
3. Ibid., 178.
4. R. Presthus, *The Organizational Society* (New York: Random House, 1962), 166, 178–226, passim 286.
5. A. Maslow, *Motivation and Personality* (New York: Harper & Row, 1954).
6. F. Herzberg, *The Motivation to Work* (New York: Wiley, 1959).
7. Paul Hersey and Kenneth Blanchard, *Management of Organizational Behavior* (Englewood Cliffs, N.J.: Prentice-Hall, 1982), 60.
8. D. McGregor, *The Human Side of Enterprise* (New York: McGraw-Hill, 1960).
9. William Ouchi, *Theory Z: How American Business Can Meet the Japanese Challenge* (Reading, Mass.: Addison-Wesley, 1981).
10. David Cooperrider et al., *Appreciative Inquiry: Rethinking Human Organization Toward a Positive Theory of Change* (Champaign, Ill.: Stipes Publishing, 2000).
11. E. E. Schattschneider, *The Semisovereign People* (New York: Holt, Rinehart, & Winston, 1960), 1–18.

Appendix
10-A

Sample Collective Bargaining Agreement

(Fictitious in all respects, for classroom use only to illustrate various aspects of contract agreement.)

COLLECTIVE BARGAINING AGREEMENT BETWEEN JGL MEMORIAL HOSPITAL AND THE CLERICAL AND TECHNICAL HOSPITAL EM-

PLOYEES' GUILD OF GREATER NEW CITY METROPOLIS, AFL-CIO AND ITS AFFILIATE LOCAL 123b.

This agreement dated January 4, 2007, to be effective as of February 1, 2007, is entered into between JGL MEMORIAL HOSPITAL (herein called the "Hospital") and Clerical and Technical Hospital Employees' Guild of Greater New City Metropolis AFL-CIO AND ITS AFFILIATE Local 123b (*herein called the "Union").

ARTICLE ONE—INTENT AND PURPOSE

1.1 Whereas, the Hospital is engaged in furnishing an essential public service vital to the health, welfare, and safety of the community and more particularly of the patients seeking and receiving service at the hospital; and

Whereas, both the Hospital and its employees have a high degree of responsibility to provide such services without interruption of this essential service; and

Whereas, both parties recognize this mutual obligation, they have entered into this Agreement to promote and improve the mutual interests of the Hospital and its employees and to establish and maintain cooperation and harmony between the Hospital and its employees;

Now, therefore, in consideration of the mutual promises and obligations herein assumed, the parties agree as follows:

ARTICLE TWO—RECOGNITION

2.1 The Hospital recognizes the Union as the sole collective bargaining Agency for all technical and clerical workers including messengers, mailroom workers, unit clerks, clerks and clerk typists, secretaries, and other technical workers as certified in the State labor relations board certification of December 11, 20NX.

2.2 The Unit specifically excludes supervisors, temporary workers, casual workers, and students.

2.3 Part-time work employees who work twenty (20) or more hours per week shall be covered by the terms of this agreement upon completion of the probationary period.

2.4 The number of part-time employees shall not exceed 5 percent of the total number of bargaining unit employees in each department as of February 1, 20N1. Temporary employees and students and independent contractual employees may not be hired for a period longer than four months per job per year.

ARTICLE THREE—UNION SECURITY

3.1 It shall be a condition of employment that all employees of the Hospital covered by this agreement who are members of the Union in good standing on the effective date of this agreement shall remain members in good standing and those who are not members on the effective date of this agreement shall, after the sixtieth (60th) day actually worked, following the date of signing this agreement, or its effective date, whichever is later, become and remain members in good standing in the Union. It shall also be a condition of employment that all employees covered by this agreement and hired on or after the date of signing or its effective date, whichever is later, shall, after the sixtieth (60th) day actually worked following such date, become and remain members in good standing in the Union.

3.2 The failure of any employee to become a member of the Union at the required time shall obligate the Hospital, upon written notice from the Union to such effect and to the further effect that Union membership was available to such employee on the same terms and conditions generally available to other members, to forthwith discharge such employee. Further, the failure of any employee to maintain his Union membership in good standing as required herein shall, upon written notice to the Hospital by the Union to such effect, obligate the Hospital to discharge such employee. Following such notification to the Hospital, the employee shall be given a period of not more than thirty (30) days during which he shall be given an opportunity to reestablish his membership in good standing with the Union.

3.3 The Union agrees that the payment of regular monthly membership dues and initiation fees shall constitute membership in good standing.

3.4 The Hospital shall for the term of this Agreement deduct union dues and initiation fees from such employees who are members of the Union and who individually and voluntarily notify the Hospital through written authorization to the Hospital for deductions from any wage paid to such employee. The Hospital agrees to make such deductions on the first payday of each month or at such other time as both the Hospital and the Union shall mutually agree and shall remit such monies promptly to the designated officer of the National Union. The Hospital shall supply the Union with a list of those employees for whom deductions were made and the amount of deductions per current month.

3.5 The Hospital will furnish the Union each month with the names, addresses, Social Security numbers, classification of work, dates of hires, names of terminated employees, together with their dates of termination, and the names of employees on leave of absence and specific kind of leave of absence. Employees shall promptly notify the Hospital of changes in their names and addresses.

3.6 The Union shall indemnify and save the Hospital harmless against any claim, demands, suits, and other forms of liability that may arise out of action taken or not taken by the Hospital for purposes of compliance with these provisions.

ARTICLE FOUR—NO DISCRIMINATION

4.1 There shall be no discrimination against or for an employee because of race, color, creed, national origin, political belief, sex, age, Union membership, or non-membership by the Hospital or by the Union.

ARTICLE FIVE—MANAGEMENT RIGHTS

5.1 Unless expressly included in this Agreement, nothing herein contained shall be construed to limit the Hospital's right to exercise the functions of management under which it shall have, among others, the right to employ, supervise, and direct the working force, to discipline, suspend, discharge employees for just cause, transfer and lay off employees because of lack of work, to require employees to observe reasonable work rules and regulations not inconsistent with this Agreement; to determine the extent to which its properties, equipment, and facilities shall be maintained and/or operated or shut down; to introduce new or improved methods and/or procedures; to determine the services to be rendered to patients and the schedules of maintaining such services; and otherwise to manage or conduct the facility, provided that these provisions shall not be used for the sole purpose of depriving any Hospital employee of work. The above rights are not all inclusive, but indicate the type of matters or rights that belong to and are inherent to Management. Any of the rights, power, and authority the Hospital had prior to entering this collective bargaining agreement are retained by the Hospital except as expressly and specifically abridged, delegated, granted, or modified by this Agreement.

ARTICLE SIX—UNION ACTIVITY

6.1 Except for Union activity expressly provided for in this agreement, no employee shall engage in any Union activity, including the distribution of literature, which could interfere with the performance of work during working time or in working areas at any time.

6.2 Union representatives (or its designee) shall have reasonable access to the Hospital for the purpose of administering the provision of this agreement, provided they obtain clearance from the designated Hospital official, who shall not unduly restrict such access.

6.3 The Hospital will provide bulletin boards for Union use for the purpose of posting only Union notices. Such bulletin boards shall be located at places readily accessible to the employees' place of work. The Union will be permitted to post on these boards such notices of a noncontroversial nature, copies to be submitted to the Labor Relations manager prior to posting.

6.4 The work schedules of employees elected as Union Delegates shall be adjusted so far as practicable as to permit attendance at regularly scheduled meetings after normal working hours, provided the Hospital's operations shall not be impaired. The Union shall give reasonable notice to the Labor Relations manager of such regularly scheduled meetings and the names of such delegates.

ARTICLE SEVEN—NO STRIKE: NO LOCKOUT

7.1 During the terms of this agreement, neither the Union nor the employees shall engage in any strike, sit-down, sit-in, slow-down, cessation, stoppage, interruption of work, boycott, or other interference with the operations of the Hospital.

7.2 The union, its officers, agents, representatives, and members shall not in any way, directly or indirectly, authorize, assist, encourage, participate in, or sanction any strike, sit-down, sit-in, slow-down, cessation or stoppage or interruption of work or other interference of the operations of the Hospital, or ratify, condone, or lend support to any such conduct or action.

7.3 Should any strike, slow-down, picketing, or other curtailment, restriction, or interference with Hospital functions or operations occur that the Union has not caused or sanctioned either directly or indirectly, the Union shall immediately:

(a) Publicly disavow such actions by the employees or persons involved.

(b) Advise the Hospital in writing that such action has not been caused or sanctioned by the Union.

(c) Post notices on the Union bulletin boards stating that it disapproves of such actions and instruct the members to return to work immediately.

(d) Take such other steps as would reasonably ensure renewed observance of provisions of this Article.

7.4 The Hospital shall have the right to discharge or otherwise discipline all employees or the Union on their behalf without having recourse to the grievance procedure and arbitration, except for the sole purpose of determining whether an employee participated in the prohibited action.

7.5 During the terms of this Agreement, the Hospital shall not engage in any lockout of any employee.

ARTICLE EIGHT—HOURS OF WORK AND OVERTIME

8.1 Eight (8) hours shall constitute a regular day's work and forty (40) hours shall constitute a regular week's work in any one day or in any one week. A work day is defined as the continuous twenty-four (24) hour period beginning at the employee's regular starting time.

8.2 All work performed by an employee in excess of forty (40) hours in any one week shall be paid for at the rate of time and one-half.

8.3 The Hospital shall distribute and allot overtime work to best suit the efficient operation of a department and will make every reasonable effort to distribute in a reasonable way the overtime work equitably among the employees of the department in which the overtime occurs, provided the employee is qualified to perform the work.

8.4 All employees shall receive a one-hour paid lunch period, which shall be counted as time worked. The Hospital will schedule this lunch period.

8.5 There shall be no pyramiding or duplicating of overtime rates. Hours compensated for at overtime rates under one provision of this Agreement shall be excluded as hours worked in computing overtime under any other provision. When two or more provisions requiring the payment of overtime rates are applicable, the one most favorable to the employee shall apply.

8.6 Employees shall be required to work overtime when assigned for the proper administration of the Hospital's operations.

ARTICLE NINE—RATES OF PAY: SHIFT DIFFERENTIALS

9.1 Job classifications and rates of pay and progression in existence on the day of this agreement are set forth in Attachment A, which is made part of this agreement.

9.2 If during the term of this Agreement new job classifications are established or substantial changes are made in existing job classifications covered by the bargaining unit, the Hospital will put the new or changed job classification into effect and establish a rate of pay therefor. Such rate will be discussed with the Union in advance, with the objective of obtaining its agreement. The Hospital may then install the rate with or without agreement; when installed after agreement, no grievance may be filed with respect to the rate. If installed without agreement, the employee(s) affected or the Union may within thirty (30) days present a grievance protesting the rate if that rate does not bear a proper relationship to existing rates. If no grievance is filed within the thirty (30) days or if the grievance is settled, the new rate will become part of Attachment A (wage scale) and shall not be subject to challenge under the grievance procedure.

9.3 Full-time employees working on a shift that begins on or after 3:00 P.M., and before 4:00 A.M., shall be paid a shift differential of $2.85 per hour. An employee who is entitled to a shift differential for work on his regular shift shall receive the shift differential for overtime hours that are an extension of the regular shift. A shift differential shall not be paid when employees are authorized to exchange shifts temporarily for personal reasons.

9.4 A shift differential shall not be gained or lost as a result of an extension of a shift caused by overtime.

9.5 If an employee is regularly assigned to a shift receiving a shift differential, the differential shall be included in calculating the employee's vacation, holiday, and sick leave pay.

ARTICLE TEN—PROBATIONARY EMPLOYEES

10.1 New employees and those hired after a break in continuity of service of more than six months will be regarded as probationary employees until they have actually worked sixty (60) days and will receive no continuous service credit during such period. During this period of probationary employment, probationary employees may be disciplined, laid off, or discharged as exclusively determined by the Hospital, and the Hospital shall not be subject to the grievance and arbitration provision of this Agreement.

Continuing employees who apply for and are accepted into another job/position are considered probationary employees for 25 working days. See Article 11.9 for related stipulations.

10.2 The rate of pay for new employees and those hired after a break in continuity of service of more than six months shall be the hiring rate for the job. The rate of pay for continuing employees shall be the grade level rate of pay.

ARTICLE ELEVEN—SENIORITY: LAYOFFS AND PROMOTIONS

11.1 Seniority is defined as an employee's length of continuous regular full-time Hospital service last date of hire. Employees who were hired the same day shall have their seniority established by lot and carried subsequently on the seniority list.

11.2 Seniority is computed from the day of last hire, upon completion of the probationary period delineated in Article Ten.

11.3 Seniority shall accrue

(a) During any authorized leave of absence with pay.

(b) During an authorized leave of absence without pay because of personal illness or accident for a period of six months or less, or maternity leave for a period of one year.

During military service, as provided by federal law, an employee will not accrue, but will not lose, seniority during an authorized leave of absence without pay.

11.4 An employee will lose seniority when he

(a) Voluntarily terminates his full-time employment.

(b) Is discharged for cause.

(c) Willfully exceeds the length, or violates the purpose, of an authorized leave of absence.

(d) Is laid off for a period of six months or the length of the employee's service with the Hospital, whichever is less.

(e) Fails to report in accordance with a notice for recall from layoff within 48 hours of the time specified in the notice sent by certified mail to the last address furnished to the Hospital by the employee. The Hospital shall send a copy of the notification to the Union.

(f) Fails to report for recall to the assigned job.

An absence from work for three consecutive work days without notice or permission shall be deemed a voluntary resignation.

11.5 An employee who is or has been promoted or transferred out of the bargaining unit and who is later transferred back into the bargaining unit by the Hospital shall be credited upon returning to the bargaining unit with the seniority he would have had if he had remained continuously in the bargaining unit.

11.6 In the event of a layoff in a department, temporary employees shall be laid off first, then probationary employees, then regular part-time employees, and then regular full-time employees on the basis of their Hospital-wide seniority. In the event a full-time permanent nonprobationary employee is scheduled to be laid off from a department he or she may either bid for a posted vacant position in accordance with the provisions of Section 7 or displace another employee within the department of equal or lesser grade on the basis of Hospital-wide seniority, provided he has the ability to perform said job within 25 days. The immediate department manager shall determine the employee's acceptability.

11.7 Recall from layoff

Employees on layoff shall be recalled as follows:

(a) To a position, if open, previously held successfully in department by the employee regardless of place on the recall list.

(b) In reverse order of layoff on a Hospital-wide basis to other open positions with the following provisions:

1. Employees may not upgrade from the recall list.

2. The employee must be acceptable to the hiring supervisor.

3. The employee must have the ability to perform the open position. The hiring supervisor shall determine the employee's acceptability for that position during the applicable probationary period for a newly hired employee in that grade level.

4. When probationary or part-time employees are laid off they shall have no recall rights.

11.8 Promotional opportunities

(a) Openings for bargaining unit positions shall be posted for five (5) work days.

(b) Employees within a department will be given preference for promotion to a higher-paying job in the department.

(c) All bids must be submitted in person and in writing to the Office of Human Resources within the five (5) days.

(d) An open position shall be defined as a position that has been posted and for which no acceptable bidders have been found.

(e) An employee who has been promoted in pay grades six (6) to ten (10) shall not be eligible for further promotion for six (6) months.

(f) An employee who has accepted a promotional opportunity shall have twenty-five (25) working days to prove that he or she can perform in the new position.

(g) An employee who has accepted a promotional opportunity and fails the probationary period shall return to his or her previous position. If this position has been filled, the employee may be offered an open equivalent position. If none is available, the disqualified employee shall be laid off, subject to recall according to the provisions of Section 11.7.

11.9 The rate of pay during the probationary period is that of the grade level of the job.

ARTICLE TWELVE—SAFETY AND HEALTH

12.1 The Hospital agrees to provide reasonable safeguards on the premises for the health and safety of its employees. Two employees from the bargaining unit mutually agreed upon by the Hospital and the Union shall serve on the Hospital Safety Committee.

ARTICLE THIRTEEN—RESIGNATION

13.1 An employee who resigns shall give the Hospital two (2) weeks advance written notice.

13.2 An employee who fails to give such notice or whose employment is terminated shall forfeit unused vacation time, provided it was physically possible for the employee to give such notice.

ARTICLE FOURTEEN—DISCIPLINE AND DISCHARGE

14.1 No employee who has completed his probationary period shall be discharged or disciplined without just cause. If disciplinary action becomes necessary in the interest of proper operation of the Hospital, care of the patients, and general employee welfare, such actions of the Hospital shall be subject to the grievance procedure. The Hospital agrees to furnish copies to the Union of disciplinary notices resulting in suspension or discharge of an employee.

14.2 Any grievance resulting from action taken as outlined in the preceding section must be filed in writing according to the grievance procedure outlined in Article Fifteen.

ARTICLE FIFTEEN—GRIEVANCE PROCEDURE

15.1 Any grievance that may arise between the parties concerning the application, meaning, or interpretation of this Agreement shall be resolved in the following manner:

Step 1. An employee having a grievance and his Union delegate shall discuss it with his immediate department head within five (5) working days after it arose or should have been made known to the employee. The Hospital shall give its response through the department head to the employee and to this Union delegate within five (5) working days after the presentation of the grievance. In the event no appeal is taken to the next step (Step 2), the decision rendered in this step shall be final.

Step 2. If the grievance is not settled in Step 1, the grievance may, within five (5) working days after the answer in Step 1, be presented in Step 2. When grievances are presented in Step 2, they shall be reduced to writing on grievance forms provided by the Hospital (which shall then be assigned a number by the Office of Human Resources at the Union's request) signed by the grievant and his Union representative, and presented to the Department Head and the Department of Personnel Services. A grievance so presented in Step 2 shall be answered in writing within five (5) working days after its presentation.

Step 3. If the grievance is not settled in Step 2, the grievance may within five (5) working days after the answer in Step 2, be presented in Step 3. A grievance shall be presented in this step to the Office of Human Resources. The Office of Human Resources shall hold a hearing within five (5) days and shall thereafter render a decision in writing within five (5) days.

15.2 Failure on the part of the Hospital to answer a grievance at any step shall not be deemed acquiescence thereto, and the Union may proceed to the next step.

15.3 An employee who has been suspended or discharged, or the Union on his behalf, may file within five (5) business days of the suspension or discharge a grievance in writing in respect thereof with the Office of Human Resources at Step 3 of the foregoing Grievance Procedure. Any prior written warnings applicable to the employee shall be mailed to the Union by the Hospital within five (5) days after the employee is notified of his or her discharge.

15.4 All time limits herein specified shall be deemed to be exclusive of Saturdays, Sundays, and holidays.

15.5 Any disposition of a grievance from which no appeal is taken within the time limits specified herein shall be deemed resolved and shall not thereafter be considered subject to the grievance and arbitration provisions of this Agreement.

15.6 A grievance that affects a substantial number of a class of employees may initially be presented at Step 2 or Step 3 by the Union. The grievance shall then be processed in accordance with the Grievance Procedure.

ARTICLE SIXTEEN—ARBITRATION

16.1 A grievance that has not been resolved may, within ten (10) working days after completion of Step 3 of the Grievance Procedure, be referred for arbitration by the Hospital or the Union to the American Arbitration Association for resolution under the Voluntary Labor Arbitration Rules of the American Arbitration Association then prevailing.

16.2 The fees and expenses of the American Arbitration Association and the arbitrator shall be borne equally by the parties.

16.3 The award of an arbitrator hereunder shall be final, conclusive, and binding upon the Hospital, the Union, and the employees.

16.4 The arbitrator shall have jurisdiction only over grievances after completion of the Grievance Procedure, and he or she shall have no power to add to, subtract from, or modify in any way any of the terms of this Agreement.

ARTICLE SEVENTEEN—HOLIDAYS

17.1 The following days are recognized as paid holidays for full-time and part-time employees who have completed their first 25 working days of employment:

New Year's Day	Thanksgiving Day
Martin Luther King, Jr. Day	Christmas Day
Memorial Day	Two additional days that
Independence Day	may be scheduled in
Labor Day	accordance with
	employee's preference

17.2 The additional days shall be taken at a mutually agreeable time and shall be requested in writing at least five (5) working days in advance. Once scheduled these days shall not be canceled by an employee without the consent of the

Hospital. These additional days must be taken within the calendar year and are not cumulative.

17.3 Employees shall receive their regular rate of pay for each holiday observed, provided they are on active pay status.

17.4 In order to be eligible for holiday benefits, an employee must have worked the last scheduled work day before and the first scheduled workday after the holiday (or day scheduled in place of the holiday) except in the case of accident or illness preventing employee from working. The Hospital may require a written certificate from a physician or other proof.

17.5 If a holiday falls during an employee's regularly scheduled day off, the employee shall receive an additional day off or an additional day's pay, as the Hospital may decide.

17.6 If an employee is required to work on a holiday, he shall be compensated at $2\frac{1}{2}$ times his regular rate of pay for time worked or shall be given a compensatory day off at regular rate of pay, as determined by the Hospital. An employee shall not be considered as working on a holiday if the shift he is working started prior to the holiday.

17.7 If the holiday falls during an employee's vacation, he shall receive an extra day's pay or an extra day off with pay, as the Hospital shall decide.

ARTICLE EIGHTEEN—VACATION

18.1 Employees shall be granted vacation with pay according to the following schedule; vacation pay rate will be at the current straight hourly rate, including shift differential, for the number of hours indicated.

Period of Uninterrupted Service		Vacation Pay
One (1) year	10 working days	80 hours
Five (5) years	12 working days	96 hours
Six (6) years	13 working days	104 hours
Seven (7) years	14 working days	112 hours
Eight (8) years	15 working days	120 hours
Nine (9) years	16 working days	128 hours
Twenty (20) years	20 working days	160 hours

18.2 Employees whose vacations occur during a period in which a holiday occurs shall receive an extra day's pay for the holiday, or an extra day off with pay, as the Hospital shall decide.

18.3 Employees must take their vacations during the twelve-month period following their vacation eligibility year. No vacations may be carried over and employees will not be compensated for vacation time not taken. No part of an employee's scheduled vacation may be charged to sick leave.

18.4 Vacations shall be scheduled by the Hospital, in order to meet the staffing needs of the Hospital. Insofar as practicable, vacations will be granted to meet the requests of employees. Employees in each department with the greatest seniority shall have first choice of vacation period. The Hospital maintains the right to limit the number of employees permitted to be on vacation at any one time. The Hospital reserves the right to change the vacation schedule as needed.

18.5 Employees shall submit their vacation request to their Department Head in writing at least two weeks before date of desired period of vacation.

18.6 Upon written request two (2) weeks in advance, an employee will be paid his or her vacation pay before starting vacation.

18.7 Employees who give two weeks' notice of voluntary termination and employees terminated involuntarily shall be entitled to accrued vacation pay.

ARTICLE NINETEEN—SICK LEAVE

19.1 "Sick Leave" is defined as the absence of an employee from work by reason of illness or accident that is not work connected or is not compensable under the Worker's Compensation laws of the state. Full-time workers are paid for an eight-hour day; part-time workers are paid for a four-hour day.

19.2 Eligibility and Benefits. An employee who has completed his probationary period is eligible for one (1) day of sick leave earned at the rate of the said day for each full month of continuous service retroactive to his date of hire but not to exceed a total of ten (10) days for any one (1) year. As of July 1 of each year, employees with at least one (1) year of service shall be credited with ten (10) days of sick leave.

19.3 Unused sick leave may be accumulated up to a maximum of 150 days. Unused sick leave will not be compensated upon termination.

19.4 Pay for any day of approved sick leave shall be paid at the employee's regular rate of pay.

19.5 Employees with accumulated paid sick leave will continue to earn vacation while out on paid sick leave. Holidays falling within an employee's paid sick leave will be treated as a holiday and a sick leave day will not be charged to that day. An employee cannot receive both holiday pay and sick leave pay for the same day.

19.6 To be eligible for the benefits of this Article, an employee must notify his or her supervisor at least one (1) hour before the start of his regularly scheduled work day unless proper excuse is presented for the employee's inability to call. The Hospital may require written certification by a physician or other proof of illness or accident. Employees who wish to return to work after sick leave may be required to be examined by a physician designated by the Hospital before returning to work.

ARTICLE TWENTY—LEAVE OF ABSENCE

20.1 Maternity leave, military leave, funeral leave, and jury duty shall be the same as described in the Employee Handbook (Nov. 20NX revision) and shall remain in effect and may not be reduced during the life of this contract.

ARTICLE TWENTY-ONE—INSURANCE AND PENSION

21.1 The provisions for life insurance, health and accident insurance, pension plan, and related benefits outlined in the Employee Handbook (Nov. 20NX revision) shall remain in effect and may not be reduced during the life of this agreement.

ARTICLE TWENTY-TWO—TERMS OF AGREEMENT

22.1 This Agreement constitutes the entire agreement between parties until and including January 20, 20N3, and shall continue in full force and effort from year to year thereafter unless and until either of the parties hereto shall give to the other party notice in accordance with applicable law, but in no case less than sixty (60) days prior to expiration of the contract. Such notice shall be given in writing.

IN WITNESS THEREOF, the parties hereto have hereunto set their hands and seals.

CHAPTER 11

Training and Development: The Backbone of Motivation and Retention

CHAPTER OBJECTIVES

- Acknowledge the importance of and necessity for employee orientation programs and ongoing training and development activities.
- Relate orientation, training, and development to the management functions of planning, organizing, directing, and controlling to employee motivation.
- Identify the components of effective employee orientation programs.
- Recommend an approach to communicating standards of conduct and behavior to new employees.
- Identify the components of employee training programs.
- Explore the availability of resources for training and development activities.

EMPLOYEE DEVELOPMENT

It is a fundamental responsibility of every manager to endeavor to shape and modify the behavior of employees so that they possess the necessary knowledge, skill, and attitude to fulfill their assignments according to the policies, rules, and regulations of the institution. Advances in technology necessitate continual retraining of experienced employees to perform new and altered tasks. Training and staff development are the fundamental means by which behavior can be changed in order to meet the immediate and long-range needs of the institution.

Training and development are continuous activities beginning with the orientation of a new employee and continuing throughout the employee's tenure with the organization. Participation in formal orientation and training programs must be documented for each employee, with copies of all reports provided to the employee for personal use and placed in the official personnel record of each employee.

Relationship of Training and Development to the Basic Management Functions

The need for sound orientation and training flows from several considerations. The mission and values of the organization usually include a commitment to quality. Certain organizational policies and practices usually reflect the intent and expectation that internal development—that is, promotion from within the organization—is the norm. Concurrently, the organization continuously seeks to meet its external mandates, which include requirements for appropriate orientation and training. The licensing and accrediting agencies include in their surveys and site visits reviews of such programs. Also, labor contracts may contain explicit provisions for training programs and related benefits, such as compensatory time for training programs attended at off-site locations.

Quality improvement programs and risk management oversight both require proper orientation and training. Management concerns such as employee evaluation or performance review, assessment of productivity measures, and the operation of merit and bonus pay programs all require, if only out of fairness to employees, that all workers be properly oriented and trained for their jobs.

The employee who knows what is expected and how to completely perform the work is likely to be a productive employee who experiences job satisfaction. When employees are generally satisfied, complaints, grievances, and job turnover decrease accordingly. The management team further assists employees in their personal development and their growth on the job by making additional training possible—

for example, through tuition reimbursement benefits, release time for educational purposes, additional stipends for incidental costs (books, fees, travel), and so on.

As a practical matter, training is necessitated by the need for workers who possess specific knowledge and skills. When the labor pool in the area does not provide a ready source of specially trained support staff, managers must engage in planned training to meet their staffing needs.

ORIENTATION

A sound beginning for each newly hired employee provides a positive atmosphere of mutual expectation between the employee and management. Ideally, the formal orientation will be brief, highly focused, and completed on the worker's first day of employment or as soon as possible thereafter. Orientation is a responsibility shared by the department head, the human resources manager, and other designated specialists such as those in employee health and safety, computer services, and public relations. The orientation program elements common to all employees are ordinarily developed and coordinated by the human resources department. Information and special practices associated with a specific department—that is, a departmental orientation—is the responsibility of that department's manager.

General Orientation

The typical content of a general orientation program includes such information as:

- A brief history of the organization along with explanation of its mission and its vision.
- The institution's ownership form, mode of governance, and administrative structure.
- An overview of the various departments and services.
- A review of specific employee policies including:
  - drug, alcohol, and substance abuse considerations
  - sexual harassment
  - nondiscrimination issues
  - conflict of interest prohibitions and gifts
  - dress codes
  - use of computers, accessing the Internet, using e-mail
  - computer security and passwords
  - privacy and confidentiality of all aspects of patient care

      – security, fire and safety, and disaster plans

      – infection control

      – review of the organization's disaster plan

An additional portion of general orientation ordinarily consists of a review of employee benefits, with direct assistance provided to new employees in signing up for such benefits.

If workers are covered under a specific labor union agreement, the provisions of the applicable contract are explained at general orientation.

The outline of the contents of a typical general orientation to a health care provider organization appears as Exhibit 11–1.

Departmental Orientation

This aspect of the new employee orientation is customized to the individual worker. The mission and goals of the department are shared. The departmental organizational chart, including names as well as job titles, is made available. The manager pays particular attention to acquainting the new worker with the other employees who will likely share common duties and work space. Preferably the manager will have made prior arrangements with an established member of the group to act as a "buddy" to the new employee to facilitate the transition into this new work environment.

Departmental policies, procedures, work standards, and productivity monitors, if any, are highlighted, with the understanding that these will be explained in detail during the formal training period. Issues relating to patient safety and privacy are reiterated, and the confidentiality statement is again reviewed and signed by the employee (if this has not already been done at time of hire or at the general orientation).

So oriented, the new employee is ready for the transition to the training phase.

The outline of one possible departmental orientation schedule appears as Exhibit 11–2. The departmental orientation may vary from one department to another depending on the nature of any given department's work.

Of Special Concern: Standards of Conduct and Behavior

An organization's code of ethics is reflected in its standards of employee conduct and behavior, which in turn are usually published in complete form in a personnel policy and procedure manual and in summary fashion in an employee handbook. There are particular behavioral expectations that should be emphasized with every

EXHIBIT 11–1

General Orientation Contents and Checklist

The following checklist is initiated in General Orientation, following which it will be permanently retained in the employee's personnel file. It is to be completed and submitted to the Human Resource representative at the conclusion of General Orientation.

Employee Name (please print)

_____

Affiliate or Division (if applicable)

_____

Department

_____

<u>Orientation Topics</u> (To initial to indicate completion of each)

_____ Organization's Mission, Vision, and Values
_____ Organization's History and Structure
_____ Overview of Operations: How all Department's Work Together
_____ Bloodborne Pathogens/TB Control
_____ Confidentiality of Patient-Related Information
_____ Domestic Violence and Its Signs
_____ Electrical Safety and the Safe Medical Device Act
_____ Emergency Preparedness (Disaster Plan)
_____ Fire Safety
_____ Hazardous Communications and the Right-to-Know Law
_____ Improving Organizational Performance
_____ Risk Management
_____ Incident Reporting
_____ Infection Control
_____ No-Smoking Policy
_____ Patient Rights
_____ Professional Misconduct
_____ Security Management and Crime Watch
_____ General Age-Specific Competencies
_____ Use of Organization's Property and Systems
_____ Introduction to Personnel Policy and Procedure Manual
_____ Received Identification Badge
_____ Completed and Submitted Confidentiality Statement
_____ Received and Reviewed Employee Handbook and Submitted Signed Receipt

EXHIBIT 11–2

Department Orientation Contents and Checklist

This form is to be initiated by the department manager or other designated individual for each new employee's department-specific orientation. Please complete the form and submit it to Human Resources following orientation; the completed form will be retained in the employee's personnel file.

Employee Name (please print)

_____

Affiliate or Division (if applicable)

_____

Department

_____

Orientation Topics (Manager, preceptor, or instructor initial upon completion of each)

_____   Welcome, tour of department, introduction to staff
_____   Department fire and life safety requirements
_____   General safety rules, specific hazards, personal protective equipment
_____   Infection control practices, if applicable
_____   Review of job description and performance expectations
_____   Reporting incidents and emergencies
_____   Department's role in emergency or disaster
_____   Age-specific competencies, if applicable
_____   Work hours, schedules, time reporting, absence reporting
_____   Dress code
_____   Parking
_____   Employee health department and annual health review requirement
_____   Pay rate, pay cycle, pay increase policy, performance appraisal process
_____   Telephone use and paging process
_____   Grievance procedure and progressive discipline process
_____   Continuing education, mandatory requirements
_____   Other considerations (if any) unique to the employee's position

I have reviewed the foregoing topics with my supervisor (or preceptor or instructor) during my orientation.

_____ Employee Signature

I have reviewed this employee's completed orientation form.

_____ Supervisor Signature

new employee, and the new-employee orientation presents the best opportunity for doing so.

Conflict of Interest

An organization's employees ordinarily retain the right to engage in outside business or financial activities as long as these do not interfere with the complete performance of their duties. It is necessary for the working health care professional to avoid both actual conflict of interest and any behavior that creates the appearance of conflict of interest.

A conflict of interest occurs when one's loyalty becomes divided between job responsibilities and some outside interest. A conflict of interest may be perceived when an objective observer of one's actions has cause to wonder whether the observed actions are motivated solely by organizational concerns or by external concerns.

Conflict of interest is the area of ethical concern likely to emerge most often in the management of a department. Some of the following guidelines apply to employees at all levels, while some are most pertinent to specific employees (for example, purchasing agents). Because many of these affect employee behavior, they are important to every department manager. Whether you are manager or nonmanager:

- Never place business with any firm in which you or your family or close outside associates have an interest.
- Derive no personal financial gain from transactions involving the organization unless the organization is advised of—and approves of—your potential benefit.
- Conduct all aspects of a personal business venture outside of the organizational environment and on non-work time. This is a guideline regularly violated and often implicitly condoned by management through failure to address the offending behavior. For example, soliciting orders for cosmetics, food containers, jewelry, and so on during work hours is in violation of ethical standards; using the organization's equipment to make photocopies for a part-time activity or other outside interest is similarly in violation.
- In situations in which you have the authority to hire or so recommend, do not employ relatives.
- Do not solicit, offer, accept, or provide any consideration that could be construed as conflicting with the organization's business interests, such as meals, gifts, loans, entertainment, or transportation.
- Do not accept gifts exceeding the maximum value established by the organization (limits may exist in amounts up to perhaps $50 but are commonly lower); never accept gifts of cash in any amount.

- Safeguard patient and provider information against access or use for financial gain by unauthorized interests.

If in doubt, disclose the situation and seek resolution of an actual or potential conflict of interest before taking what might later be seen as an improper action. Questions concerning potential conflicts of interest can usually be addressed with the organization's human resource department.

Finally, in many organizations managers and professionals are asked to sign a conflict-of-interest statement either indicating the presence or absence of potential conflicts. This statement is usually the same as that executed by members of the board of directors.

Use of Organizational Assets and Information

It is the responsibility of all employees to protect the assets of the organization against loss, theft, and misuse. The organization's property may not be used for personal benefit, nor may it be loaned, sold, given away, or disposed of in any manner without appropriate authorization.

The organization's assets are intended for use for business purposes only during legitimate employment. Improper use ordinarily includes unauthorized personal appropriation or use of tangible assets such as computers and copiers and other office equipment, medical equipment, vehicles, supplies, reports and records, computer software and data, and facilities. Intangible assets such as intellectual property, trademarks and copyrights, proprietary information including computer programs, confidential data, business plans, and such must be protected as vigorously as tangible property.

It also is necessary to protect patient property and information in accordance with established policies requiring patient information to be shared only with those who are authorized to receive it and have a legitimate need for it.

The responsibility for protection also extends to proprietary information entrusted to the organization by vendors, referral sources, contractors, service providers, and others. This standard includes the requirement to use only legally licensed computer software, with the use of bootleg or pirated software considered illegal as well as unethical.

Concerning information, an organization's ethical standards of conduct may set forth the following principles:

- It is prohibited to disclose proprietary information to anyone external to the organization, whether during or after employment, except as specifically authorized.

- All organizational property and information in your possession must be surrendered upon termination of employment.

Referral Practices

The laws governing Medicare, Medicaid, and other federally sponsored programs prohibit payment in any form in return for the referral of patients. The federal anti-kickback statute imposes criminal penalties for knowingly and willfully seeking or receiving payment for referring patients. The kinds of payments prohibited by the statute include kickbacks, bribes, and rebates. The Self-Referral Law (known as the Stark law) prohibits physicians holding a financial interest with an entity providing any designated health service from referring Medicare and Medicaid patients to that entity. The law also prohibits billing federal health care programs for items or services ordered by a physician who has a financial relationship with the billing entity.

The foregoing and additional consideration may be incorporated in an organization's ethical standards of conduct in the following manner:

- No employee shall solicit, receive, offer to pay, or pay remuneration of any kind in exchange for referring or recommending referral of any individual to another person, department, or division of the organization for services or in return for the purchase of goods or services to be paid for by a federal program.
- No employee shall offer or grant benefits to a referring physician or other referral source to secure the referral of patients or patient business.
- No physician shall make referrals for designated health services to entities in which the physician has a financial interest through either ownership or a compensation arrangement.
- No physician shall bill for services rendered as a result of an illegal referral.

Political Activity

An organization's code of conduct will often include an expectation that employees who participate in political activity will ensure that they are not doing so as representatives of the organization. There is, in fact, a legal prohibition against political activity by not-for-profit hospitals and nursing homes, and participating in political activity can jeopardize the employer's tax-exempt status.

Employee Privacy

Although personnel files remain the property of the employer, the organization will have a privacy policy limiting access to these files to those having a legitimate need for the information. The policy will usually state that personnel information will be released externally only upon employee authorization or in response to a subpoena or other legal order

Patient Confidentiality

Records relating to or concerning individuals to whom the organization is providing or has provided service should be held in the strictest confidence. It is a violation of the ethical code of conduct to reveal patient information to anyone outside of the organization without the express written authorization of the patient (or the patient's guardian, administrator, or executor), or a court order or other appropriate legal instrument. Within the organization, patient information is to be retained in confidence and revealed on a need-to-know basis only.

Employee Relationships

The following is a suggested model for the portion of an organization's ethical standards of conduct addressing relationships with employees:

> Every employee will be treated and judged as an individual on the basis of individual qualifications without regard to race, gender, sexual orientation, religion, national origin, age, disability, veteran status, or other characteristic protected by law. This pledge extends to all areas of the employment relationship including hiring, promotion, benefits, training, and discipline.
>
> [The organization] will conscientiously observe all federal, state, and local laws and regulations applicable in any way to the employment relationship.
>
> [The organization] is committed to providing a work environment in which employees are free from harassment, sexual or otherwise. No employee will be made to feel uncomfortable in the work environment through exposure to coarse, profane, or sexual language or derogatory comments.
>
> Employees are encouraged to express themselves freely and responsibly through established channels and procedures. Complaints will be treated as confidential information and will be revealed only to those who need to know as part of a process of investigation or resolution. Interference, retaliation, or coercion by any employee against an employee who registers a concern or complaint will not be tolerated.
>
> We will observe the standards of our professions and exercise judgment and objectivity at all times. Significant difference of professional opinion will be referred to the appropriate management for prompt resolution.
>
> We shall show respect and consideration for one another regardless of position, status, or relationship.

Latter-Day Concerns: E-mail and the Internet

Electronic mail (e-mail) and the Internet have been experiencing increasingly widespread business use for a number of years, and it is clear that their use will likely continue to expand for some years to come. These particular business tools have brought about significant increases in efficiency in a number of activities, but they have also given life to a number of practices that are contrary to reasonable expectations of employee conduct; that is, these modern computer-based conveniences are highly susceptible to considerable abuse. Therefore, it is necessary to establish rules for their use.

Policy

The organization's Internet facilities, including e-mail systems, are to be used for business purposes only by employees and other authorized users, subject to the following standards and requirements.

Internet   Only authorized employees are allowed Internet access and then only for valid business reasons. Assigned account numbers and access codes are personal to each user and must not be shared with others. Management reserves the right to deny or terminate access to the Internet at its own discretion.

Employees do not have an expectation of privacy with respect to their use of the organization's Internet facilities. Any and all messages, data, images, or other information received, transmitted, or archived using the Internet facilities may be accessed, copied, and used by systems administrators and management. Also, any messages, data, or images may be disclosed to legally entitled third parties such as regulators, law enforcement agencies, and courts. The organization reserves the right to monitor, log, and filter Internet access by employees.

Prohibited uses of Internet facilities include but are not limited to:

- viewing, displaying, copying, or communicating libelous, threatening, or sexually explicit material, material that fosters a hostile work environment, or material that fosters discrimination of any kind as defined in the Civil Rights Act of 1964 and subsequent antidiscrimination laws
- supporting an outside activity, whether a commercial venture, charitable or political cause, or other private undertaking
- developing personal home pages
- recreational "surfing" during work hours
- playing games

Electronic Mail   All employees are advised that electronic mail (e-mail) is available within the organization for business use only. Transmitting jokes, cartoons, recipes, personal messages, and other non-business-related information constitutes misuse of the organization's communications capacity and misuse of work time.

All users of e-mail should also be aware that in spite of individual accounts and passwords, an individual's e-mail can be readily accessed by unauthorized persons and may also be subject to monitoring internal to the organization. There is no expectation of e-mail privacy; all e-mail messages are potentially public.

TRAINING

An organized formal training program to meet certain objectives is the most effective method of changing the behavior of employees. To establish such a program, the manager and those individuals involved in the organized training program must (1) identify the training needs, (2) establish training objectives, (3) select appropriate methods and techniques, (4) implement the program, and (5) evaluate the training outcomes. (See Appendix 11–A for excerpts from a training program designed for release of information specialists.)

Identification of Training Needs

The manager reviews various aspects of the work, including individual employee performance, to determine training needs. Such detailed review might include the following:

1. Comparison of specified job requirements (as stated in the job descriptions) with current or new employee skills.
2. Analysis of performance ratings. Where are workers having difficulty meeting accuracy or productivity standards? Where are errors concentrated? Is there a pattern of difficulty in some technical aspects of the work?
3. Analysis of personnel records and reports. Is there a pattern of lateness, absenteeism, accidents, safety violations, client complaints, or equipment damage?
4. Analysis of short- and long-range plans. These often indicate the need for training in new procedures or in skills for dealing with new client groups.
5. Analysis of current trends and changes in laws, regulations, accrediting standards, and new technologies. When new regulations or standards are promulgated (e.g. The False Claims Act required reporting) or new tech-

nological support becomes available (e.g., a new software program), re-training is required.

A director of health information systems used an analysis of grievances over five months (Exhibit 11–3), a quarterly audit of the storage and retrieval function (Exhibit 11–4), and a four-year long-range plan excerpt (Exhibit 11–5) to determine training needs.

The first aspect of this overall analysis focused on the question, is this a systems problem or a training problem? Notice that six incidents involved work standards and procedures, indicating a systems problem. Then notice that there are several

EXHIBIT 11–3 Analysis of Grievances (May to October)

Substance/Issue	Employee	Outcome for Mgt.
1. Harassment by supervisor: inconsistent application of late/absentee docking	File clerk	Lost
2. Arbitrary and excessive work standards in file area	File clerk	Lost
3. Excessive work standards in file area	File clerk	Sustained
4. Firing for unauthorized release of record	File clerk	Sustained
5. Arbitrary change in procedure for delivery of records to outpatient clinics	File clerk	Lost
6. Excessive work standard for transcription	Transcriber	Lost
7. Arbitrary employee evaluation	Transcriber	Lost
8. Inconsistent merit money allocation	Release of Info. clerk	Sustained
9. Harassment: inconsistent application of work rules re: dress code	Release of Info. clerk	Lost
10. Arbitrary selection of candidate for job promotion	File clerk	Lost
11. Firing for failure to meet work standards for chart retrieval	File clerk	Lost
12. Unequal rate of pay	Coder	Sustained
13. Harassment for failing to meet work standard	Transcriber	Sustained
14. Suspension for insubordination	File clerk	Sustained

EXHIBIT 11–4

Audit of Storage and Retrieval System (July to September)

Percentage of misfiles: active records; terminal digit, color-coded system	14%
Percentage of missing or incorrectly place outguides	11%
Percentage of loose reports misfiled in records	8%
Percentage of "permanently lost" records	4%
Percentage of records unavailable at time of appointment (appointment request had clear patient ID)	33%

# of Accidents/Incidents:

Falls from ladder	3
Back strain: moving/accessing boxes of emergency room reports	1
Eye injury: hit in eye by falling outguide	1
Bruised hip due to file cabinet drawer jammed open	1

Other Problems Noted

20% turnover rate

All employees in unit = entry level

Poor "housekeeping" in inactive area; active storage = o.k.

Active storage area: terminal digit and color coded

Inactive storage area: middle digit and different color-coded record jackets

---

incidents that indicate a specific training need: e.g., worker unable to meet work standards; the series of misfiles in the storage/retrieval area; the supervisor and the uneven application of department policy.

The audit of the storage and retrieval system leads the manager to review the system itself (dual system for historic reasons; available space and possible overcrowding; lighting; general "housekeeping"). The manager then notes that there are specific training needs: to make certain that the workers understand the two different filing systems and to review safety and ergonomics to prevent injury.

The short- and long-range plans for the organization and the department provide yet another series of training needs. For example, as the health care organization undergoes its expansion of specialties (home care, hospice, sports medicine) there will be a need to train the health information specialists in the related aspects

EXHIBIT 11–5

2007–2010 Long-Range Plans (excerpt)

Organizational Expansion:

Sports medicine outpatient clinic	July 2008
Participation in regional tumor registry program	July 2008
Affiliation with local university's college of health professions	September 2007
Home care program	July 2009
Hospice program	January 2010

Departmental Objectives (in addition to plans
stemming from organizational expansion):

Conversion to outsourced transcription	September 2007
Conversion to ICD-10 coding system	September 2009
(dependent on status of ICD-10 development)	

of documentation, coding, and registries appropriate to those services. There is a training need that is still conditional: the new coding system, depending on the external mandate to implement ICD-10. The manager would revisit the long-range plan periodically as this, or similar training needs, become certain.

Once training needs have been identified, the manager must establish the objectives for the program. The objectives should be written in measurable terms and should state the specific outcomes to be achieved at the conclusion of the training program. For example, if a training program for physical therapists is to introduce the SOAP (subjective, objective, assessment, plan) format for writing notes, the manager must establish an objective that states, "Record physical therapy progress notes using the SOAP format for all patients receiving treatment in the department." This objective is specific and stated in measurable terms, since the desired results can be factually determined through recordkeeping. Written objectives serve as the fundamental guide for organizing the program and evaluating the desired outcomes.

Training objectives are stated in stylized language. Usually each objective contains:

- the statement of the main focus (what is to be demonstrated or stated)
- the level of mastery or an acceptable performance level (e.g., "error-free" or "with 100 percent accuracy"); when mastery-level performance is adopted, a realistic time limit to obtain mastery (e.g., after a certain number of practice sessions) may be stated

- any conditions, such as use of specific regulations or use of designated equipment
- a time frame/performance standard, which may be presented in stages, with an initial phase of untimed performance followed by progressively increased performance levels until the work standard is met

These training objective elements may be stated in whole or in part at the beginning of the training design for each unit and need not be repeated. For example, the various activities or processes that the trainee carries out must be in "accordance with the specified policies and procedures. Having stated this condition initially, the training specialist need not repeat it for each learning objective."[1]

Training Module Content

Detailed content is developed for each sequence of the training module. The manager takes care to use materials consistent with professional standards. Materials made available from professional associations are reliable and up to date. There is an advantage to using such resources: these training materials represent best practices and widely accepted methods. They have been developed and vetted by teams of experts and supported by research. They are revised on a regular basis to reflect changes in requirements. The testing materials have been developed by experts in testing design. The materials reflect the body of knowledge required for certifications at various levels.

The manager augments these standardized materials with information specific to the organization. Finally, the manager sequences the training modules in logical order. For example, a training module on the release of information would follow a training module on HIPAA.

Training Methods and Techniques

The manager has many training methods available to achieve the desired outcomes. The methods most often used are as follows:

Job Rotation

This is a popular approach to staff training and development. Under a rotating schedule, job assignments usually last anywhere from three to six months. This approach gives an employee the opportunity to acquire the broad perspective and diversified skills needed for professional and personal development. Job rotation can also be used to introduce new concepts and ideas into the various units within the department and to help individual employees to think in terms of the whole program rather than their immediate assignments.

> Selma manages a department of occupational therapy in a large urban acute care hospital. After years of rapid staff turnover, Selma decided to rotate staff every six months. There was overlap between new assignments so "old" staff trained the "new" staff. Staff enjoyed the change and felt that they were gaining invaluable experience and increased knowledge and skills. Selma noticed that staff turnover was reduced.

Formal Lecture Presentations

The lecture method is one of the oldest techniques used in training and development programs. The fundamental purpose of the lecture is to inform. The lecture format saves time because the speaker can present more material in a given amount of time than can be presented by any other method. The lecture should be supplemented by visual aids, however, or the results are likely to fall short of the instructional goals. During the lecture, employees are passive. Outside disturbances or mental wanderings frequently distract individuals and render the lecture ineffective.

> Alice had two years of therapy experience and wanted to change her area of practice. She had three interests: pediatrics, hand therapy, and sports medicine. She found that she could get a job in any one of these areas and wondered how she could begin to narrow her choices. As she glanced through her professional newspaper, she discovered an announcement for a lecture on hand therapy. She attended the one-hour presentation and was excited by the description offered by the physician and therapists. Based on her new experience, Alice searched for a hand therapy position.

Seminars and Conferences

The major purpose of seminars and conferences is to allow for the exchange of ideas, the discussion of problems, and the finding of answers to questions or solutions to problems. The opportunity for employees to express their own views and to hear other opinions can be very stimulating. Employees who actively participate are more committed to decisions than they would be if the solution were merely presented to them. Remember that learning takes place in direct ratio to the amount of individual involvement in the discussion process.

> James owned a private practice group. To keep the staff informed and up to date, he mandated that each employee must attend at least three seminars and one conference each year. He urged the attendees to discuss ideas with other professionals at the conference and to bring the ideas back so they could be shared with other members of the practice group.

Role Playing

Acting out situations between two or more persons is a training method used successfully with all levels of employees. Interviewing, counseling, leadership, and human relations are a few of the content areas in which role playing has been used. By playing the role of others, employees gain valuable insight not only from their own action but from the comments of observers.

> Jan was surprised when she heard David, a recent graduate, talking to an elderly patient as if she were deaf when, in fact, she had Alzheimer's disease. Jan set up a role-play situation at the next staff meeting and asked David to play the patient. Almost immediately, David realized that he was stereotyping the patient by assuming that she could not hear.

Committee Assignments

Through committee assignments, employees can explore a topic or problem to gain a broader or new perspective, experience situations involving the resolution of different ideas, learn to adjust to someone else's viewpoint, and practice reaching decisions. Committee assignments also offer opportunities for employees to assume positions of leadership that they would not otherwise have.

> The State Association needed help with justifying a renewal of the Sunset Clause of its licensure act. The task of proving the importance of licensure to a new group of legislators seemed overwhelming. One member spoke up and suggested dividing the work into tasks that could be assigned to several committees. Each committee was given a portion of the work and the State Association officers noted the increased interest in the renewal process since members were helping rather than standing on the sidelines.

Case Studies

Based on the premise that solving problems under simulated conditions enables employees to solve similar problems in an actual work situation, the case study method requires employees to become actively involved in a problem-solving situation, either hypothetical or real. The case studies used in developing problem-solving skills should be carefully selected and pertinent to the job so that their use meets the training and development requirements of the employees.

> Glen had no idea how to treat a patient who was wearing an unusually elaborate wrist splint. Then he remembered a case study that was presented during one of the conferences he attended. The case study reminded him of the correct protocol to use during treatment. The human example stuck in his mind and promoted better application of the knowledge.

Program Implementation

Throughout the implementation phase, the physical and psychological environment must be constantly monitored. For example, the time schedule, the learning environment, and the pace need to be checked periodically.

The primary consideration in any training program is to establish a time schedule to provide the greatest educational impact possible without reducing work output or, in health care institutions, patient care. The training program and the methods to be used should be announced well in advance. This allows everyone involved sufficient lead time to arrange individual schedules so that work assignments can be adequately covered during the employee's absence.

The arrangement of the room in which the training is to occur can either promote or handicap the process of learning. It is important to ensure that each participant see and hear each member of the group. The traditional classroom setting in which the "teacher" sits in the front of the room and the participants are seated in neat rows should be avoided whenever possible because it creates a stiff and formal atmosphere. One of the best arrangements for a training session is to put the tables in an open-ended rectangle, with chairs placed only on the outside perimeter. In addition, the room should be well lighted and adequately ventilated.

The pace and timing of each session are also important during the implementation phase of a training program. The function of pace is to maintain interest; therefore, the pace should be quickened when interest begins to wane, or it should be slowed if individuals are having difficulty absorbing content. A training session should not last longer than two hours. In fact, a one-hour session is believed to produce better results. If a two-hour session is necessary, a break should be allowed at the midpoint. Common sense and individual attention spans dictate how long adults accustomed to active work can be kept relatively immobile.

Evaluation of Outcomes

Probably the most difficult aspect of a training program is evaluating the outcomes to determine whether they are or are not what was desired. This is so because there are no concrete and precise measuring tools for assessing changes in behavior and attitudes. Outcomes must be measured indirectly and conclusions based on inference. The evaluation is not just a single act or event but an entire process. Evaluation is made easier, however, if objectives have been clearly stated in measurable terms.

A before-and-after comparison may be a useful way of evaluating change. If the manager and those individuals involved in the training program assess the behavior factors they wish to change before training and examine the same factors after training has been concluded, they can determine if a change occurred.

For material of a factual nature, where precise knowledge should be demonstrated, fact tests are used. More commonly, trainees are evaluated through performance tests. Each trainee has activities to carry out; these are drawn from the usual work of the job. The final evaluation may be carried out in stages: practice activity, followed by real work activity under immediate supervision, followed by real work activity with diminishing levels of immediate supervision.

The evaluation brings the training process full circle. Each trainee has been given specific objectives to attain, appropriate didactic and practice materials have been explained, and practice activities with appropriate feedback and correction have been provided. The evaluation, therefore, consists of determining the trainee's capacity to perform the work outlined in the job description and specified through the detailed policies and procedures of the department.

Resources for Training

The manager should be endeavoring to provide timely and thoroughly developed training materials. The cost of training materials and the time to be expended are also factors to consider. The manager can use to advantage the many programs developed by professional associations. For example, AHIMA has developed training programs for coding, making it easier for health information department employees to enhance that particular skill set. Distance learning is yet another option in which both technical and professional-level courses are readily available.

Some topics are common to several disciplines, thus enabling the management team to share resources and split the cost. The training material for HIPAA implementation represents one such training program that is suitable for interdepartmental use.

Training, while desirable as well as necessary, can be costly. Budget decisions and justification for such expenditures may be systematized by reviewing training resources against a set of criteria. Exhibit 11–6 reflects such an assessment.

MENTORING

Professional practitioners may find themselves in the special teaching role of mentor. Mentoring is a process in which a more experienced and usually older person guides and nurtures a younger or less experienced employee. The mentoring re-

EXHIBIT 11–6

Budget Justification for Training Resource

Title of Resource:	*Confidentially Speaking: Keeping Patient Information Private*
Sponsor:	Norton and Collins, Inc.
Target Population:	New employees of Health Information Services
	Students accepted for clinical internship in Health Information Services
	Employees needing a refresher course in basic principles
Job Skill:	Fostering and maintaining confidentiality of patient information

Cost:

2-part video:	$104.00
Shipping and handling:	11.00
Total cost:	115.00

Additional notes:

1. Video can be reused within the department
2. Video can be loaned to other departments
3. Video content has been reviewed by experts in the field of HIPAA compliance
4. Content meets continuing education approval by national association

lationship may be informal and limited—for example, in the instance of a senior practitioner encouraging a visiting student during the student's part-time job. The relationship may be formal and limited, as in the relationship of the clinical supervisor during training rotation or in assisting with thesis supervision. The relationship may then become informal and ongoing, as in a partnership of interest, leading to shared projects, co-presenting at workshops and co-authoring papers.

Network

A network is a group of individuals who communicate through formal and informal channels and willingly promote each other for mutual benefit. The network members trade services, ideas, recommendations, and "tips" to further their own development and success. The various state and national professional associations are examples of networks.

Peer Pals

Peer pals boost each other's careers by sharing information and strategies. They share each other's strengths and weaknesses since they are on the same developmental level.

EXERCISE: WHAT TO DO WHEN BUDGET-CUTTING THREATENS?

Any department manager who has been through a financial belt-tightening exercise has undoubtedly collided with one of the fundamental contradictions to be encountered in organizational life, and especially in health care organizations. That contradiction is that on one hand, education receives a considerable amount of verbal support from top management people who speak of its importance and their belief in education; on the other hand, as department managers frequently discover, after the first budgeting pass, when it becomes evident that trimming is needed to bring projected revenue and expenses into line, education is one of the first line items to be reduced or eliminated.

You are to explain why you believe the fundamental contradiction described above exists, and describe what arguments you might use in defense of your education budget.

Also, by many who tend to view all expenditures in terms of cost versus benefits, education comes up short by very nearly defying cost-benefit analysis. In defense of your education budget, which the budget director has said must be reduced by half or more, you are to:

- Develop an argument for keeping as much of your education budget as possible.
- Describe how you would go about attempting to measure the results of education.

CASE: THE DEPARTMENT'S "KNOW-IT-ALL"

Several weeks ago physical therapist Willis Patrick said to his boss, Glen Jones, director of physical therapy, "Glen, the way that we develop the budget in this department doesn't make much sense. We just take last year's actual expenses and stick an inflation factor onto it and make some other guesses. We really ought to be budgeting from a zero base, making every line item completely justify itself every year."

Glen said something about simply following the instructions issued by the finance department and doing it the way all the managers were told to do it. He pursued the matter no further.

A few days later Willis approached Glen, saying, "Don't you think the way we do performance appraisals ought to change? Surely most smart managers know it's better to evaluate employees on their anniversary dates than all at once, the way we do it now."

Glen again answered to the effect that he was simply doing what he had to do to comply with the policies and practices of the organization. They discussed the matter for perhaps five minutes, and although Glen was not going to start working to inspire change in the performance appraisal system, he nevertheless felt led to concede that Willis had brought up a number of good points. It struck Glen that his employee was idealizing an appraisal system in almost textbook terms; it seemed flawless in theory, but Glen had been through enough actual systems to be able to recognize a number of potential barriers to thorough practical application.

In the ensuing two to three weeks Willis had more and more to say to Glen about how the organization should be managed. And it took Willis only a matter of days to get beyond generalized management techniques like budgeting and appraisal and start offering specific advice on the management of the department.

Glen quickly came to realize that he could count on Willis to offer some criticism of most of his actions in running the department and most of administration's actions in running the hospital. Glen did not appreciate this turn in his relationship with an otherwise good employee. Glen had always seen Willis as an excellent physical therapist, perhaps somewhat opinionated but not to any harmful extent. Recently, however, he had come to regard Willis as a sort of conscience, a critical presence who was monitoring his every move as a manager.

The worsening situation came to a head one day when Willis attempted to intercede in a squabble between two other physical therapy employees and, when Glen entered the situation, proceeded to criticize Glen's handling of the matter in front of the other employees.

Glen took Willis into his office for a private one-on-one discussion. He first told Willis that although he was free to offer his suggestions, opinions, and criticisms regarding management, he was never again to do so in the presence of others in the department. Glen then asked Willis, "It seems that lately you have a great deal to say about management and specifically about how I manage this department. Why this sudden active interest in management?"

Willis answered, "Last month I finished the first course in the management program at the community college, a course called Introduction to Management

Theory. Now I'm in the second course, one called Supervisory Practice. I know what I'm hearing—and quite honestly, it's pretty simple stuff—and when I see things that I know aren't being handled right, I feel that I have an obligation to this hospital to speak up."

Glen ended the discussion by again telling Willis that he expected all such criticism and advice to be offered in private and never again in front of other employees. Overall, the conversation did not go well; more than once Glen felt that Willis's remarks were edging toward insubordination. Because of the uneasy feeling the discussion left with him, Glen requested a meeting with the hospital's vice president of human resources.

After describing the state of the relationship between him and Willis in some detail, Glen spread his hands in a gesture of helplessness and said, "I'm looking for advice. Apparently on the strength of a course or two of textbook management, this guy suddenly has all the answers. What can I do with him?"

Questions:

1. If Willis does indeed act as though he has all the answers, what can Glen do to encourage modification of this attitude?
2. If you were Willis, how should you best proceed in applying your newly acquired knowledge of management? Explain and provide an example.
3. What are the possible reasons behind Glen's growing aggravation with Willis? List a few possible reasons and comment on the validity of each.

NOTE

1. Joan Gratto Liebler, *Medical Records: Policies and Guidelines* (Gaithersburg, Md.: Aspen Publishers, 1991).

Appendix
11–A

Training Design: Release of Information

Note: this phase of training follows successful completion of HIPAA training unit.

CONTENTS

ASSUMPTIONS*

The learning objectives presented in this training design are based on the following four assumptions.

1. Performance condition: the activity is carried out according to the prescribed policy and procedure.

---

*Reprinted with permission from Aspen Publishers, Inc. Joan Gratto Liebler, *Medical Records: Policies and Guidelines,* 1991.

2. Acceptable level of performance:
   a. alternative one: 100 percent accuracy is attained.
   b. alternative two: mastery-level competence is attained (no stated accuracy level is given).
3. Time frame/performance standard:
   a. during training: the activity is accomplished at [60 percent] of the established performance [time] standard.
   b. final, comprehensive evaluation: the trainee meets fully the stated performance [time] standard.
4. These learning objectives relate to the release of information; therefore, this phrase is not repeated in each objective or evaluation statement.

OVERALL LEARNING OBJECTIVE

At the conclusion of this training sequence, the trainee/employee will demonstrate the ability to process written and oral requests for the release of information:

- according to the standard policies and procedures of this facility
- with 100 percent accuracy
- within the performance [time] standards established for this work

The training sequence that follows is intended to develop the trainee's capacity to meet this comprehensive objective.

GENERAL ORIENTATION AND INTRODUCTION

Purpose

To acquaint the trainee with the general content and scope of the release of information processes.

Content

- review of job description: release of information specialist
- overview of policy and procedure manual
- explanation of learning objectives:
  – performance conditions
  – accuracy level (or mastery level)
  – performance standards

Methods

- In-basket activity: The trainee is given a representative sample of the various types of requests in the usual form in which such requests are received. (Note: All examples used at this stage of orientation and training are fictitious.)
- Discussion: The trainee has a brief discussion with the trainer in order to answer immediate questions and concerns and to present the outline for the detailed training to follow.

Evaluation

None: at this stage of the orientation, the trainee will not carry out activities.

GENERAL REQUIREMENTS FOR AUTHORIZATION

Purpose

To acquaint the trainee with general principles relating to the need for patient authorization.

Learning Objectives

- Given [___] written requests containing various types of written requests, the trainee will determine the need for authorization for each request.
- Given the same set of written requests and a mix of authorizations, the trainee will determine the adequacy/validity of each authorization for those requests needing authorization.

Content

- general underlying principles used to determine need for authorization
- the patient's capacity to authorize
- designated representatives of a patient who may authorize on behalf of the patient
- circumstances in which no authorization is needed
- requirements for valid authorization
- formats of authorizations:
  - insurance claim form
  - patient's own wording
  - facility's recommended form

Methods

Lecture is followed by practice activity. The trainee is given a representative sample of written requests, including a variety of authorization formats and a mix of both adequate and inadequate authorization statements.

Evaluation

A performance test consisting of fictitious written requests and a mix of authorizations is used.

- The trainee will determine which requests require authorization.
- The trainee will determine which authorizations are adequate/valid when compared to the listing of the required content for an authorization.

ADMINISTRATIVE AND PROCEDURAL STEPS

Purpose

To acquaint the trainee with the detailed administrative and procedural steps for the release of information from patient's medical records.

Learning Objective

Given [____] written requests, the trainee will process each request in an eight-step sequence established in the procedure manual.

1. performing preliminary sorting and processing
2. making entries in the release of information log
3. determining patient status
4. requisitioning the patient's medical record
5. preparing the cover letter
6. determining and calculating the fees
7. photocopying and reassembling the medical record
8. processing outgoing mail

Content

- examples of types of written requests:
  - U.S. mail
  - interdepartmental mail
  - fax

- categories of requests:
  - direct patient care
  - third-party payers
  - government agencies
  - review agencies
  - attorneys
- initial processing:
  - sorting and date-stamping
  - handling confidential mail
  - routing mail for further processing
- priority matrix: purpose and use
- release of information log:
  - purpose and use
  - content
  - staged entries: initial logging through final entry
  - computer security safeguards
- determining patient status:
  - accessing the patient master index
  - interpreting information in the patient master index
  - recording information on the request/inquiry
- requisitioning the patient health information record:
  - preparing the requisition form
  - coordinating with the Storage and Retrieval unit
- preparing the cover letter:
  - purpose
  - sample formats
  - appropriate response statements and cover letters
- processing fees:
  - fee schedule and guidelines
  - determining applicable fees
  - calculating the fee
  - handling money received
  - transmitting fees to accounts receivable
- photocopy process
- equipment use:
  - safeguards to prevent misfiling during processing
- reassembling the chart:
  - chart order

> – problem and misfile identification: notification of Storage and Retrieval-unit and correction of misfile or problem
> – inclusion of original request, authorization, and record of material released
> – return of record to Storage and Retrieval unit
> • final preparation for mailing the completed response

Methods

- lecture and demonstration of each step
- immediate practice activity following the lecture and demonstration of each step

Evaluation

Stage 1: The trainee will be given one standard request to process through the complete procedural cycle.

Stage 2: The trainee will be given one nonstandard request to process through the complete procedural cycle.

Stage 3: The trainee will be given [____] written requests reflecting a mix of materials typically received. The trainee will process these requests through the complete procedural cycle.

12

Authority, Leadership, and Supervision

CHAPTER OBJECTIVES

- Differentiate among the terms *power, influence,* and *authority.*
- Recognize the importance of authority for organizational stability.
- Identify the sources of power, influence, and authority.
- Relate the sources of power, influence, and authority to the organizational position of the line manager.
- Recognize the limits placed on the use of power and authority in organizational settings.
- Recognize the importance of delegation of authority.
- Identify the styles of leadership.
- Identify the relationship of leadership to the supervisory activities of issuing orders and directives and taking disciplinary action.

The manager gives an order or directive, and there is compliance; why did the employee obey? Is it correct to use the term *obey* to describe this compliance? What bases of authority are operative in superior–subordinate transactions? What are the limits of a manager's authority? What if a particular supervisor is seen as a weak manager? Are there any remedies to problems related to weak or ineffective management leadership? Of what value to the organization is the authority structure?

What are the consequences to organizational life if there is not a general, untested compliance most of the time? When such actions of compliance are described, which term is the proper point of reference: *power, authority,* or *influence*? Are these terms mutually exclusive or are they synonymous when used in the context of organization relationships? These questions arise when discussion of authority in organizations is undertaken.

Organizational behavior is controlled behavior, directed toward goal attainment. The authority structure is created to ensure compliance with organizational norms, to suppress spontaneous or random behavior, and to induce purposeful behavior. No matter how the work within the organization is divided, no matter what degree of specialization, departmentation, centralization, or decentralization is formalized, there must be some measure of legitimate authority if the organization is to be effective. The concept of formal authority is supported by the two related concepts of power and influence. These concepts may be separated for analytical purposes; in actual practice, however, the two concepts are intertwined.

THE CONCEPT OF POWER

Power is the ability to obtain compliance by means of coercion, to have one's own will carried out despite resistance. Power is force or naked strength; it is a mental hold over another. Like authority and influence, power aims at compliance, but it does not seek consensus or agreement as a condition of that compliance.

Power is always relational. An individual who has power over another person can narrow that person's range of choice and obtain compliance. The power holder does not necessarily force the compliance by physical acts but may operate in more subtle ways, such as an implicit threat to carry out sanctions. Latent power is frequently as effective as a show of power. Power attaches to people, not to official positions. The formal authority holder (i.e., the person who has the official title, organizational position, and grant of authority) may or may not have power in addition to this formal grant of authority.

An imbalance in superior–subordinate relationships can occur when a nonofficeholder has more power than the official officeholder. This can even be seen in family life. For example, when a two-year-old shows signs of an incipient temper tantrum in the middle of the annual family gathering, the power balance clearly is in favor of the child if the tantrum pattern has developed. The child does not have to carry out the explosive behavior; the mere threat of doing so brings about some desired behavior from the parent caught in the situation. In the privacy of the home, however, the parent–child power balance shifts.

Workers have power over line supervisors and managers. A worker with specific technical knowledge can withhold that key information from a manager or can develop a relationship that is personally favorable. The information may not actually be withheld; the mere possibility that the manager cannot rely on an individual is enough to shift the balance, at least temporarily, in favor of the worker. Groups of workers can control a manager when it is well known that the manager is responsible for meeting a deadline or quota; the manager's ability to do this is dependent on the cooperation of the workers. The normal, steady output may be reached routinely, but that extra push needed to go over the quota or to reach a special level of output rests more with the workers than with the manager. Strikes by workers are classic examples of mobilized power, but the power shifts back in favor of management if striking workers are terminated during a strike.

When an individual can supply something that a person values and cannot obtain elsewhere in a regular manner, or when the individual can deprive this person of something valued, then there is a power relationship. This implicit or explicit power relationship may or may not be perceived by one or both parties.

THE CONCEPT OF INFLUENCE

Like power, influence is the capacity to produce effects on others or to obtain compliance, but it differs from power in the manner in which compliance is evoked. Power is coercive; influence is accepted voluntarily. Influence is the capacity to obtain compliance without relying on formal actions, rules, or force. In relationships of influence, not only compliance but also consensus and agreement are sought; persuasion rather than latent or overt force is the major factor in influence. Influence supplements power, and it is sometimes difficult to distinguish latent power from influence in a situation. Does the individual comply because of a relationship of influence or because of the latent power factor? Together, power and influence supplement formal authority.

THE CONCEPT OF FORMAL AUTHORITY

Authority may be termed legitimate power. It is the right to issue orders, to direct action, and to command or exact compliance. It is the right given to a manager to employ resources, make commitments, and exercise control. By a grant of formal authority, the manager is entitled, empowered, and authorized to act; thus, the manager incurs a responsibility to act. Authority may be expressed by direct command or instruction or, more commonly, by suggestion. Through the authority delegation, coordination is secured in the organization.

The authority mandate is delineated and reinforced in several ways, such as organizational charts, job descriptions, procedure manuals, and work rules. Although the exercise of authority in many situations tends to be similar to transactions of influence, authority differs from influence in that authority is clearly vested in the formal chain of command. Individuals are given a specific grant of authority as a result of organizational position. Power and influence may be exercised by an individual authority holder, but they may also be exercised by individuals who do not have a specific grant of authority.

Authority is both complemented and supplemented by power on one hand and influence on the other. It is within the realm of formal authority to exact compliance by the threat of firing a person; however, this may be such a rare occurrence in an organization that such a threat is really an exercise of power more than an exercise of authority. However, formal aspects of authority may be so well developed that the major transactions remain at the influence level, with the influence based largely on the holding of formal office. The infrequent use of formal authoritative directives to evoke compliance may indicate organizational health.

THE IMPORTANCE OF AUTHORITY

When a subordinate refuses to accept the orders of a superior, the superior has several choices, each carrying potentially negative consequences for the attainment of organizational goals. The superior could accept the insubordination, withdraw the order, and seek to find others to carry out the directive. This action would probably further weaken authority, however, because the superior would be perceived as lacking the subtle blend of power and authority to exact compliance on a predictable basis. A chain reaction of insubordination could occur. If other workers are asked to carry out a directive that had been refused by a worker, resentment could build up with negative consequences. If the order is withdrawn completely, the work will not be accomplished.

The manager who decided to enforce compliance may suspend or fire the insubordinate worker. The superior still must find a worker to carry out the directive. If there is a chain reaction of insubordination, it may become impractical to suspend or fire the entire work force. The situation moves from one of authority to one of power. Therefore, managers must identify and widen their bases of authority to help ensure a stable work climate.

SOURCES OF POWER, INFLUENCE, AND AUTHORITY

The manager's organizational relationships flow along the continuum of power, influence, and authority, varying in emphasis at different times and in different situations. In order to more fully understand the dynamics of the power-influence-authority triad, it is useful to examine the sources or bases of authority in formal organizations. The wider the base of authority, the stronger the manager's position; with a wide base of authority, the manager can work in the realm of influence and need not rely only on the formal grant of authority that flows from organizational position.

The sources of formal authority have been studied by several theorists in the disciplines of social psychology, management, and political science. A review of the literature suggests several sources or bases of authority: (a) acceptance or consent, (b) patterns of formal organization, (c) cultural expectations, (d) technical competence and expertise, and (e) characteristics of authority holders. The limits or weaknesses of each theory are offset by the approach taken in another.

The Consent Theory of Authority

The concept that authority involves a subordinate's acceptance of a superior's decision is the basis for the acceptance or consent theory of formal authority. A superior has authority only insofar as the subordinate accepts it. This theory implies that members of the organization have a choice concerning compliance, when often they do not. It remains important to recognize the concepts of acceptance and consent in order to identify the centers of more subtle and diffuse resistance to authority, even when there is no overt and massive insubordination.

The zone of indifference and the zone of acceptance are two similar concepts in the acceptance or consent theory of authority. Chester Barnard used the term *zone of indifference* to describe that area in which an individual accepts an order without conscious questioning.[1] Barnard noted that the manager establishes an overall setting by means of preliminary education, prior persuasive efforts, and known inducements for compliance; the order then lies within the range that is more or less anticipated by the subordinate, who accepts it without conscious questioning or resistance because it is consistent with the overall organizational framework. Herbert Simon used the term *zone of acceptance* to reflect the same authority relationship. The zone of acceptance, according to Simon, is an area established by subordinates within which they are willing to accept the decisions made for them by their superior.[2] Simon noted that this zone is modified by the positive and negative sanctions in the authority relationship, as well as by such factors as community of purpose, habit, and leadership.

Coupled with these factors is the concept of the rule of anticipated reactions, which Simon included in his discussion of zone of acceptance.[3] The subordinate seeks to act in a manner that is acceptable to the superior, even when there has been no explicit command. The authority system, including anticipated review of actions, is so well developed that the superior needs only to review actions rather than issue commands. The past organizational history in which positive and negative sanctions were enforced is recalled; the expectation of the review of actions is fostered so that the subordinate's zone of acceptance is expanded.

Another approach to the concept of authority as a relationship between organizational leaders and their followers is described by Robert Presthus, who posited a transactional view of authority in which there is a reciprocity among individuals at different levels in the hierarchy.[4] Compliance with authority is in some way rewarding to the individual, and this individual, therefore, plays an active role in defining and accepting authority. Everyone has formal authority in that each has a formal role in the organization. There is, Presthus stated, an implicit bargaining and exchange of authority, each individual deferring to the other.

The notion of reciprocal expectations in authority relationships is further supported in Edgar Schein's discussion of the psychological contract.[5] As in Barnard's concept of the zone of indifference and in Simon's rule of anticipated reactions, the premise of member acceptance of organizational authority and its attendant control system is basic to the psychological contract. The workers' acceptance of authority constitutes a realm of upward influence; in turn, the workers expect the authority holders to honor the implicit restrictions on their grant of authority. The workers expect the authority holders to refrain from ordering actions that are inconsistent with the general climate of the given organization and from taking advantage of the workers' acceptance of authority. The workers also expect as part of this psychological contract the rewards of compliance (i.e., positive sanctions readily given and negative sanctions kept at a minimum).

The Theory of Formal Organizational Authority

In his classic study of bureaucracies, Max Weber discussed three forms of authority: charismatic, traditional, and rational-legal. Charisma, as defined by Weber, is a "certain quality of an individual personality by virtue of which he is set apart from ordinary men and treated as endowed with supernatural, superhuman, or at least specifically exceptional qualities."[6] The social, religious, and political groups that form around charismatic leaders tend to lack formal role structure. The routines of bureaucratic structure are not developed and may even be disdained by the group. Charismatic authority figures function as revolutionary forces against established systems of leadership and authority. Charismatic authority is not bound by explicit rules; the authority remains invested in the key charismatic individual. Personal devotion to and an almost irrational faith in the leader bind the members of the group to each other and to the leader.

Since charismatic authority is linked to the individual leader, the organization's survival is similarly linked. If the organization is to endure, it must take on some of the characteristics of formal organizations, including a formalized authority pattern. In this area, two developments are possible. The charismatic leadership may evolve into a traditional system of authority, or it may develop into the rational-legal system of formal authority. In traditionalism, a pattern of succession is developed. A successor may be designated by the leader or hereditary/kinship succession may be established; then a system of transferring the leadership to the legitimate designated individual or heir must be developed. This, in turn, leads to a system of roles and formal authority. Weber uses the term *routinization of charisma* to describe this transformation of charismatic authority into traditional and then into rational-legal authority.

Rational-legal authority is the authority predicated in formal organizations. It is generally assumed that formal organizations come into being and derive legitimacy from an overall social and legal system. Individuals accept authority within the formal organizational structure because the rights and duties of members of the organization are consistent with the more abstract rules that individuals in the larger society accept as legitimate and rational.

Within the formal organization, a system of roles and authority relationships is carefully constructed to enable the organization to survive and move toward its formal goal on a continuing, stable basis. Authority has its basis in the organizational position, not in any individual. Weber described in detail the major characteristics of bureaucratic structures; the following characteristics relate to the rational-legal authority structure:[7]

1. There is the principle of fixed and official jurisdictional areas, which are generally ordered by rules—that is, by laws or administrative regulations.
   a. The regular activities required for the purposes of the bureaucratically governed structure are distributed in a fixed way as official duties.

   b. The authority to give the commands required for the discharge of these duties is distributed in a stable way and is strictly delimited in a fixed way as official duties.

   c. Methodical provision is made for the regular and continuous fulfillment of these duties and for the execution of the corresponding rights; only persons who have generally regulated qualifications to serve are employed.

2. The principles of office hierarchy and of levels of graded authority mean a firmly ordered system of superiority and subordination in which there is supervision of the lower offices by the higher ones.

The theory of formal organizational authority rests on this rational-legal system of formal office, impersonality of the officeholder, and a system of rules and regulations to constrain the grant of authority. Delegation of formal authority from top management to each successive level of management is the basis for formal organizational authority. Authority is derived from official position and is circumscribed by the limits imposed by the hierarchical order.

Cultural Expectations

Both the consent theory of authority and the theory of formal organizational authority include an implicit assumption that individuals in a society are culturally induced to accept authority. Furthermore, the acceptable use of authority in organizations is defined in part by the larger societal mores as well as by union contract, corporate law, and state and federal law and regulation.

Acceptance of the status system in a society is learned as part of the general socialization process. General deference to authority is ingrained early in the psychosocial development of the child, and social roles with their sanctions are accepted and reinforced throughout adult life. The role of employee carries with it both formal and informal sanctions; insubordination is not generally condoned. Even as a group cheers the occasional rebel, there is an attendant discomfort because something is out of order in the relationship. When the insubordination of an individual begins to threaten the economic security of the group, there is counterpressure on that individual to bring about reacceptance of authority. Fear of authority may bring about a similar response of renewed acceptance of authority and counterpressure on any dissidents.

The expected zone of acceptance or zone of indifference varies with different social roles. These variables are rarely spelled out in great detail; they are learned as much through the pervasive cultural formation process as through the formal orientation process in any one organization. There is a kind of group mind that includes the general realization that a particular behavior pattern is part of a given role, and the entire role set reinforces this general acceptance of authority.

Technical Competence and Expertise

Three terms reflect the organizational authority that is derived from or based on the technical competence and expertise of the individual, regardless of what office or position the individual holds in the organization. These terms are *functional authority, the law of the situation,* and *the authority of facts.*

Functional authority is the limited right that line or staff members (or departments) may exercise over specified activities for which they are responsible. Functional authority is given to the line or staff member as an exception to the principle of unity of command. For the purposes of this discussion on the sources of authority, it is useful to emphasize the special character of functional authority: It is given to a line or staff member primarily because that individual has specialized knowledge and technical competence. For example, the human resource manager normally assists all other department heads in matters of employee relations, although this manager has no authority to intervene directly in manager–employee relations. The situation changes when there is a legally binding collective bargaining agreement; the human resource manager, with special training in labor relations, may be given functional authority over all matters stemming from the union contract because of specialized knowledge. Another example is that of computer technical support staff who, because of technical competence, are given authority to make final decisions over certain aspects of data collection. The authority is granted because of the technical competence of the staff members.

Mary Parker Follett, a pioneer in management thought, introduced the terms *law of the situation* and authority of facts.[8] Follett described the ideal authority relationship as that stemming from the situation as a whole. Each participant in the organization, who is assumed to have the necessary qualifications for the position held, has authority tied to position. Orders become depersonalized in that each participant in the process studies and accepts the factors in the situation as a whole. Follett stated that one person should not give orders to another person but that both should agree to take their orders from the situation.[9] She developed this concept further; both the employer and the employee should study the situation and should apply their specialized knowledge and technical competence through the principles of scientific management. The emphasis shifts, in Follett's approach, from authority derived from official position or office to authority derived from the situation. The individual who has the most knowledge and competence to make the decision and issue the order in a particular situation has the authority to do so. The staff assistant or a key employee potentially has as much authority in a particular situation as does a holder of hierarchical office.

Closely tied to the concept of the law of the situation is that of authority of facts. Follett stressed that, in modern organizations, individuals exercise authority and leadership because of their expert knowledge.[10] Again, the leadership and authority shift from the hierarchical position to the situation. The one with the knowledge demanded by the situation tends to exercise effective authority.

Both of these concepts place emphasis on the depersonalization of orders. At the same time, the source of the authority is highly personal in that knowledge and competence for the exercise of authority belong to an individual. Underlying the concepts of functional authority, law of the situation, and authority of facts is the theme that authority is derived from the technical competence and knowledge of individuals in the organization who do not necessarily hold formal office in the line hierarchy.

Characteristics of Authority Holders

Authority rests in individuals. The talents and traits of the individual may become the source of authority, as in the case of the charismatic leader. A person holding power may use this as a base for gaining legitimate authority; a group may invest the person of power with legitimate authority as a protective measure and seek to impose the limits and customs of authority. They may also accept the power holder as formal officeholder as a means of accepting the situation without further conflict. Technical competence and knowledge are also personal characteristics that become the basis of authority in certain situations.

The Manager's Use of Sources of Authority

In practice, managers should recognize all the potential sources of authority and should weigh the contribution of each theory to obtain as complete a picture of the authority nexus as possible. They should assess their own grant of authority and try to determine which elements tend to strengthen their authority and which tend to erode it.

The base of authority shifts from time to time. For example, an individual is offered the position of department head of the health information service because of that individual's competence in the administration of record systems; this specialized knowledge and technical competence is the first pillar of authority. When the individual accepts the position, the formal authority mandate of that official position is added. This authority, in turn, is shaped by the prevailing organizational climate, which includes a wide or narrow zone of acceptance on the part of employees. The personal traits of the authority holder complete the authority base for that office.

The individual with a participative management style may emphasize those aspects of authority that widen the zone of acceptance. The setting itself may dictate the predominant authority base, as in the law of the situation; in a highly technical setting, those with the most technical knowledge use this knowledge as the base of authority. Although there is a tendency to downplay internal politics in organizations such as health care institutions, some individual managers may use power as a major source of authority. Astute managers regularly assess the several bases of authority available to them in order to enhance the authority relationships and thereby contribute more effectively to the achievement of organizational goals.

RESTRICTIONS ON THE USE OF AUTHORITY

Several factors restrict the use of authority. Some constraints stem from internal factors, such as the limits placed on authority at each organizational level; others stem from external factors such as laws, regulations, and ethical considerations. The following is a systematic summary of these factors:

1. *Organizational Position.* Each holder of authority receives a limited delegation of authority consistent with the position held in the organization. An individual has no legitimate formal authority beyond that accorded to the organizational position.
2. *Legal and Contractual Mandates.* Authority is limited by the federal, state, and municipal laws and regulations relating to safety, work hours, licensure, and scope of practice; by internal corporate charter and bylaws; and by union contract.
3. *Social Limitations.* The social codes, mores, and values of the overall society include both implicit and explicit limits on the behavior of individuals. Authority holders are expected to act in a manner consistent with the predominant value system of the society. These social limitations are major factors in shaping the zone of acceptance and the general cultural deference of individuals who are members of organizations.

4. *Physical Limits.* An authority holder cannot force a person to do something that is simply beyond that person's physical capabilities, nor can an authority holder escape the natural limits of the physical environment, such as climate or physical laws.

5. *Technological Constraints.* The advances and the limitations of the state of the art must be considered in the exercise of authority; no amount of power or authority can bring about a result that is beyond the technical ability of the individuals.

6. *Economic Constraints.* The scarcity of needed resources limits the behavior of formal authority holders.

7. *Zone of Acceptance of Organization Members.* Both authority and power have their limits in that the net cost of using either must be calculated. When a weak manager is faced with a strong employee group, as in a strong union setting, the cost of using even legitimate authority may be too high; the authority grant is actually diminished.

Although many employees do not have complete freedom to choose what they will or will not do, they may resist authority in subtle ways, such as adherence to job duties exactly as stated in the job description, passive resistance, and failure to take initiative in any area not specifically designated by the supervisor. The manager must move into a distinct leadership position to develop a wide zone of acceptance, as leadership becomes an essential adjunct to the exercise of authority.

IMPORTANCE OF DELEGATION

Although the manager retains overall responsibility and authority for the work of the department or service, he or she must necessarily delegate authority to specific workers under his or her jurisdiction. Simply put, it is not possible for the manager to carry out every task. Therefore, each worker receives delegated authority from the manager to proceed on a day-to-day basis. Managers set up the parameters for action through several means: the development of policies and procedures; the promulgation of known work rules and codes of behavior; the development of job descriptions with job duties and expectations well delineated; and the presentations of formal orientation and training programs associated with job duties. The manager consciously selects an appropriate style of leadership and communication to further enhance an atmosphere in which workers accept responsibility for their part in meeting the organizational goals.

A manager who is new to the role set may experience some uneasiness with delegating. First of all, there is simply that natural tendency to think, "I can do this better or faster myself." Second, a manager may harbor some fears: if the worker fails at the task, the responsibility still rests with the manager; it is the manager who will take the heat, so to speak. There is also a certain loss of satisfaction and recognition; managers are often removed from day-to-day interaction with patients and their families and their own professional peers who remain in the arena of active, hands-on practice. Recognition of these inner barriers to delegation is the first step to overcoming resistance to this necessary aspect of authority.

Do's and Don'ts of Delegation

1. Know when to delegate: in most day-to-day circumstances, delegation of responsibility is the norm. Routine tasks such as employee scheduling, for example, are easily accomplished by the supervisor closest to the unit. Certain highly specialized tasks such as revenue-cycle/compliance reviews are best delegated to a member of the department team who specializes in the area. Such a person would have the most up-to-date knowledge in the topic. Workflow coordination along with routine problem solving between or among working units are best accomplished by the immediate unit supervisors who are in continual interaction. Delegation is also a part of team development: the manager builds capability and confidence in the assistant managers, unit supervisors, and specialists. Delegation is part of the intentional training and mentoring goals of the manager.

2. Know when not to delegate: certain activities remain the primary responsibility of the manager and normally are not delegated, such as hiring, disciplinary action, and termination. Throughout each process there will be input from unit managers and supervisors, but the final action is that of the manager. Complex or volatile employee or client situations sometimes arise; these too are the manager's responsibility. Overall systems and workflow, along with equipment and layout, are the manager's concerns, although there is input from unit managers and supervisors.

3. Avoid common pitfalls associated with delegation: two common pitfalls can occur inadvertently; the manager takes care to avoid these. First, a manager might undermine a unit supervisor by countermanding, even informally, a decision made by the supervisor. For example, a unit supervisor might deny a request for a schedule change by an employee, due to workflow or

staffing considerations. The employee might informally ask the manager to approve the desired schedule change; managers who allow themselves to override a unit manager's decision undercut the authority/responsibility grant of this intermediate manager. (This is not the same thing as the normal appeals process during which an employee may meet with a higher-level manager at designated steps in the appeal.) Another pitfall is associated with the best of intentions: the manager solicits information on a regular basis, perhaps daily, from unit managers. The casual but purposeful question, "how are things going in your unit today?" may lead to on-the-spot reports of one or another workflow or staffing problem. The concerned manager might readily respond, "I'll look into that and get back to you," instead of assisting the unit manager in solving the problem.

Set up a balanced system of availability and support. The manager remains available to unit supervisors through a mix of formal and informal interactions:

- Formal, periodic meetings with individual supervisors for in-depth feedback about a specific function. These meetings focus on workflow and related problem solving.
- Formal development meetings with individual supervisors or the team of supervisors. The focus is development of supervisory skills, mentoring, and career path development.
- Informal day-to-day "prn" interaction.
- A combination of formal and informal daily briefing, sometimes referred to as "the huddle." This practice involves a brief daily meeting, about 15 minutes, held early to midday. By this time, any immediate concerns have surfaced, yet there is sufficient time remaining in the day to solve most problems. The team usually remains standing while each supervisor summarizes the particular concerns in his functional unit, allowing each member of the team to become aware of workflow impact, employee issues, and "news of the day." Team members are able to make immediate plans to deal with intradepartmental concerns without the manager having to mediate such coordination. An administrative assistant also attends, bringing materials for distribution on the spot, which eliminates the piling up of materials in the inbox for each team member. The manager comments on such materials if some follow-up is required. The secretary's presence also facilitates actions to keep things moving without further instruction—e.g., he or she will follow up on a purchase order or check on a question relating to a payroll matter. The manager rotates

the location of "the huddle" among the different units of the department unless confidential information is involved. In such a case, the unit supervisor of that department leads a roundtable briefing. This action provides visibility of the authority-responsibility mandate entrusted to that supervisor. The employees of the unit see their unit supervisor as a member of the team. Furthermore, this experience of leading a roundtable briefing provides additional training in leadership for each team member. "The huddle" takes place daily, even when the manager is unable to attend, thus reinforcing the role set of the supervisors as designated agents of the manager.

Recognition of the benefits of proper delegation and, conversely, awareness of the consequences of poor delegation further enhance a manager's ability to delegate. Just as proper delegation increases the zone of acceptance on the part of employees, failure to delegate demoralizes workers, thereby shrinking their field of cooperation. Morale suffers; turnover rates increase; loss of productivity results. When workers in regular contact with clients cannot easily take immediate and effective action, client groups become alienated and unhappy and seek services elsewhere. The organization develops a reputation for being wrapped in bureaucratic red tape. Finally, without proper delegation, a manager must remain constantly present to authorize action; this is time consuming and wasteful of managerial resources. It is also unrealistic because a manager's duties frequently require being out of the department or office and even away from the premises. With solid management practices in place, and with a manager's commitment to delegation, the day-to-day activities flow toward accomplishing the overall mission of the organization.

LEADERSHIP

Professionals frequently describe a leader as a powerful person who made it to the top of his or her field. The successful health professional does not seem to share familiar and common habits with the average practitioner. We imagine the person as a romantic figure that is not human. Drucker describes leadership in reality as "mundane, unromantic and boring. Its essence is performance."[11] Yet leadership is vital for the future growth and development of health professions. This section is designed to address the leadership qualities that everyone has buried within. Rather than define leadership as distant and unusual, this section describes it as a set of characteristics that emerge from individuals who are able to get things done within an organization.

Leaders are not born, they develop. In fact, leaders are not extraordinary except that they can match organizational goals to the abilities and interests of their work groups. This talent is mercurial and one finds that some leaders are effective in one set of circumstances but not in others. Leadership is not based on impossible characteristics possessed by few; rather, it is a collection of abilities.

Definition of Leadership

A leader is a person who can organize tasks and make things happen. Using the unique interests and needs of every member of the work group, effective leaders inspire goal-directed behavior that is consistent and efficient. The leader cajoles, rewards, punishes, organizes, stimulates, strengthens, communicates, and motivates. There is no set standard for leadership behavior as individuals must match their own characteristics to the needs of the organization.

The personal characteristics of leaders are a strong self-image, a vision of the future, a firm belief in the goals of the organization, the ability to influence the behavior of subordinates, and the ability to relate to and influence individuals in parallel or superior positions of authority.

Leadership exists both informally and formally. Informal leadership is exerted in many settings, including formal organizations. Within any formal organization, there are subunits and even paraorganizations, such as a collective bargaining unit, that are led by individuals who do not hold formal hierarchical office. Leadership is implied, even explicitly included, in the role of the manager whose function is to achieve organizational objectives by coordinating, motivating, and directing the work group. For the remainder of this discussion on formal leadership, the presumption is made that the manager is a leader in addition to being a holder of formal authority.

Leadership Qualities

To influence and induce others to strive toward a goal, the leader must possess not only a deep vision of that goal but also the ability to render the goal meaningful to the group. The knowledge, insight, and skill of the leader are greater than those of other members of the group. At an obvious level, the leader leads but does not drag, coerce, or push the group; the group members are steadily induced to move toward the goal. They are influenced in a pervasive way so that the overall goal becomes their own goal. The leader does not achieve the work alone but instead successfully coordinates the work of the group. The leader inspires confidence through both emotional and knowledge ties with the followers.

Leadership Functions

In formal organizations, the leader has certain functions that are tied to the organizational need for leadership. The leader is expected to influence, persuade, and control the group. As the individual with vision, the leader is expected to take calculated risks and to be a catalytic agent in the change process.

The leader carries out important functions on behalf of group members through the role of representative; for example, employees look to their unit or department head to speak for them and to seek or to obtain advantages for them. The leader may be cast in several roles by followers, especially at the symbolic level, and may even be seen as the father figure who shields the individual from difficulties. The leader may also be the scapegoat; as the management representative closest to the rank-and-file worker, the leader-manager bears the brunt of anger when the organizational situation is less than optimal.

The leader is presumed to embody the values of the group. As such, the leader becomes the focal point in the motivational process. Leaders foster the development of the climate and conditions that favor individual involvement in group effort. Leadership is a process more than a structure; the leader creates the climate for change so that the organization will have the adaptability needed for its survival.

In its 1996 accreditation standards the Joint Commission placed renewed emphasis on the role of department heads as members of the leadership team.

From Theory to Practice: A Leader's Plan of Action

The manager must make a conscious commitment to the exercise of leadership through specific action. Leadership activity clusters natural groupings which, in turn, are intertwined. Here are some examples of leadership action relating to health information management.

1. The leader starts and sustains the conversation: by being out in front of the trends, the leader studies the big challenges, "digests them," "talks them up," and translates them into an action plan within the organization. Examples include encouraging employee development through the attainment of additional specialty credentials; promoting participation in regional health information exchange and eHealth initiatives.

2. The leader uses professional and technical competence to promote the health information professionals as the authoritative sources for clinical documentation systems and practices. Activities would typically include monitoring the federal initiatives concerning the Nationwide Health Information Network (NHIN); disseminating of information about the

current changes in electronic discovery civil rule and the related topic of the definition of the electronic legal record; serving as Electronic Health Record (EHR) project manager or team member.

3. The leader partners with key players in the organization. The leader identifies individuals whose support is critical to successful implementation of major systems—e.g., the EHR, speech recognition technology, or computerized provider order entry (CPOE). The leader takes the initiative in interdepartmental collaborative action such as:
   - policy and procedure affecting joint action
   - clinical pertinence review protocols
   - inservice training needs
   - compliance reviews and billing audits
   - risk management reviews
   - interorganization peer review

4. The leader is actively engaged in the life of the organization. The leader recognizes and accepts that the work extends well beyond the routine 9-to-5 day and well beyond the borders of the department. The leader's attitude is one of loyalty to and enthusiasm for the work of the organization. This visible support of the mission might take on a variety of forms:
   - participation in organizational events to honor employees or volunteers—e.g., employee recognition ceremonies and receptions
   - participation in outreach activities such as career days, health fairs, fund-raising events
   - attendance at events sponsored by other departments—e.g., the open house celebrating a designated professional week (such as Physical Therapy Week or National Nurses Week)
   - participation in the organization's Speakers Bureau
   - hosting regional meetings of one's profession to bring attention to the organization's areas of excellence

5. The leader passes on the praise and the pride. Employees are not taken for granted. Their accomplishments are noted within the department and the organization. The leader takes care to nominate employees for appropriate awards such as employee of the month. Departmental activities are included in the internal newsletter, with its customary "spotlight on" column. The leader submits entries for trade and professional association newsletters featuring the department. The leader finds opportunities for employees to participate in extradepartmental events, such as the annual disaster/

emergency preparedness drills, thereby raising the visibility and involvement of the group.

Styles of Leadership

The manner in which a manager interacts with subordinates reflects a cluster of characteristics that constitute a style of leadership. While any manager uses several styles of leadership—choosing the style most appropriate for a given situation—one style generally emerges as that manager's predominant mode of interaction.

Autocratic Leadership

Also referred to as authoritarian, boss-centered, or dictatorial leadership, autocratic leadership is characterized by close supervision. The manager who employs this style gives direct, clear, and precise directions to employees, telling them what is to be done and how it will be done; there is no room for employee initiative. Employees do not participate in the decision-making process. There is a high degree of centralization and a narrow span of management. The chain of command is clearly and fully understood by all. Autocratic managers use their authority as their principal, or only, method of getting work done because they feel that employees could not properly or efficiently carry out work assignments without detailed instruction.

Although this style of leadership apparently gets results, it can be fatal over the long run. Employees easily lose interest in their assignments and stop thinking for themselves, since there is no occasion for independent thought. Under certain conditions and with specific employees, however, a degree of close supervision may be necessary. Some employees prefer to receive clear and precise orders, because close supervision reassures them that they are doing a good job. Even so, it can generally be assumed that the autocratic, close leadership style is the least effective and least desirable method for motivating employees.

Bureaucratic Leadership

Like the autocratic leader, the bureaucratic leader tells employees what to do and how to do it. The basis for this leadership style is almost exclusively the institution's rules and regulations. For the bureaucrat, these rules are the laws. The bureaucratic manager is normally afraid to take chances and manages "by the book." Rules are strictly enforced, and no departures or exceptions are permitted. The bureaucrat, like the autocrat, allows employees little or no freedom.

Participative Leadership

In participative leadership, the contribution of the group to the organizational effort is emphasized. This style is the opposite of autocratic, close supervision. The manager who employs the participative method involves the employees in the decision-making process and in the maintenance of cohesive group interaction. The manager consults with employees concerning goals and objectives, work assignments, and the extent and content of a problem before making a final decision and issuing directives or orders. This approach is an attempt to make full use of the talents and abilities of the group members; the manager is the facilitator of this process. It is difficult for employees who have participated in the consultative process not to accept the resulting decision.

Some managers use a pseudoparticipative method of leadership to give employees the feeling that consultation has taken place. Employees quickly sense that the manager is manipulating people, however, and that their participation in the decision-making process is not real. The manager who employs the participative style of leadership must take it seriously and must be willing to listen to and evaluate employees' opinions and suggestions before making a final decision.

Participative management does not weaken a manager's formal authority, since the manager retains the right to make the final decision. The obvious advantage of the participative style of leadership revolves around the meaningful involvement of the employees, which greatly enhances the implementation of the decisions that have been made.

Laissez-Faire Leadership

Laissez-faire or "free rein" leadership is based on the assumption that individuals are self-motivated. Employees receive little or no supervision. Employees, as individuals or as a group, determine their own goals and make their own decisions. The manager, whose contribution is minimal, acts primarily as a consultant and does so only when asked. The manager does not lead but allows the employees to lead themselves. Some managers consider this approach true democratic leadership, but the usual end result is disorganization and chaos. The lack of leadership permits different employees to proceed in different directions.

Paternalistic Leadership

The manager who is paternalistic treats employees like children. The manager tells employees what is to be done but does so in a nice way. It is the paternalistic manager's belief that employees do not really know what is good for them or how to make decisions for themselves. In this approach, everyone is watched over by the benevolent manager—the benign dictator—and the employees eventually become extremely dependent on their "paternalistic boss."

Continuum of Leadership Styles

Another way to view leadership behavior is on a continuum ranging from highly boss-centered to highly group-centered. The relationship between the manager and the employee in the continuum ranges from completely autocratic, in which there is no employee participation in the decision-making process, to completely democratic, in which the employee participates in all phases of the decision-making process. The following is a brief description of the seven gradations along the continuum:

1. *Manager makes decision and announces it.* The manager identifies a problem, considers alternative solutions, selects a course of action, and tells employees what they are to do. Employees do not participate in the decision-making process.
2. *Manager "sells" decision.* The manager again makes the decision without consulting the employees. Instead of announcing the decision, however, the manager attempts to persuade the employees to accept it. The manager details how the decision fits both the goals of the department and the interests of group members.
3. *Manager presents ideas and invites questions.* The manager has made the decision but asks the employees to express their ideas. Thus, the manager allows for the possibility that the initial decision may be modified.
4. *Manager presents tentative decision subject to change.* The manager allows the employees the opportunity to exert some influence before the decision is finalized. The manager meets with the employees and presents the problem and a tentative decision. Before the decision is finalized, the manager obtains the reactions of employees who will be affected by it.
5. *Manager presents problem, gets suggestions, makes decision.* Up to this point on the continuum, the manager has always come before the employees with at least a tentative solution to the problem. At this point, however, the employees get the first opportunity to suggest solutions. Consultation with the employees increases the number of possible solutions to the problem. The manager then selects the solution that he or she regards as most appropriate in solving the problem.
6. *Manager defines limits; asks group to make decision.* For the first time, the employees make the decision. The manager now becomes a member of the

group. Before doing this, however, the manager defines the problem and the limits and boundaries within which the decision must be made.

7. *Manager permits subordinates to function within limits defined by superior.* For the maximum degree of employee participation, the manager defines the problem and lists the guidelines and boundaries within which a solution must be achieved. The limitation imposed on the employees comes directly from the manager, who participates as a group member in the decision-making process and is committed in advance to implementing whatever decision the employees make.

In summary, the manager's relationship with the employees influences morale, job satisfaction, and work output. Employee satisfaction is positively associated with the degree to which employees are permitted to participate in the decision-making process. In contrast, poor supervision causes employee dissatisfaction, high turnover rates, and low morale.

Factors That Influence Leadership Style

No one style of leadership fits all situations. A successful manager selects a method appropriate for a given situation. Before selecting a style of leadership or deciding to blend several styles, the manager must consider a number of factors:

1. *Work Assignment.* If the work assignment is repetitious, the properly trained employee does not need constant or close supervision. If the assignment is new or complex, however, close supervision may be required.

2. *Personality and Ability of the Employee.* Employees who are not self-starters react best to close supervision. Others, by reason of their personality and work background, can take on new and important responsibilities on their own; these individuals react best to participative leadership. The occupational makeup of a department may also influence the leadership style used by the manager. For professional people (e.g., physical therapists, occupational therapists, health information personnel) or other highly skilled employees, the employee-centered participative leadership style is often most effective. When employees are unskilled or unable to act independently, the boss-centered or autocratic style of leadership may produce better results.

3. *Attitude of the Employee Toward the Manager.* Managers cannot begin to lead or influence behavior unless they are accepted by the group. Employees give managers their authority only when they believe that the goals and objectives of the managers are consistent with their own personal and professional interests.

4. *Personality and Ability of the Manager.* The manager's personality has a very definite effect on the behavior and performance of employees. The manager must treat employees' opinions and suggestions with respect and must sincerely encourage employee participation.

When faced with different work group encounters and situational factors, the good manager shifts from one style of leadership to another, often without conscious recognition of a shift in style. Table 12–1 shows examples of the adjustments in leadership style that a manager makes in order to stimulate maximum effort from employees.

ORDERS AND DIRECTIVES

The manager's role is to direct the employees toward achieving the goals and objectives of the department and the institution. Regardless of the leadership style employed, the manager must issue orders and directives to indicate what must be

Table 12–1 Variables in Leadership Style

Work Group	Key Activites	Leadership Style
Hospital transporters	Transport of patient Safety considerations Schedule considerations Mode of transport	Bureaucratic—policies and procedures must be followed
Staff physical therapist with experience	Patient evaluation "Need evaluation today" Neurological case Conference at 10:00 A.M.	Laissez-faire—manager does not need to tell physical therapist such typical evaluation elements as motor, sensory, and cognitive tests
Total physical therapy professional staff (5 physical therapists)	Vacation schedules Consideration of patients, students, and overall coverage One staff resignation in July	Participative—manager consults with employees concerning vacation schedule and the need for proper coverage during the summer months
Staff physical therapist	Call from physician to staff therapist; wishes to see therapist at patient's bedside promptly at 9:15 or "Sorry to interrupt but just had a call from Dr. Jones and he requests you be at the patient's room #343 in 5 minutes" (*Note:* Even, nice tone)	Autocratic, nonnegotiable

done. The terms *orders* and *directives* may be used interchangeably, although *orders* has a more autocratic tone.

Giving orders is a major function of the manager's day-to-day operation of the program. Too often, it is taken for granted that every manager knows how to give orders. Unfortunately, this is not true. The manager must remember to convey to the employees *what* is to be done, *who* is to do it, and *when, where, how,* and *why.* At times, some of the components are implied or omitted. For example, "Effective July 1, John Doe will be the Senior Physical Therapist of the Amputee Service." This statement answers the *what, who, when,* and *where* but omits the *how* and *why.*

Verbal Orders versus Written Orders

The form of an order depends on the situation. The verbal order is the most frequently used. Because it is given on a one-to-one basis with immediate feedback, the manager can observe the employee's reaction, ask questions, and appraise the degree of understanding. Disagreements can be handled immediately. Observation of the employee's body language provides additional feedback.

When permanence is important, written orders are more appropriate. This form is most effective when information is to be disseminated to employees as a group. Written orders are more carefully thought through, since there is less opportunity for explanation. The use of long sentences, excessive adjectives, and involved word patterns should be avoided. The written order also carries a degree of formality not present in the verbal order. It is difficult, however, to keep written material up to date and impossible to clear up obscure meanings.

Making Orders Acceptable and Effective

The issuing of effective orders requires attention to timing and language. Planning to issue the order involves content, format (oral or written), and the manner in which the order is actually issued. When there is rapport between the manager and employee, a simple request may be suitable; an implied order is sometimes given with the same informality. When certain action must be taken, precision is involved, or misunderstanding must be avoided, the written, direct order is the best method. The sense of command may be foreign to many managers, yet commands may be needed on some occasions, such as emergencies. Although policies, work rules, and procedures may not be considered orders, they do set required courses of action as determined by management.

Since a critical aspect of the manager's function is communicating, effort must be given to making orders acceptable and effective. Acceptability is enhanced by the general processes of leadership that the manager has developed over time. In effect, the manager prepared the employees in many ways so that when orders are actually given, they are normally both acceptable and effective in terms of essential communication.

DISCIPLINE

The attitudes, emotions, and motivations of each employee within an organization not only affect the degree to which goals and objectives are attained but also influence the behavior of other employees. The manager of any unit or department must be concerned with the conduct or behavior of all employees within that unit or department. A manager's guidance of a work group can best be facilitated by first establishing reasonable standards of conduct, or work rules, and informing employees of these standards, and second, by enforcing all rules consistently and humanely.

The word *discipline* has acquired different and sometimes less-than-welcome connotations over the years. In the military context we usually associate discipline with order, consistency, and unquestioning obedience. In the context of the work organization, however, the word *discipline* is immediately associated with the use of authority and thus it carries the disagreeable connotation of punishment. However, a brief foray into the origins of the word reveals that discipline comes from the same root as disciple and as such actually means *to teach so as to mold*. So at one time teaching was the primary intent of discipline, the process of shaping or molding the disciple. But for the most part, in the context of the work organization we have come to associate discipline—and therefore disciplinary *action*—with punishment.

The primary objective of disciplinary action should never be punishment. Rather, the principal purpose of disciplinary action should be *correction of behavior*. Therefore it is a requirement of disciplinary action that the transgressing party be afforded the opportunity to correct the offending behavior. There are of course apparent exceptions in the form of those instances of behavior that are sufficiently serious to prompt "correction" of a situation by removing (that is, terminating) the offender without a second chance. These exceptions arise in a relative minority of disciplinary situations; for the greatest part, disciplinary action is properly directed toward correcting errant behavior.

In addition to using disciplinary action to improve employee behavior, at times it can help to motivate employees so they become self-disciplined and thus more effective in the performance of their jobs. However, no matter how skillfully it is applied, disciplinary action will always carry something of a negative connotation for many employees, so in the long run calling attention to correct behavior is more effective in promoting self-discipline and cooperation than calling attention to incorrect behavior. In other words, disciplinary action is necessary and it has its place, but praise ultimately proves more powerful in inspiring acceptable performance and behavior. Even in an organization where employees exhibit a high degree of independence and self-discipline, a manager must occasionally apply disciplinary action of some kind because rules have been broken.

At this stage of the discussion it is necessary to make a distinction between two kinds of employee problems with which the manager may be confronted: problems of performance and problems of conduct or behavior. When we speak of taking disciplinary action we are talking of addressing problems of conduct or behavior—that is, problems that involve the breaking of rules or the violation of policies. In addressing these kinds of problems, although it is usually our purpose to correct the errant behavior, the process frequently involves "warnings" of various kinds. Thus the process can acquire a negative connotation and be perceived as including "punishment." Most if not all problems of conduct or behavior involve violations that are willful or that at least result from carelessness or indifference. Such violations are considered the fault of the perpetrators.

Problems of performance, however, are an entirely different matter. The warnings and suspensions and such described within a progressive disciplinary process are inappropriate for problems of performance. Such problems, usually encompassing an employee's failure to meet the minimum expectations of the job, are not considered willful violations of rules. Therefore, problems of performance must be addressed through counseling and retraining as necessary, utilizing a process that is entirely corrective in nature and not punitive in any respect. The progressive disciplinary process, then, is applicable only to problems of conduct or behavior and not at all to problems of performance.

Distasteful as the application of disciplinary action may be, it is the manager's responsibility to act promptly, firmly, and consistently when action is called for. Disciplinary action should follow the misconduct as closely in time as possible. The only significant reasons for ever delaying disciplinary action even briefly are to allow tempers to cool, perhaps to investigate a situation and decide how to proceed, or to take the time and opportunity to secure a private one-on-one meeting with the offending individual. Every instance of disciplinary action must be treated as a confidential matter, handled in private; it is, quite bluntly, nobody's business but that of the offending employee and the manager.

Progressive Disciplinary Action

Several steps constitute the progressive disciplinary process. Not all of these steps will be applicable in all instances; at which step the process is entered and how many steps are applied will depend on the nature of the specific infraction. The steps composing a complete progressive disciplinary process are described as follows.

Counseling

The initial step taken to address a number of kinds of noncritical errant behavior should be counseling. In a one-to-one meeting with the manager, the employee should be told the nature of the perceived problem, why it is a problem (or how it can *become* a problem), what the rules are concerning this behavior (with specific reference to handbooks and policy manuals), what the possible consequences of this kind of behavior are, and the period of time within which correction is expected. This should be accomplished without reference to any kind of "warning"; it is simply an important, job-related discussion between manager and employee.

The manager should document each counseling session. Some organizations use a specific form for documenting counseling sessions, but a simple handwritten note retained in departmental files should be sufficient.

Oral Warning

Repeated problem behavior following counseling should be addressed using the more formal early stages of the progressive disciplinary process, specifically the oral warning. The oral warning stage, often regarded as involving a "counseling" session itself, should be utilized only after the employee has failed to respond to informal counseling.

The oral warning should be documented by the manager, preferably on a form created for that purpose. Exhibit 12–1 presents an example of a simple oral warning form.

Often someone will argue that if the "oral" warning is documented, it is actually a *written* warning. It may seem so, but the difference between a written and oral warning lies in what goes into the employee's personnel file. The record of an oral warning should be retained in department files; it should go into the official personnel files only as part of a subsequent warning for the same kind of behavior.

One might logically ask that if it is truly to be an "oral" warning, why document it at all? This is done because the oral warning is a step in the published progressive disciplinary process, and when an employment relationship breaks down and legal

EXHIBIT 12–1

Record of Oral Warning

Employee Name _____ ID No. _____

Department _____ Hire Date _____

Job Title & Grade _____ Job Date _____

Infraction or incident; policy reviewed and discussed:

Dates of counselings or discussions concerning the same policy:

The employee must take the following action:

Employee Signature _____ Date _____

Manager Signature _____ Date _____

This record will be maintained in departmental files. If further action is required for the same offense, it will be forwarded to Human Resources for inclusion in the personnel file.

problems result, it can become necessary to provide evidence that every step in the process was followed.

Written Warning

The written warning follows the oral warning as necessary, with this documentation automatically included in the employee's personnel file. Exhibit 12–2 is an example of a written warning form.

An employee whose improper behavior has not been corrected following counseling, oral warning, and written warning is in a position in which failure to change will lead to loss of income via suspension and perhaps eventual loss of employment. By this stage the manager and employee have been together on the subject of the

---

EXHIBIT 12–2

Written Warning

Employee Name _____ ID No. _____

Department _____ Hire Date _____

Job Title & Grade _____ Job Date _____

Infraction or incident; policy reviewed and discussed:

Dates of previous actions related to the foregoing:

The employee must take the following action:

Employee Signature _____ Date _____

Manager Signature _____ Date _____

This record puts the employee on notice that additional violations will result in more serious disciplinary action such as suspension without pay or discharge.

---

employee's behavior problem at least three or more times. It is time for the supervisor to bring other resources into the process.

Before Suspension

Before proceeding to the suspension step, the manager should consider referring the employee to one of two available sources of assistance: the employee health service or the human resources department.

If in any of their numerous contacts the employee has given the manager reason to believe he or she may be experiencing health problems of any kind, a referral to the employee health service is in order. If the problem appears to possibly lie in employee attitude or in other difficulties unrelated to health, the referral should be to human resources. In the ideal system the human resource department will include an employee relations specialist or employee ombudsperson, but in the absence of such specialists most human resource generalists can fill the employee relations role.

This referral puts the employee in contact with someone who may be able to point the way toward resolution of some underlying problem. Also, a knowledgeable person other than the manager is brought into the process, and this new participant may be able to get through to the employee where the manager could not. This step provides the employee with more distinct opportunity to correct the problem behavior. Also, the involvement of human resources can be helpful in instances in which tension or strain exists between department manager and employee.

Suspension and Discharge

If the referral step described above proves unsuccessful, suspension without pay, which in many systems ranges from one to five days, may follow. Eventually, discharge will likely be necessary if nothing up to and including suspension without pay is successful in changing behavior. Exhibits 12–3 and 12–4 are examples of forms used to document suspension and discharge respectively. However, a well-functioning referral program for employee behavior problems will significantly reduce the use of the clearly punitive steps of suspension and discharge.

There is an important point to address concerning suspension without pay. Note that in Exhibit 12–3, there is the option for the manager to waive the time-off requirement of a suspension. The manager is permitted to use this option on occasions when the enforced time off of a suspension would leave an important job untended or an area critically understaffed. However, the employee must be strongly advised that waiver of time off does not lessen the severity of the disciplinary action as far as the official record and future actions are concerned.

The manager who believes to have cause to discharge an employee should take the case to the human resources department for thorough review before taking action. Given the legal environment of the times, most organizations today require human resources or administrative review and concurrence for most discharges. This review will attempt to determine whether all bases have been covered from a legal perspective and whether the record clearly demonstrates that the employee was given the opportunity to correct the inappropriate behavior. Because of the time required to accomplish it, this review serves another extremely important function in assuring that no employee is ever fired on the spot or otherwise terminated in the anger of the moment.

EXHIBIT 12–3

Suspension Without Pay

Employee Name _____ ID No. _____

Department _____ Hire Date _____

Job Title & Grade _____ Job Date _____

Infraction or incident; policy reviewed and discussed:

Specific problem or incident, and rule or policy reviewed and discussed.

Previous Disciplinary Actions:
   Date: Action Taken:

Suspended for _____ days from the above date. Report back on regular shift on _____.

Or

_____ Time off waived by manager for the following reason (waiver does not lessen the severity of the action.):

Employee Signature _____ Date _____

Manager Signature _____ Date _____

This is a final warning. Failure to respond appropriately may result in discharge.

EXHIBIT 12–4

Notice of Discharge or Dismissal

Employee Name _____ ID No. _____

Department _____ Hire Date _____

Job Title & Grade _____ Job Date _____

Your employment is being terminated for the following reasons:

Previous Disciplinary Actions:
    Date: Action Taken:

_____ Check here to indicate whether the employee desires an exit interview to discuss benefits status. If this opportunity is declined, continuation-of-benefits information will be mailed to the employee's home address.

Employee Signature _____ Date _____

Manager Signature _____ Date _____

Some severe infractions must of course be dealt with as they occur. However, immediate firing is never the answer. The offending employee should instead be sent home on indefinite suspension pending investigation and resolution.

Not all kinds of infractions will require the application of all the foregoing steps. A mild infraction, such as tardiness (within a few minutes of starting time) may, if it becomes chronic, eventually require all of the steps described above. A more serious infraction, such as sleeping on duty, may call for a written warning or suspension on the first violation and discharge on the second violation.

The organization's human resource department ordinarily provides guidance for determining the severity of disciplinary action for specific infractions. Differences exist among organizations as to what kind of action applies to what sort of infraction, but guidelines might include the following:

- For a typical minor infraction such as chronic tardiness, absenteeism, or perhaps discourtesy, for multiple offenses the progression might consist of, first, oral warning, second, written warning, then one-day suspension, then three-day suspension, and finally discharge.
- For a more serious infraction such as, for example, conducting personal business on work time, unexcused absence, or failure to report for work when scheduled, the progression might consist of written warning for the first offense, then three-day suspension, and finally discharge.
- For still more serious infractions such as insubordination, falsification of records, or violation of confidentiality, the complete progression might consist of a written warning for an initial offense and discharge for a second offense.
- For the most serious infractions there is no progression; these call for discharge upon the first and only offense. Typical serious infractions include theft, fighting on the job, possessing or using alcohol or illegal substances on the job, bringing weapons onto the premises, deliberate destruction of property, and absence without notice for three consecutive scheduled days (considered job abandonment).

Heading Off Infractions Before They Occur

The manager who observes an employee apparently headed toward a point where disciplinary action will be necessary is advised to introduce counseling before true progressive discipline is necessary. If the manager, for example, sees that a particular employee is developing a poor attendance record and is closing in on the point at which disciplinary action is called for, the manager should address this via counseling with the employee before such action is necessary. It is the unfeeling manager who, observing that an employee is approaching the point where disciplinary action is necessary, will allow the circumstances to continue until action is unavoidable. Better by far for both manager and employee to use counseling in an effort to head off the problem before it fully develops.

Appeal Procedure

Numerous organizations utilize appeal procedures to address employee complaints about work-related matters. Such matters can include, for example, disciplinary actions, performance evaluations, and decisions based on specific interpretations of policy. A typical appeal procedure might include the following steps or some variation of them. The time frames given are simply what one organization might specify.

- An employee with a complaint should first address the issue with the immediate supervisor.
- If the employee is not satisfied with the supervisor's response, within a week of the meeting he or she may complete a simple appeal form (obtained from human resources) and schedule a meeting with the appropriate department head (the manager to whom the supervisor reports). If the department head *is* the immediate supervisor, this step and the following step are omitted.
- Within two weeks the department head will review all facts and circumstances, investigating as necessary, and render a decision in writing on the appeal form.
- If not satisfied with the department head's response, the employee may take the appeal to the member of administration to whom the department head reports. As in the previous step, within two weeks the administrative representative will render a decision in writing.
- If the employee remains unsatisfied with the response, the appeal is then taken to the director of human resources, who will convene a three-party ad hoc appeal committee consisting of one staff employee, one management employee, and one human resource representative. Within two weeks this committee will submit a confidential recommendation to the director of human resources.
- As necessary the director of human resources will review the complaint and recommendation with administration or legal counsel for legal or other significant implications. Once cleared at this level, the recommendation becomes final and binding.
- The employee does of course have external options such as the Equal Employment Opportunity Commission (EEOC) and the State Division of Human Rights (DHR). However, if the organization's representatives have applied the appeal procedure honestly and impartially, the chances of a successful external challenge are severely limited.

Grievance Procedure

The word *appeal* was used throughout the foregoing procedure to differentiate the process from that which might be embodied in a collective bargaining agreement (union contract). Collective bargaining agreements invariably use the term *griev-ance* in the same sense that *appeal* might be used in a non-union context. As in the non-union appeal process, a union grievance procedure will utilize several steps that take the complaint up through succeeding levels of consideration. The essential differences arise from the involvement of union officials and perhaps outside arbitrators or mediators.

One form of grievance procedure is presented in Appendix 10-A, Sample Collective Bargaining Agreement, Article Fifteen, Grievance Procedure.

CASE: AUTHORITY AND LEADERSHIP: RISING FROM THE RANKS

Background

After working eight years as a staff nurse on a general medical/surgical unit, Julie Davis was appointed nurse manager of that unit. Following a staff meeting at which her promotion was announced, Julie found herself surrounded by three longtime coworkers offering their congratulations and making other observations and comments.

"I'm really happy for you," said Sarah Johnson. "This sounds like a terrific career step. But I suppose this means our carpool is affected, since your hours are bound to be a lot less predictable from now on."

Elaine Rowe said, "And I guess that shoots the lunch bunch, too. Management commitments, you know." The emphasis on management was subtle though undeniable, and Julie was not at all sure that she was pleased with what she was hearing.

Jane Davidson offered, "Well, maybe now we can get some action on a few age-old problems. Remember, Julie, you used to gripe about these things as much as the rest of us."

"We've all complained a lot," Sarah agreed. "That's been sort of a way of life around here." The tone of her voice shaded toward a suggestion of coolness and her customary smile was absent when she added, "Now Julie's going to be in a position where she can do something, so let's hope she doesn't forget who her friends are."

Elaine and Jane looked quickly from Sarah to Julie. For an awkward 10 seconds or so nobody spoke. At last someone passing by said something to Julie, and as Julie turned to respond, Elaine, Jane, and Sarah went their separate ways.

Instructions

1. Identify the potential advantages Julie might enjoy in becoming manager of a group of which she has long been a member, and contrast these with the possible disadvantages that might present themselves because she has long been a member of this group.

2. Describe how you believe Julie will have to proceed in establishing herself as the legitimate possessor of supervisory authority on the unit, and describe the sources and forms of Julie's authority.

CASE: DISCIPLINE AND DOCUMENTATION—HERE SHE GOES AGAIN

Background

"I've come to the end of my patience with Roberta Weston," said accounting manager Sam Best. "The position she's in is so important to us that we simply can't afford any more of her omissions or mistakes. For the sake of the hospital and the department, I believe she's got to go."

"What's the problem?" asked human resource director Charlene Harrison.

"Problems, plural," Best answered. "She's so late in posting receipts on rentals in the medical arts center that we wind up double-billing a number of physicians every month. Actually, it's the same with just about all miscellaneous income—since she's responsible for all receipts except third-party reimbursement. We're losing control of income, and I get three or four complaints a week from people who claim they've been billed again for charges they've already paid."

Best shook his head and added, "I've really tried to give her every chance to turn around, but nothing seems to work. At least not for very long."

Harrison said, "I've reviewed Roberta's file. The only evidence of a problem I found was your rather detailed performance improvement review of two months ago. In that process, you're supposed to give the employee detailed direction aimed at correcting the problem. You did that, and you also provided a warning that task performance would be monitored closely for 30 days and that she could be let go by the end of that period if her work didn't come up to satisfactory levels. You did the review well, but I didn't see anything about any follow-up."

Best said, "That's because she had shaped up by the end of the 30 days."

"But now she isn't working up to the requirements of the job?"

"No. Her work was just marginally okay at the end of the 30 days, but within two weeks after that the bottom dropped out again and the mistakes started rolling in."

Harrison asked, "What do you mean by 'again'?"

"This is the third time I've been through this with her. I go over the areas in which she's not working up to standard, she puts on a burst of effort and does better, and a month or so later she falls back into her old ways." Best frowned and added, "I can't put up with it any longer. Three strikes—she's out."

Harrison said, "According to her file it's just one strike. The only documentation is your single performance improvement review. What about the other two times?"

"Strictly verbal."

"You didn't write up anything? You're supposed to cover oral warnings with a counseling form or at least a memo for the record."

Best said, "If I wrote up one of those every time I had to talk to an employee, I'd never get done writing. It's a lot of work."

"I know it is," responded Harrison, "but you've got to have your documentation. As it stands right now, if we terminate her she could probably give us a real hard time with a couple of outside agencies."

"So what should I do?" Best asked.

Instructions

1. Describe the ways in which the employee might be able to give the organization a "real hard time" if she is terminated now.
2. Develop a plan of action that you would recommend Sam Best to follow in dealing with employee Roberta Weston.

NOTES

1. Chester Barnard, *The Functions of the Executive* (Cambridge, Mass.: Harvard University Press, 1968), 167–69.
2. Herbert Simon, *Administrative Behavior* (New York: Macmillan, 1965), 12.
3. Ibid., 129.
4. Robert Presthus, "Authority in Organizations," in *Concepts and Issues in Administrative Behavior,* edited by Sidney Mailick and Edward H. Van Ness (Englewood Cliffs, N.J.: Prentice-Hall, 1962), 122.
5. Edgar H. Schein, *Organizational Psychology* (Englewood Cliffs, N.J.: Prentice-Hall, 1965), 11.

6. H. H. Gerth and C. Wright Mills, *From Max Weber: Essays in Sociology* (New York: Oxford University Press, 1946), 196–204.

7. Ibid.

8. H. C. Metcalf and L. Urwick, eds., *Dynamic Administration: The Collected Papers of Mary Parker Follett* (New York: Harper, 1942).

9. Ibid.

10. Ibid.

11. P. F. Drucker, "Leadership: More Doing than Task," *Wall Street Journal* (January 6, 1988).

13

Human Resource Management: A Line Manager's Perspective

CHAPTER OBJECTIVES

- Outline the functions of human resources and indicate how these functions relate to the role of the manager.
- Overview the individual manager's responsibilities in the management of human resources.
- Describe a number of actions the manager can take to ensure that he or she will obtain appropriate service from human resources when needed.
- Guide the manager toward the establishment of a working relationship with human resources that will lead to improved human resource service to the department.
- Review pertinent areas of legislation that the manager should know and that generally influence the manager's relationship with human resources.

"PERSONNEL" EQUALS PEOPLE

As a professional managing the work of others you are charged with the task of facilitating the work performance of a number of people. Quite literally you are, in large part, there to make it possible for your employees to get their work done better than they could without your presence. In this role you are expected to ensure that the efforts of your group are applied toward the attainment of the organization's objectives. This must be done in such a way that the group functions more effectively with you than it would without you. And as a first-line manager, there are some days when you can use all the help you can get in fulfilling your basic charge. Help is where you find it in your organization, and one place where the manager can find appropriate help in many instances of need is the human resource (HR) department.

Human resources is today's more all-encompassing title for what most organizations once called "personnel." Whatever the label, however, the true operative word is people. Management is frequently described as getting things done through people. People do the hands-on work and other people supervise them, and still other people oversee those who supervise and manage.

As surely as the most sophisticated piece of medical equipment requires periodic maintenance to ensure its continued functioning, so too do the human beings who supply patient care require regular maintenance. Given that the human machine is generally unpredictable and varies considerably from person to person in numerous dimensions, the manager's maintenance will encompass many activities.

There are many places in the organization where the manager can go for help with various tasks and problems. For people problems, however, and for some straightforward people-related tasks that cannot yet be described as problems, the manager's greatest source of assistance is the human resource department. It remains only for the manager to take steps to access that assistance. It is to the individual manager's distinct advantage to know exactly what should be expected from human resources and how to get it when needed.

A VITAL STAFF FUNCTION

As a service department, human resources should be prepared to offer a variety of employee-related services in a number of ways. Human resources should anticipate numerous kinds of difficulties and needs and should communicate the availability of assistance throughout the organization. For example, a personnel policy manual dispenses advice and guidance in employee matters, and top management's instructions to managers to seek one-on-one guidance from human resources in matters of disciplinary action are essentially "advertising" for human resource services.

Even though human resources should be prepared to help in a variety of ways and should have so advised all levels of management, the human resource department cannot anticipate every specific need of each individual supervisor or manager. To truly put the human resource department to work, the supervisor must be prepared to take his or her needs to the HR department and expect answers or assistance.

The terms *human resources* and *personnel* are still often used interchangeably and are currently used about equally as the designation for this particular service. This organizational function sometimes exists under other names, for example: employee services, employee affairs, and people systems. Fairly common among a few other designations are *employee relations* and *labor relations*. These latter two labels have also found use as descriptors of subfunctions of modern HR, with *employee relations* referring to dealing with employee problems and *labor relations* referring to dealing with unions. Regardless of label, however, the mission of this particular service department should remain the same—to engage in acquiring, maintaining, and retaining employees so that the objectives of the organization may be fulfilled. As a critical staff function, HR does none of the actual work of the health care organization; rather, human resources facilitates the work of the organization by concerning itself with the organization's most important resource.

A SERVICE OF INCREASING VALUE

The HR department has long been a resource of increasing value to the organization at large and the individual manager in particular. Its value has increased because of rational responses to a number of forces, both external and internal to the organization, that have resulted in additional tasks for someone. Two major forces have been the expansion in the number and kinds of tasks that have fallen to HR and the proliferation of laws affecting aspects of employment. A third major force is the trend toward organizational "flattening" evident among present-day health care organizations.

Increase in Employee-Related Tasks

Like the majority of departments in a modern organization, there was a time when HR did not exist, and also like other departments, HR arose to fill a need. The earliest human resource departments were commonly known as employment offices, created as businesses grew large enough to see the advantages of centralizing much of the process of acquiring employees. Employment and employment-related record-keeping initially comprised all the work of the employment office.

When wage and hour laws came into being, the employment office absorbed much of the concern for establishing standard rates of pay and monitoring their application relative to hours worked. These tasks mark the beginnings of the compensation function.

As organizations, in response to new laws and other pressures both internal and external, began to provide compensation in forms other than wages, the employment office took over the administration of what became known as *fringe benefits*. As organizations responded to labor legislation and to labor unions themselves, labor relations functions were added to the growing list of activities that shared a common theme: all had something to do with acquiring, maintaining, or retaining employees.

Other people-related activities were added as needed, and what had once been the employment office became personnel—the body of people employed by the organization. During the last quarter of the 20th century the term *personnel* was increasingly replaced by the term *human resources*, but the essential meaning remains the same. All the while, the HR function grew in value as it took on an increasing number of employee-related functions.

Proliferation of Laws Related to Employment

A number of laws were of course primary in causing much of the increase in employee-related tasks. For example, the establishment of Social Security, Workers' Compensation, and unemployment benefits all created tasks for HR, and much labor relations activity was brought about by laws affecting relationships with unions. In addition, various antidiscrimination laws, including the Civil Rights Act of 1964, the Age Discrimination in Employment Act, and the Equal Pay Act, brought with them much new work for HR.

The antidiscrimination laws have forever changed the way many organizations do business. They have created a strongly legalistic environment in which lawsuits and other formal discrimination complaints have become routine HR business. They have also turned employee recruitment in general, and specific processes such as employee evaluation and disciplinary action, into legal minefields filled with traps and pitfalls for the unwary. In the process these laws have created more work for HR and have created myriad reasons for the individual manager to turn to HR on more occasions.

The Effects of Flattening

The tendency toward organizational flattening and its attendant elimination of entire layers of management has not appreciably added tasks to HR or increased the inherent importance of the HR function in and of itself; however, it has markedly increased the importance of human resources to the individual manager.

Recent years have seen financially troubling times overtake many of the nation's health care provider organizations. As hospital reimbursement is tightened and income grows at a lesser rate than costs, the resultant financial pinch is often felt in staffing, including numbers of management personnel. Usually the first managers to suffer, whether in health care of other kinds of settings, are middle managers.

Financial problems have caused significant reductions in middle management positions, but all such reductions have not occurred solely because of money problems. Increasing reliance on management approaches calling for increased employee participation and decision making also have resulted in the necessity for fewer middle managers.

Regardless of how it occurs, a reduction in the number of middle managers means that more decisions must be made closer to the bottom of the organization. This means that certain decisions that might once have been made by a middle manager—such as, for example, sanctioning an employment offer at above the normal entry rate or deciding how far to proceed in a situation that includes a high degree of legal risk—are forced down to the level of the individual first-line manager. The more employee-related decisions are forced to the first line of management, the more the first-line manager has to depend on the guidance and support of the human resource department. Thus the tendency toward flattening has increased the value of HR to the manager.

LEARNING ABOUT YOUR HUMAN RESOURCE DEPARTMENT

To be able to get the most out of your organization's human resource department, it is first necessary to understand the nature of the HR function, know how HR relates organizationally, and be familiar with the functions performed by your particular HR department.

The Nature of the Function: Staff versus Line

Human resources has already been described in this chapter as a staff function. As opposed to a line activity, a function in which people actually perform the work of the organization (for example, nursing or clinical laboratories), a staff function enhances and supports the performance of the organization's work. The presence of a staff function should make a difference to the extent that the organization's work is more effectively accomplished with the staff function than without it.

The distinction between line and staff is critical to appreciate because a staff function cannot legitimately make decisions that are the province of line management. Operating decisions belong to operating management; they must be made within the chains of command of the line departments. The primary purpose of human resources in enhancing and supporting work performance is to recommend courses of action that are (1) consistent with legislation, regulation, and principles of fairness and (2) in the best interests of the organization as a whole.

It is not unusual for some managers to blame human resources for decisions other than those they would have made by themselves. Complaints such as "This is the HR department's decision" are not uncommon from managers whose preferred decisions are altered because of HR's recommendations. In general, however, human resources does not—and should never—have authority to overrule line management in any matter, personnel or otherwise. If, as occasionally is the case, a personnel decision of line management must be overruled for the good of the organization, the overruling is done by higher line management. Human resources may have to reach out and bring higher management into the process when a manager insists on pursuing a decision that HR has recommended against, but it must remain line management that actually decides.

As to whether line management really listens to its advisers in human resources depends largely on the apparent professionalism of the HR function and HR's track record in making solid recommendations.

The Human Resource Reporting Relationship

The modern HR department will report to one of the two top managers in the organization. Depending on the particular organizational scheme employed, human resources might report to the president or chief executive officer (CEO) or perhaps to the executive vice president or to the chief operating officer (COO). Generally, human resources should report to a level no lower than the level that has authority over all of the organization's line or operating functions.

Human resources must be in a position to serve all of the organization's operating units equally and impartially. This cannot be done if HR reports to one particular operating division that stands as the organizational equal of other divisions. If, for example, HR reports to a vice president for general services who is the organizational equal of three other vice presidents, HR cannot equally serve all divisions because of being ultimately responsible to just one of those divisions.

Be wary if your HR department reports in the undesirable manner just described. Regardless of how well the HR function might be managed, at times of conflict, when inevitable differences arise concerning personnel decisions, you may conclude that the division that "owns" HR is usually the division that wins. Independence and impartiality are essential for human resources to function effectively for the whole organization, and independence and impartiality are impossible in perception and unlikely in actuality if HR is assigned to one of several operating divisions.

Be wary also of the occasionally encountered practice of duplicating HR functions within the same facility. For example, one will encounter the occasional hospital in which the department of nursing has its own HR function while another HR office serves all other departments. Although there are sometimes advantages to be gained from basing some recruiting activity in the nursing department, splitting or subdividing other HR activities tends to create duplication of effort while increasing the organization's exposure to legal risks.

The Human Resource Functions

There are almost as many possible combinations of human resource functions as there are HR departments. A great many activities that may generally be described as administrative can find their way into the human resource department. For the purposes of this book, however, the discussion will center on the significant activities or groups of functions that are often identified as the tasks of human resources. These basic human resource functions are as follows:

- Employment, often referred to as recruiting. This is the overall process of acquiring employees—advertising and otherwise soliciting applicants, screening applicants, referring candidates to managers, checking references, extending offers of employment, and bringing employees into the organization.
- Compensation, or wage and salary administration. This is the process of creating and maintaining a wage structure and ensuring that this structure is administered fairly and consistently. Related to compensation, as well as to

other HR task groupings, are job evaluation, the creation of job descriptions, and maintenance of a system of employee performance evaluation.

- Benefits administration. This activity is a natural offshoot of wage and salary administration, since benefits are actually a part of an employee's total compensation. Benefits administration consists of maintaining the organization's benefit structure and assisting employees in understanding and accessing their benefits.

- Employee relations. Generally, this activity may be described as dealing with employees and their problems, needs, and concerns. It may range from handling employee complaints or appeals through processing disciplinary actions to arranging employee recognition and recreation activities.

These four general activities are at work in essentially every human resource function regardless of size and overall scope. In a very large organization these will be separate activities or groups within HR, each with its own head and its own staff and perhaps including multiple subdivisions. In a very small organization these are likely to be the tasks of a single person who has other duties as well.

One additional basic function that might be encountered is labor relations. Although labor relations may be a functional title that identifies a whole department or simply a human resource department activity, it is also a relatively generic label that applies to the maintenance of a continuing relationship with a bargaining unit—that is, a labor union. Again, depending on size, labor relations may be a subdivision of HR in its own right or simply one of several responsibilities assigned to one person.

Other activities that might be found within human resources include the following:

- Employee health. Often part of HR, in health care organizations it sometimes will be a part of one of the medical divisions.

- Training for both managers and rank-and-file employees. With the exception of nursing inservice education, traditionally a part of the nursing department, if a formal training function exists it is most often part of human resources.

- Payroll. In the past it was often a part of personnel, in recent years payroll has usually resided in the finance division; however, a working interrelationship of personnel and payroll has always been essential, and recent years, bringing integrated personnel/payroll systems, have seen the beginnings of payroll's organizational shift back toward HR.

- Security and parking. With increasing frequency these services, because of their strong employee relationships, are becoming attached to HR. At present, however, they are more likely to be found attached to an environmental or facilities division.
- Safety. As with security, safety is becoming increasingly attached to HR but is just as likely to be found in the facilities division.
- Child care. As an activity characterized largely as an employee service, an organization's child care function is most likely assigned to human resources.

Rounding Out Your Knowledge

Using the foregoing paragraphs as a guide, determine exactly which functions are performed by your organization's human resource department. Further, take steps to attach a person's name to each function. Strive to be in a position to understand how the HR department is organized—that is, who does what, who reports to whom, and who bears overall responsibility. Moreover, it is important to know the organizational relationships of the sometimes-HR functions (for example, security) that belong elsewhere in your particular organization, in order to ensure that matters are taken to the correct department.

Next, take the time to make a list of the management activities or activities that can lead you to seek information or assistance from human resources. The lists of most managers may have a great deal in common.

- Employment—finding sufficient qualified candidates from whom to fill an open position
- Benefits—providing information with which to answer employees' benefits questions
- Compensation—providing information with which to answer employees' questions related to pay
- Employee problems—determining where to send a particular employee who is having difficulty with a given problem
- Job descriptions/job evaluations—determining how to proceed in questioning the salary grade of any particular position
- Policy interpretations—determining the appropriate interpretation of personnel policy for any particular instance
- Disciplinary actions—determining how to proceed in dealing with what appear to be violations of work rules

- Performance problems—determining how to proceed in dealing with employees whose work performance is consistently below the department standard
- Performance appraisals—securing guidance in doing appropriate performance appraisals, and finding out how much to depend on human resources to coordinate the overall appraisal process

The foregoing list can be expanded by each manager who may refer to it. One helpful method of expanding the list includes leafing through your organization's personnel policy manual and employee handbook: this will bring to mind additional areas of concern.

PUTTING THE HUMAN RESOURCE DEPARTMENT TO WORK

A Universal Approach

The first, simplest, and most valuable advice to be offered for getting the most out of the human resource department involves the age-old two-step process of initiation and follow-up. It is but a slight variation on a practice followed by most successful managers. The successful manager knows that any task worth assigning is worth a specific deadline. Planning on doing things when you "have a little time to spare" or whenever you happen to think of something that needs doing breeds procrastination, delay, and inaction. An assignment—necessarily a well-thought-out, specific assignment—must be accompanied by a target for completion, a deadline that although perhaps generous or even loose leaves no doubt as to expected completion. When that deadline arrives and no results have been forthcoming, the manager then exercises the most important part of the total process—faithful follow-up. Faithful follow-up is the key; the manager who always waits a week beyond the deadline is behaviorally telling the employees that they always have at least an extra week.

Anything needed from the human resource department should be addressed in a similar manner. Relative to the HR department, the process might be summarized as follows:

- Make certain the function of interest is part of HR's responsibilities, and determine, if possible, who in HR would be the best person to approach on the topic.

- Refine your question or need so that it is sufficiently specific to permit a specific response.
- If an answer is not immediately available, ask when one will be supplied.
- If the promised reply date occurs later than your legitimate need date, negotiate a deadline agreeable to both you and HR.
- If your agreed-upon deadline arrives and you have not received your answer, follow up with the HR department. Follow up politely, follow up diplomatically, but follow up faithfully. Never let an unanswered deadline pass without following up.

  This process should be applied not only to problems, issues, and concerns that you as a manager would consider taking to human resources. It should also—and especially—apply to questions and concerns that employees bring to you. If an employee's question in any way involves human resources concerns and you are unable to respond appropriately, then take the question to HR as though it were your own.

Taking the Initiative

The human resources department exists to assist individual managers and their employees—to assist, in fact, all employees from the chief executive officer to the newest entry-level hire. Human resources can be of considerable help to the department manager, but only if the manager is willing to reach out and request assistance when needed.

Expect the human resource department to house the organization's resident experts on all organization-wide personnel practices. Respect HR's knowledge of personnel policy and procedure and never hesitate to ask HR for clarification of any policy or practice that relates to employment and employee relations in any way. In those occasional instances when HR cannot immediately and completely respond to an inquiry—say, for example, the issue is one that requires input from legal counsel as well as HR—you should nevertheless expect HR to secure the answer.

When a personnel question has legal implications, as the majority of such questions do, there is all the more reason to take it to HR to minimize management's exposure to the potential results of a faulty decision. It is far better to ask than to inadvertently put the organization at risk.

Often human resources has exactly the information the department manager needs, and HR is more than willing to share this information. Take the initiative to reach out and ask human resources. And expect answers.

SOME SPECIFIC ACTION STEPS

Any number of management needs present opportunities to put the human resource department to work. The more frequently encountered of these are described here.

Finding New Employees

There are any number of points in the employment process at which the manager and HR must work together. Fulfill your end of the working relationship, and expect HR to fulfill theirs. For example, if none of the candidates HR has supplied for a particular position is truly appropriate, ask for more; do not settle for only what is given if it is genuinely not enough. For your part of the arrangement, do not continue to call for more applicants in a search for the "perfect" candidate if you have already seen two or three who meet the posted requirements of the job. Also, stay in touch with HR concerning the extending of offers, the checking of references, and the scheduling of preemployment physical examinations and starting dates. Do not be unreasonable: recognize that these activities take time. By making your interest and attention known, however, you will encourage completion of the process.

Bringing Job Descriptions Up to Date

The manager ordinarily has a significant responsibility in maintaining current job descriptions for the department. The HR department usually has the responsibility for associating a pay level with each job and for maintaining central files of up-to-date job descriptions. Job descriptions should be written in large part by those who do the work and those who supervise the doing of the work; however, it is important to involve HR deliberately in contributing consistency to every necessary job description and ensuring that each job is properly placed on a pay scale. Once again, your visible interest in the process will encourage timely completion of HR's activities.

Disciplining Employees

Regardless of the extent of human resource involvement in the disciplinary process, it is not the HR department that decides on disciplinary action. The HR department disciplines nobody except employees of the HR department, as necessary. Any employee deserving of disciplinary action must be disciplined through his or her immediate chain of command. In most organizations it is a requirement for the manager to take proposed disciplinary actions—at least those entailing actions more severe than oral warnings—through human resources before implementation. Whether or not this is true for your organization, you are advised to always take your best assessment to HR and ask for advice. Expect sound advice, whether in the form of a single recommendation, complete with rationale for doing so, or as two or more alternatives, each with its own possible consequences fully explained. The decision is theoretically all yours, and if it is a poor decision you will bear much of the blame. Never let HR avoid responsibility by failing to provide specific direction; insist on complete HR participation in deciding upon disciplinary action.

Evaluating Employees

One of the most important tasks of the supervisor is the appraisal of employee performance. No formal system of performance appraisal can function consistently throughout the organization without the central guidance usually provided by human resources. Although it is certainly possible to evaluate employees' performance without the assistance of HR, you can do a much more consistently acceptable job of evaluation with HR involvement. Most of human resources' involvement in evaluation should occur automatically as far as the manager is concerned. The HR department should provide forms, instructions, schedules, and reminders throughout the process. If, however, the HR department is not always on top of the manager's employee appraisal needs, according to the needs of the moment the manager should

- keep track of scheduled review dates and ask HR for forms and timetables if not supplied automatically
- ask for periodic instruction in how to apply rating criteria, especially if criteria have changed and refresher instruction is not supplied
- keep HR advised of how changing job requirements may be affecting the application of criteria based on previous requirements
- periodically ask HR for rating profile information that reveals patterns in the manager's rating practices and shows whether those patterns are changing with time, and perhaps also shows how this specific manager's rating patterns compare with those of other managers

Dealing with Training Needs

If the human resource department has responsibility for any employee training—and in most health care organizations there is a better-than-even chance that this is so—do not wait for needed training. If there are training needs in your work group, take them to HR. If, for example, several employees require training in basic telephone techniques, take your well-defined needs to human resources, negotiate a timetable for providing the training, and offer to become personally involved in the training. (With appropriate HR involvement, every manager is a potentially valuable instructor in some topic.)

The foregoing are presented as a few specific suggestions but are offered primarily to convey a general idea to the manager. This idea is that the human resource department exists as a service function for all employees and that it remains for the supervisor to take each legitimate personnel-related need to HR and to ask for—and expect—an honest response.

FURTHER USE OF HUMAN RESOURCES

In addition to the above-mentioned activities, there are occasionally other times when the manager is well advised to turn to HR. These include:

- examining staff turnover patterns and attempting to determine what might be done to increase the chances of retaining key employees
- planning for potential future staffing needs
- periodically examining staff pay rates relative to the community, the region, and the occupations employed
- using human resources as a sounding board, a "safe harbor" for venting frustrations without involving employees, peers, or superiors
- looking for confidential guidance in addressing difficult situations experienced with others
- drawing upon HR experience and resources in celebrating individual employees as appropriate (for example, employee of the month) and in periodically recognizing various occupations (for example, National Nurses Week, Physical Therapy Week)

WANTED: WELL-CONSIDERED INPUT

The most effective human resource departments are not one-way dispensers of information and assistance. Effective HR departments are responsive to the needs of the organization's work force; however, the HR department can go only so far in anticipating needs and meeting them within the limits of available resources. To be fully effective, the HR department must learn of employees' needs from employees and managers and must in turn go to top management with solid proposals for meeting the most pressing needs.

Some employees, usually a minority, take their own questions, concerns, and suggestions to the human resource department. But most employees will never do so for themselves; their needs, whether conveyed through words, actions, or attitudes, must find their way to human resources and eventually to top management through their managers.

Among the kinds of information that the manager should pass along to human resources are:

- reactions to various personnel policies, especially when policies seem to have become less appropriate under changing conditions
- employee attitudes concerning pay and benefits, especially perceptions of inequities and alleged instances of unfair treatment
- complaints—and compliments as well—about employee services such as cafeteria and parking
- comments on the appropriateness of various employee benefits, and perceptions of benefits needed or desired as opposed to those currently given
- potential changes in any or all means of acquiring, maintaining, or retaining employees that might afford the organization a competitive edge in its community

UNDERSTANDING *WHY* AS WELL AS *WHAT*

It is relatively easy to determine what human resources as a department does within the organization; however, it is necessary to go beyond *what* and develop an appreciation of *why* this department does what it does and why HR sometimes must espouse a position in opposition to a line department's position. Consider the case of a manager who appeals to the HR department to help her resolve a seemingly unending series of difficulties by agreeing to the termination of a particular employee. As the manager says, "I simply can't do any more with this person. She's chronically late in spite of all my warnings. Her absenteeism disrupts staffing; she uses up her sick time as fast as she earns it. Her attitude is absolutely terrible; she's been rude to patients and families, and the way she talks to me borders on insubordination most of the time. Her clinical skills are just average at best, and she's a disruptive influence within the group. I've been patient longer than anyone has the right to expect me to be, but nothing has changed. I want to discharge her."

As often occurs in such circumstances, the human resource practitioner hearing the manager's request briefly reviews the employee's background and immediately recommends against termination. This may understandably disappoint and upset the manager and leave her displeased with the HR department. She may complain, with some justification, that she ought to be supported in her efforts to get rid of an unsatisfactory employee. She may well view HR as obstructive and adopt an adversarial position, perhaps even attempting to solicit the assistance of her own higher management in opposing the human resource position.

Why would human resources be automatically protective of any employee whose relationship with work is as bad as described above? The differences lie in, first, the manager's perspective versus the human resource perspective, and second, the frequently cited employee personnel file—"the record."

The manager is legitimately focused on the good of the patients and the good of the unit, and the employee in question threatens both. By contrast, human resources must view the issues in two ways that conflict with the manager's perspective: in micro terms, HR must be concerned with the rights of the individual; in macro terms, HR must be concerned with the good of the total organization. The organization is of course no more than the sum total of a number of individuals, but in focusing on the one and the all, the HR perspective fails to match that of the manager, which is necessarily a focus on more than one but much less than all.

Then there is "the record" to consider. In the foregoing case it turns out that all of the manager's "warnings" concerning tardiness were informal oral warnings of which no record was made; likewise for warnings for absenteeism, except for a single written warning that was far too old to give weight to current disciplinary action. No other warnings appeared in the personnel file, and although in the mind of the manager this employee had always been less than satisfactory, the personnel file included several performance evaluations that, although not glowing with praise, suggested at least minimally acceptable performance. In short, there was no basis for termination existing except perhaps in the manager's mind. Concerning problems such as that just described, the HR department is

- defending the rights of the individual, not only because doing so arises from a sense of fairness but also because there are many laws requiring the organization to do so
- protecting the total organization from a multitude of legal risks

Whenever there is a risk that an employee problem or complaint will be taken outside of the organization, it is best to think of any criticism of employee conduct or performance in a single light: if it is not reflected in the record, it never happened. Except in instances of termination for major infractions calling for immediate discharge (and these days even many of these actions are successfully challenged), a discharge must be backed up with a paper trail describing all that occurred leading up to the termination. It is legally necessary to be able to demonstrate that the employee was given every reasonable opportunity to correct the offending behavior or improve the unsatisfactory performance.

LEGAL GUIDES FOR MANAGERIAL BEHAVIOR

A number of areas of legislation—federal, state, and in some instances local—define how work organizations must deal with employees in certain respects. Any work organization is of course subject to many laws that bear on essentially all aspects of the conduct of business. A great many laws applicable to business are essentially invisible to the individual manager; for example, nothing done in the normal course of business by the manager of rehabilitative services has any bearing on corporate compliance with certain financial reporting laws. However, some laws directly shape the relationship between employer and employee. It is this collection of laws affecting employment that concerns the manager, and it is this general area of employment legislation for which human resources is the source of most of the individual manager's guidance.

Labor Relations

The National Labor Relations Act (NLRA) of 1935, known originally as the Wagner Act, provided the basis for most labor law in the United States. It was significantly amended in 1947 by the Labor Management Relations Act, otherwise known as Taft-Hartley. It is Taft-Hartley that is the primary reference applicable when discussing aspects of union organizing. There are numerous references to the NLRA that are actually references to the NLRA as amended by Taft-Hartley, which provides the framework for all modern labor law.

Before 1975, not-for-profit hospitals were exempt from all provisions of Taft-Hartley; however, in 1975 the act was amended to remove the not-for-profit hospital exemption. Before 1975, hospital employees were covered only in special sections of the labor-relations laws of some states. The 1975 amendments provided hospitals, because of the nature of their business, with certain legal protections not available to other industries. For example, there is a requirement that 10 days' notice be provided prior to any picketing, strike, or other concerted refusal to work, a requirement not applicable in other industries. Overall, however, the effect of the removal of the exemption essentially made not-for-profit hospitals and certain other health care institutions equally subject to union organizing as organizations in other industries.

The individual manager needs to know the general impact of labor law as it applies to day-to-day operations within the department. If the organization's employees are not unionized and if there is no active threat of union organizing, labor law will be of little immediate concern and commonsense management will prevail. If there is a union in place, much of the manager's behavior concerning employees will be governed by a collective bargaining agreement (contract). If there is no union but there is active organizing, the manager's conduct in regard to employees will be governed by provisions of the NLRA. In either case, the manager's primary source of guidance will be the human resource department.

Wages and Hours

Of primary interest is the Fair Labor Standards Act (FLSA), the federal wage and hour law and as such the model for the wage and hour laws of many states. Occasional points that might not be addressed in federal law may be covered by pertinent state laws. Generally, if the same points are covered by both state and federal laws but differences exist between the two, the more stringent legislation will apply.

In general the wage and hour laws spell out who is to be paid for what and how. They specify who can be exempt and who must be considered nonexempt—with exempt literally meaning exempt from the overtime provisions of the law. Exempt employees—certain executive, administrative, and professional employees who meet special legal requirements—do not have to be paid overtime pay. Nonexempt employees as defined under the law must receive time-and-one-half the regular rate of pay for hours in excess of 40 in a week.

In 2004 a number of changes were made in the rules used for determining who is or is not eligible for overtime pay. Some significant issues surrounding these rules remain controversial and, in a practical sense, are not yet completely resolved. Many agree that the FLSA is antiquated and confusing, particularly the portions addressing overtime pay. The new rules mandate overtime pay for more low-income workers but at the same time appear to render certain white-collar workers and professionals ineligible for overtime pay. For example, those benefiting include the likes of restaurant and store managers, and those losing overtime eligibility include emergency medical technicians, licensed practical nurses, dental hygienists, and many registered nurses.

The entire overtime question can sometimes be confusing to the individual manager, but the status of overtime regulations at any given time is usually known in the human resource department.

Human resources and the organization's payroll department are usually the manager's two primary sources of advice and assistance concerning the wage and hour laws. At the very least the individual manager should be aware of the status (exempt or nonexempt) of each person in the work group and how time reporting and wage payment are handled for each. The wage and hour laws are actually extremely detailed and extensive, and fortunately only a relative handful of regulations will apply to any individual manager's situation.

Equal Pay

A specific section of the Fair Labor Standards Act, as augmented by the Equal Pay Act of 1963, requires covered employers to provide equal pay for men and women performing the same work. In 1972, coverage of this act was extended beyond employees covered by FLSA to an estimated 15 million additional executive, administrative, and professional employees, including academic and administrative personnel and teachers in elementary and secondary schools, and to outside salespeople.

Civil Rights

Title VII of the Civil Rights Act of 1964, as amended by the Equal Employment Opportunity Act of 1972, prohibits discrimination because of race, color, religion, sex, or national origin in any term, condition, or privilege of employment. As enforced through the Equal Employment Opportunity Commission (EEOC), Title VII covers:

- all private employers of 15 or more persons
- all educational institutions, public as well as private
- state and local governments
- public and private employment agencies
- labor unions with 15 or more members
- joint labor-management committees for apprenticeship and training

The EEOC investigates job discrimination complaints, and when it finds reasonable cause that charges are justified, attempts, through conciliation, to eliminate all aspects of discrimination revealed by the investigation. If conciliation fails, the

EEOC has the power to take the employer to court to enforce the law. Discrimination charges may be filed by individuals, job applicants as well as active employees, and also by organizations on behalf of aggrieved individuals.

Title VII was modified and strengthened by the Civil Rights Act of 1991 in an effort to reverse the effects of several Supreme Court decisions that had the effect of weakening the law. The 1991 act also made possible increased financial damages against organizations found guilty of discriminatory practices. It is civil rights legislation that causes the most potential difficulty for working managers. Therefore, it is in this area of concern that the human resource department, usually backed up by the organization's legal counsel, is most prepared to advise and support department management.

Americans with Disabilities

Passed in 1990 and largely made effective in 1992, the Americans with Disabilities Act (ADA) affirmed the right of persons with disabilities to equal access to employment, services, and facilities available to the public, including transportation and telecommunications. The ADA requires employers to provide "reasonable accommodation" for disabled individuals who are capable of performing the essential functions of the positions for which they apply. This may include altering physical facilities to make them usable by individuals with disabilities, restructuring jobs about their essential functions, and altering or eliminating nonessential activities so that disabled persons can perform the work. The EEOC is responsible for dealing with complaints filed under the Americans with Disabilities Act.

Family and Medical Leave Act

The Family and Medical Leave Act (FMLA) of 1993 makes it possible for an eligible employee (one who has been employed at least one year and has worked at least 1,250 hours) to take up to 12 weeks of unpaid leave in a 12-month period for certain specified reasons without loss of employment. Qualifying reasons are: for the birth of the employee's child or the care of that child up to 12 months of age; for placement of a child with the employee for adoption or foster care; for the employee to care for spouse, child, or parent having a serious health condition; and for the employee's own serious health condition involving the employee's inability to perform the essential functions of the job. An employee returning to work within the 12-week limit must be returned to his or her original position or to a fully equivalent position in terms of pay and benefits and overall working conditions.

The FMLA can be relatively complex in its interrelationships with other laws, conflicting in instances with the Americans with Disabilities Act, the Fair Labor Standards Act, and various states' workers' compensation laws. Once again, however, human resources, backed up with corporate legal counsel, stands ready to advise the manager.

Sexual Harassment

Sexual harassment has been prominent in society for a number of years, and it continues to be an active concern in work organizations and elsewhere. The number of sexual harassment complaints filed with the EEOC and various state agencies continues to increase, as do the numbers of employers involved and the monetary penalties. In recent years sexual harassment has been one of the two leading causes of legal complaints against employers (the other is age discrimination).

Sexual harassment is in fact a form of sex discrimination under Title VII of the Civil Rights Act of 1964. It consists of unwelcome sexual advances, requests for sexual favors, or other conduct of a sexual nature if submission is either an actual or implied condition of employment, if submission or rejection is used as a basis for making employment-related decisions, or if the conduct interferes with work performance or creates an offensive work environment. A key concern in the foregoing resides in the word *unwelcome*; conduct is considered unwelcome if the employee neither solicits nor invites it and regards it as undesirable or offensive. Whether a particular occurrence is or is not sexual harassment may depend largely on the perception of the victim.

Sexual harassment can take a number of forms. Sexually explicit pictures or calendars, offensive sexually related language, sexual humor, other sexual conduct that creates a hostile environment, sexually explicit behavior, indecent exposure, sexual propositions or intimidation, offensive touching, and participation in or observation of sexual activity are all examples of sexual harassment. Also considered sexual harassment is something as seemingly innocent (to some) as repeatedly asking a coworker or subordinate for a date after having been turned down. This adds the dimension of repetition to some harassing behavior; asking a time or two might be considered reasonable, but asking repeatedly after having been turned down may be considered harassing.

Sexual harassment is not limited strictly to the workplace; it is also sexual harassment if it occurs off-premises at employer-sponsored social events and at private sites if it involves people who have an employment relationship with each other. In addition to involving employees, sexual harassment can involve visitors, vendors, patients, and others as either potential perpetrators or victims.

To limit liability for sexual harassment it is necessary for the employer to promptly and confidentially investigate all complaints, take appropriate corrective action, and create and retain complete and accurate records.

A sound prevention program is vital where sexual harassment is concerned. At a minimum such a program should include a published sexual harassment policy and a detailed procedure for investigating complaints. All employees, and especially all managers, should be educated in the recognition and prevention of sexual harassment.

Violence in the Workplace

Violence in the workplace often results from stress. It frequently occurs when a person becomes stressed to what for that individual is an unbearable level. When stress becomes unbearable some people become ill, some break down, some walk away from the sources of stress, and some become violent. Violence is similar to other forms of human behavior in that it is action in response to a condition, need, or demand.

Every change that alters employees' expectations becomes fertile ground for chronic anger, which can lead to reduced productivity and quality, increased fatigue, burnout, depression, and violence. One of every six violent crimes occurs in the workplace. Motor vehicle accidents are the leading cause of death for working men, but murder is the leading cause of death for working women.

The highest risk areas for nonfatal assaults are the retail trades, such as grocery stores and eating and drinking establishments, and the service organizations, such as hospitals, nursing homes, and social service agencies. During the late 1990s almost two-thirds of nonfatal assaults occurred in hospitals, nursing homes, and residential care facilities, and most cases involved patients assaulting nurses.[1]

The department manager's best approach to workplace violence is awareness and prevention. There is no consistent profile to describe a person who commits violent acts in the workplace, but violence may be perpetrated by someone who

- is experiencing family problems
- has problems related to the abuse of alcohol or drugs
- has a history of violence
- is a known aggressive personality
- is experiencing certain mental conditions (for example, depression)
- possesses a poor self-image or low self-esteem

People commit violent acts for a variety of reasons, which have been known at times to include:

- the inability to cope with what to the person is extreme stress
- drug reactions
- problems involving job, money, or family
- reaction to the loss of employment
- reaction to the loss of a relationship
- frustration with long waits or rude or indifferent treatment
- confusion or fear
- perceived violation of privacy

We can never tell for certain who may resort to violence. However, there are steps to consider for preventing violence.

- treat everyone with respect and consideration
- keep all potential weapons stored beyond the reach of patients and visitors
- take threats seriously and report them immediately
- know your security procedures, alarms, and warning codes

Be extra alert to the possibility of violence if a person

- appears to be under the influence of alcohol or drugs
- appears to have been in a fight
- is brought into the facility by the police
- is already being restrained

Visible indicators of potential violence include:

- obvious possession of a weapon
- nervousness or abrupt movements
- extreme restlessness, such as pacing and obvious agitation

When observing an individual who appears to be on the edge of losing control

- notify other staff and call security
- stay alert but remain calm
- maintain a safe distance, giving the person plenty of space; do not turn your back and do not touch the person
- keep obstacles between you and the individual
- be certain you have a way out; avoid dead-end corridors or corners
- listen; do not display anger or defensiveness and do not argue; speak slowly and quietly

Some departments, such as the emergency room, are more prone to violence than others, but violence is possible anywhere. Every department's staff should have some orientation in how to deal with violent behavior. If violence does occur:

- protect yourself to the extent necessary
- sound the alarm or call the appropriate code
- help remove others from the vicinity, if necessary
- do not try to disarm or restrain the person yourself
- give the individual what he or she is demanding, if possible

AN INCREASINGLY LEGALISTIC ENVIRONMENT

Although the issues just described are those of greatest concern to the manager (especially civil rights, wage and hour, and possibly labor relations), there are many other federal, state, and local laws that can impact the employment relationship. It may seem at times as though this is excessive legislation and that all of these rules and regulations may not be truly necessary. Remember, however, that managers are employees as well and that the protections afforded employees under legislation such as equal pay and civil rights also extend to managers.

All working managers should be willing to recognize that the laws affecting employment represent a well-defined part of management's boundaries, those outside limits within which it is necessary to learn to work in the fulfillment of management's responsibilities.

As a staff function, human resources is organized as a service activity. Service activities render no patient care; they do not advance the primary work of the organization. Rather, they support the performance of the organization's work and in a practical sense become necessary. For example, if a pure service such as building maintenance did not exist, the facility's physical plant would gradually self-destruct. Similarly, without human resources to see to the maintenance of the work force, the overall suitability and capability of that work force would steadily erode. Recognize human resources for what it is: an essential service function required to help the organization run as efficiently as possible.

EMPHASIS ON SERVICE

Learn what the HR department does, and especially learn why the department does what it does. Provide input and forge a continuing working relationship with the HR department, making it clear that you expect service from this essential service department. Challenge HR to do more, to do better, and to continually improve service—and put the human resource department to work for you and your employees.

CASE: WITH FRIENDS LIKE THIS . . .

Background

One morning, well before the start of your department's normal working hours, you were enjoying a cup of coffee in the cafeteria, shaping up your calendar of tasks and appointments for the day, when you were approached by one of your employees. The employee, Millie Norman, one of your two or three most senior professionals in terms of service, seated herself across from you and said, "There's something going on in the department that you need to know about, and I've waited far too long to tell you." You reacted internally with both impatience and annoyance—you were not prepared to interrupt what you were doing, and you had not even invited Millie to join you.

Millie proceeded to tell you ("In strictness confidence, please, I know you'll understand why") that another long-term professional employee, Cathy Johnson, had been making a great many derogatory comments about you throughout the department and generally questioning your competence.

For 10 minutes Millie showered you with criticism of you, your management style, and your approach to individual employees, all attributed to Cathy Johnson. On exhausting her litany, Millie proclaimed that she did not ordinarily "carry tales" but that she felt you "had a right to know, for the good of the department—but please don't tell her I said anything."

Although Millie's comments were filled with "she saids" and "she dids," she being Cathy, and generally twice-told tales without connection to specific incidents, something extremely disturbing clicked in your mind while you were listening. Recently your posted departmental schedule had been altered, without your knowledge, in a way indicating that someone had tried to copy your handwriting and forge your initials. Two separate, seemingly unconnected comments by Millie together revealed that only one of two people could have altered your schedule. Those two people were Cathy Johnson and Millie Norman herself.

As Millie finally fell silent you were left with an intense feeling of disappointment. You wondered if you could ever again fully trust two of your key employees.

Instructions

Write at least a fully developed paragraph in response to each of the following questions:

1. What should be your immediate response to Millie Norman? Why?
2. Do you believe you have the basis on which to proceed with disciplinary action against someone? Why or why not?
3. How can the human resource department help you in your present concern?

CASE: THE MANAGERIAL "HOT SEAT"

Background

Carol Greely had been a registered nurse for 25 years and a nurse manager for more than 10 years when she was asked to take over as nurse manager of a particular medical/surgical unit known throughout the hospital, none too affectionately, as the "hot seat." Although she had heard a few things about this floor, because of the size of the hospital and her recent assignment in a relatively removed area, Carol had little information about why the hot seat was so designated. After three months on the job, however, Carol had formed some strong opinions regarding the bases of many of the unit's problems. To her, the majority of staff on the unit exhibited a complete lack of professionalism. Carol became convinced of this for a number of reasons, including the following:

- There were many appearance problems and many violations of the department's none-too-often-enforced dress code. If there were a worst-dressed list maintained, Carol concluded, surely her nurses would be on it.
- The unit's rate of absenteeism was the worst of any unit within the nursing department.
- Two (thankfully unsuccessful) attempts by unions to organize the hospital's nurses had apparently originated with the nurses in Carol's unit.
- Carol had never before seen a unit with such a high level of schedule juggling—shift trades, requests for specific days off, and especially changes to the schedule at the last minute.

It was not long before Carol found herself becoming highly cynical about the unit and its future. It seemed to her that nursing meant no more to many of these people than the paycheck and that they constantly put their social lives and personal preferences before the needs of the patients.

When she had been on the job six months, Carol received a startling piece of secondhand information from a friend in the nursing department who swore her to secrecy as to the source. It was apparently a closely guarded secret in nursing administration that her particular unit was deliberately maintained as a concentration of marginal employees. It was, in the words of Carol's friend, "to keep the butterflies and malcontents all in one place as much as possible, so they wouldn't disrupt other units." Carol was further led to believe that she could expect to be reassigned after about 18 months on the job, when it would then be someone else's turn to sit in the hot seat.

Carol's initial reaction to what she had learned was anger; however, the more she thought about the position in which she found herself, the more she became determined to do something with the time left to her in the unit. She decided she was going to do everything in her power to turn the hot seat into a real nursing unit.

Instructions

Develop a fairly detailed plan of action for Carol Greely to follow in attempting to accomplish her admittedly difficult objective or to go as far toward accomplishing it as possible. Highlight those steps in her plan for which the human resource department can probably provide positive advice or assistance, and describe the likely nature of the human resource involvement.

NOTE

1. Preventing Violence in the Workplace, "Group Insurance Agency, Inc., Healthcare Association of New York State," Albany, N.Y., May 9, 1997.

14

Communication: The Glue that Binds Us Together

CHAPTER OBJECTIVES

- Provide a working definition of communication.
- Address the critical manager's role in employee communication.
- Review the common means of communication used in the work setting.
- Provide guidelines for the proper use of electronic mail (e-mail).
- Examine the components of individual and small-group communication, including verbal (oral) and nonverbal communication.
- Enumerate the essential components of successful interpersonal communication.
- Review a number of means of fostering, enhancing, and improving interpersonal communication and overcoming barriers to individual communication.
- Provide guidelines for personal improvement in using written communication in its various forms.
- Present the fundamentals of organization communication, including both formal and informal communication.
- Differentiate between formal and informal communication in the organizational setting.
- Review the commonly encountered barriers to effective communication in the organizational setting.

A COMPLEX PROCESS

It is necessary to begin this chapter with an important disclaimer: what follows is no more than a once-over-easy treatment, an effort to hit the high spots of a topic of extreme importance to every manager, professional or otherwise. Each heading and subheading in this chapter could be the subject of an entire book in its own right and yet leave much unaddressed. We have endeavored here to provide an introduction to the basics of communication within the health care organization as experienced from the perspective of the individual manager.

In a relatively large health care organization—for example the average hospital—decisions are frequently presented as orders or instructions, and members whose activities are affected are expected to comply. Organizational roles may be specialized, and much communication occurs through relatively formal channels such as memos, policies, procedures, or regulations.

In a relatively small organization like a group medical practice of fewer than 20 employees, the communications environment may be considerably different. In the small organization, work roles overlap and are likely to be far less specialized. In this setting communication is less formal and the opportunity for the direct sharing of information is greater than in a large organization. Formal communication in the small organization may be minimal. The single factor of size can influence the quality and kinds of communication employed within an organization.

There are, however, many factors other than organization size to consider. Communication is a complex process requiring particular skills on both individual and group levels. Also, as an individual interacts with more and more people the overall complexity of the interactions increases. Whether considered in an individual or organizational context, communication is a far more complex process than many at first imagine. Therefore, to be optimally successful, communication requires considerably more conscious effort than most people give to it.

Communication may be described as the exchange of ideas, thoughts, or emotions between or among two or more people. It may be literally described as the transfer of meaning or, in a somewhat broader sense, the development of mutual understanding. Concerning the transfer of meaning, the intent is to take information that exists in a specific form in one person's mind and ensure that it is duplicated in another's mind. In the broader sense, the development of mutual understanding, the intent is for two or more people to share whatever information they have about a specific subject and arrive at an agreed-upon meaning, whether that meaning is an opinion, a decision, or a course of action.

From the perspective of the individual manager, communication in the organizational setting ranges from the highly informal to the strictly formal, from on-the-run spoken remarks to structured presentations, from quick e-mail or voice mail messages to formal reports, and from one-on-one contacts to the necessity to address large groups. In other words, as experienced by the individual manager, communication in the organizational setting can occur in nearly any form or format.

COMMUNICATION AND THE INDIVIDUAL MANAGER

Many of the problems encountered in communicating with others arise because the majority of human beings take their communications capacity for granted. After all, communication is basic to all human activity; except when asleep, most people are usually in one of four fundamental communicating modes: talking or writing (that is, sending information out) or reading or hearing (that is, receiving information). Note that the fourth mode was identified as *hearing* rather than *listening*, suggesting the source of a great many problems and misunderstandings: one can hear without truly listening. In any case, one who is awake is in one of the four fundamental communicating modes, with hearing being the "default" mode.

Whether in the workplace or any place, people cannot function adequately without communicating. For the individual manager, communication in any of several forms is essentially constant. Consider communication in the context of the essential management functions of planning, decision making, organizing, staffing, directing, coordinating, and controlling. Once formulated, plans mean nothing unless they are communicated; once made, decisions never see implementation unless they are communicated in some form; likewise, to be complete, organizing, staffing, coordinating, and controlling all require communication. And the basic function of directing is itself largely communication. Truly, communication holds everything together.

In day-to-day activity the manager must be involved in communication in one form or another for reasons that include:

- receiving orders, instructions, and direction from above
- delivering orders, instructions, and direction to employees
- coaching, counseling, and disciplining employees as necessary
- interviewing and selecting candidates for employment
- relating to managers and employees of other departments

- relating to patients, visitors, clients, customers, vendors, and others from outside as necessary
- reporting to higher management on departmental activities
- responding to questions and requests coming from any of a number of sources

Depending on the situation, the manager's communication under the foregoing various circumstances might be spoken or written, or formal or informal. And it might make use of any of several common communications practices or media, described as follows (along with the significant advantages and disadvantages of each):

Face-to-Face

This is potentially the strongest means of communication available to the manager, "potentially" because far too many face-to-face contacts are neither efficient nor effective. Properly utilized, the face-to-face contact has some important characteristics going for it. A message is transmitted not only in words but with vocal tone and facial expression and other body language. Because it occurs in the here and now, the opportunity for feedback is immediate; questions and answers can flow back and forth until understanding is achieved. Properly used, the face-to-face contact is the most effective means of fulfilling most of the communication needs that arise during the workday; it appeals to multiple senses, offers immediacy of feedback and response, and ensures the maximum likelihood of establishing mutual understanding.

The disadvantages of this method are few. Face-to-face contact is frequently more time-consuming than other means because it involves bringing the parties together physically. Because it is immediate, there is always some risk of instant disagreement. Also—and this may be a minor consideration in most instances but once in a while can become extremely important—there is no physical record resulting from the conversation unless positive steps are taken to create one.

The Telephone

As an aid to business communication, the telephone offers several advantages. A telephone call provides for immediate feedback and response; views can be exchanged and mutual understanding can be achieved without delays between messages. A message comes through not only as words themselves but also as vocal tone and general manner of speaking. And for many purposes the telephone is faster than most other means.

Consider, however, what is lost in using a telephone call instead of meeting face-to-face. What can often be a significant part of one's "message"—the facial expressions and other body language—are completely lacking. Since one's body language is not always communicating the same message as the words one uses, the telephone call is generally less reliable than the face-to-face conversation. Also, unless a record is deliberately created or a call is recorded, there is no record of the transaction.

Voice Mail

Voice mail represents the telephone call with one critical omission: immediacy of feedback and response, extremely important in interpersonal communication, is absent. A clear advantage of voice mail, frequently accessed, is speed of transmission; a message is quickly left in a voice mail box and the originator moves on to other matters. (Undoubtedly some also see it as an "advantage" to speak to a voice mail system rather than a live person; when delivering bad news, criticism, or something controversial, many a caller is happy to simply "drop it and run.") One clear advantage of voice mail is that many issues can be successfully addressed via messages and responses without the parties having to connect directly.

One disadvantage, of course, lies in having to wait for someone to respond to a message. Also, as noted, there is no immediacy of feedback and response so voice mail is a still weaker means of communication than the telephone. Again, there is no record unless positive steps are taken to create one.

Letters and Memos

When a communication takes the form of a letter or memo, everything has been removed except the words themselves: there is no vocal tone, facial expression, or body movement, there is no immediacy of feedback and response. The words are made to carry the entire message, so to do so with reasonable accuracy the words must be well thought out. The primary advantage of a letter or memo is the creation of a record that can be read again, shared with others, and retained in a file. And often the permanent record is important because of legal implications.

The principal disadvantage, as already noted, is the absence of all the dimensions of an effective communication except the words themselves. Another disadvantage lies in time; it invariably takes longer to write an effective letter or memo than to use most other means. And we might also state that the disadvantages include the dislike of writing shared by many in the work force and the carelessness with which so many apply the written word.

Written communication is addressed further in a later section of this chapter.

E-mail

E-mail has probably become the most actively used means of message transmission, for messages both from person to person and from individuals or groups to other individuals or groups. In some respects, however, it is one of the weaker means available. Response to e-mail is generally faster than response to a letter or memo, but as with letters and memos e-mail is dependent on words only. And often—although certainly not always—e-mail messages are prepared with considerably less care than their paper counterparts and are thus more susceptible to misinterpretation.

E-mail is rapid as far as message transmission is concerned, and feedback can—but does not reliably—occur quickly. There is also the availability of instant messaging that can offer very nearly the same advantages as the telephone call except for the voice.

Other aspects of e-mail are addressed later in this chapter.

Consideration of the characteristics of these several communication methods provides some guidance for structuring one's communications according to need. That is, the means chosen for a particular communication may be governed by:

- the time available; that is, how quickly resolution is needed
- the importance of the issue
- the complexity of the issue
- the sensitivity of the issue
- the need for negotiation or problem-solving
- the need for documentation (a paper trail)

VERBAL (ORAL) COMMUNICATION

Spoken communication, which may be correctly referred to as either "oral" or "verbal" communication, is of critical importance in all aspects of health care. The understanding of the thoughts and ideas of others is essential to the delivery of quality patient care. The principal parts of a verbal exchange are the voice, the content of the message and response, and the method used to transmit the information. The voice conveys emotions; the tone used for delivery, the use of silences, the choice of words, the accents and intonation, and the speed of delivery are all factors in a verbal exchange.[1] Some of these factors (for example, voice quality) are genetic, and certain others (like speed of speech) are cultural. Health practitioners must also understand that their professional education has trained them to express ideas in a selective fashion.

The unconscious aspects of verbal communication are frequently overlooked. Conscious information is volitional because the speaker is aware of the content, direction, and reasons for the exchange. In greetings, information sharing, confrontations, and discussions, for example, the speaker can identify the reasons for the communication. However, there may be unconscious motives behind a given verbal communication, such as thoughts, aspirations, desires, anxieties, fears, or emotions that influence behavior but are hidden from the person's conscious thoughts. A slip of the tongue is an example of an unconscious verbalization.[2]

Nonverbal Communication

Nonverbal communication is included in the discussion of verbal communication because the two are inseparable parts of many interpersonal exchanges. Composed of movements, gestures, expressions, and silences, nonverbal communication may or may not be an important accompaniment to verbal communication. People may not speak, and yet ideas are exchanged. Although telephone conversations, for example, are largely dependent on the voice alone, intonation and silences frequently convey information beyond the spoken words. Two people who share a "knowing" look while waiting for a third have shared an idea without uttering a word.

Nonverbal communication can have both conscious and unconscious aspects. Conscious information is available for analysis and scrutiny. Unconscious thoughts also influence behavior, but these thoughts, feelings, or emotions are not part of the person's awareness. Analysis of the content of thoughts is difficult because the forces are hidden.

Body language, at the heart of nonverbal communication, is a series of conscious or unconscious postures that convey information to others. Many studies, both popular and scholarly, have been undertaken to explore this topic. Some popularized versions seem to convey the belief that gestures are universal; however, most gestures are, in fact, culturally bound. A nod of the head may mean yes in one society but it may mean no in another. Interpretations of human gestures, expressions, silences, and body movement must be rendered cautiously. It is best to check perceptions with the other person.

Communication levels can be clearly portrayed in a matrix. Table 14–1 is based on the Johari Window, which was developed by Joseph Luft and has appeared in many group dynamics texts and courses in the past 20 years.[3]

Table 14–1 Examples of Personal Communication

	Verbal	Nonverbal
Conscious	Speeches, greetings	Wave hello; nod head to affirm interest
Unconscious	Slip of the tongue, mistake in verbalizing	Cross legs away from speaker, smirk while hearing suggestion

Communication Distance

Hall discussed four levels of distance that are used by humans during communication.[4] His research was based on observations and interviews with middle-class adults from the northeastern seaboard of the United States. These crude observations are merely a first attempt to develop approximate categories. The four distance zones are as follows:

1. Intimate Distance (from 1 to 18 inches). Individuals are involved in love-making, wrestling, or comforting or protecting each other.
2. Personal Distance (from $1\frac{1}{2}$ to 4 feet). Individuals can hold or grasp each other. Visual images are distorted, but they begin to normalize as the person moves to arm's length.
3. Social Distance (from 4 to 12 feet). Individuals are less intimate. Voice level is normal, and conversations can be overheard. Impersonal business is conducted at this distance, but the interaction becomes more formal as the persons involved move toward the 12-foot distance.
4. Public Distance (from 12 to beyond 25 feet). Voice volume is increased, and details about the person are not noticed. Verbalization is formal.

Components of Communication

Communication includes four principal components: initiation, transmission, reception, and feedback. For communication to occur, there must be a sender, someone who begins the interaction. Initiation, which includes the preparation for the interaction, might begin on a nonverbal level and move to a verbal exchange. Transmission is the movement of the communication from one party to another; it depends on verbal and nonverbal sharing methods. Reception is the manner in which the message is received. The receiver's perception shapes the way in which a message is decoded and acted upon. To ensure that the sender and the receiver are truly sharing ideas, the receiver offers feedback, which is a verbal or nonverbal signal that acknowledges the message. Acknowledgments include modification, suppression, or nonacceptance of the information.

Interpersonal communication depends on assumptions, perceptions, feelings, past experiences, and present surroundings. Although people frequently talk, communication may prove taxing and difficult. People must transcend personal and cultural barriers that obstruct their understanding of an exchange.

Methods of Improving Communication

Communication is improved by observing, attending, responding to requests, and checking information. Each of these strategies depends on an objective analysis of an exchange. Observation is the activity of perceiving events, objects, and people. Skilled observers are objective and can separate their own inner world from outside reality. Accurate observation is dependent on self-knowledge, because inner reality can make someone "see" an event that did not occur. An event can be "real" in the mind of the person who really wants to "see" it.

Attending helps people hear or see events as they are. During a conversation, instead of planning their next remark, those who are attending direct their energy toward listening or empathizing with the other person. Attending is also referred to as active listening. Responding is the behavior an individual selects to address the needs or requests of the other person. The behavior may be verbal or nonverbal, and the quality of the response shapes the remainder of the communication. If a person asks for the time and receives a pleasant answer, that person may decide to continue the exchange. In contrast, unpleasant replies may inhibit further communication.

Active listening can also help an individual decode less obvious requests. Sometimes a sender makes an indirect request, which may be symbolic or may indicate unconscious desires. A perceptive listener should try to "hear" the request and bring the buried topic into the conversation. For example, Allie asked Mary for her pathology notes. Mary responded by saying that she would be glad to duplicate the notes, and she began to rummage in her purse. Allie handed Mary a tissue. Mary seemed grateful and quickly wiped her nose. Allie then handed Mary some money to cover the cost of duplicating the notes. A less perceptive listener may have mistaken Mary's action as a hint for payment or as a rejection of the request. In reality, Mary's nose was running, and she was distracted for a minute while she attended to it.

Communication is also improved by checking information. Listeners can check information by matching their perceptions of a situation with the sender's intention. In the example given earlier, Allie could have asked Mary if she needed a tissue. Listeners can examine the validity of their perceptions by paraphrasing the sender's message and asking for feedback.

People must be aware of symbols that may be archetypal, cultural, or idiosyncratic.[5] A symbol can be almost anything that is used to represent something else. Archetypal symbols are shared by humans and extend back in history; for example, a circle means unity throughout the world. Cultural symbols are specific to a subgroup (e.g., a thumb extended upward means a victory or a good job). Idiosyncratic symbols are specific to an individual or small group. Symbolic meanings contribute to the variety and breadth of communication by forcing listeners to move beyond their personal understanding of gestures, body movements, expressions, and silences.

Personal Tools to Foster Communication

There are six personal tools to be applied in promoting interpersonal communication:

1. *authenticity*: the ability to be true to one's own feelings
2. *acceptance of feelings* (based on authenticity): people who accept their own feelings can extend this acceptance to the feelings of others
3. *disclosure*: the ability to share feelings, both positive and negative, with others (honest people are able to share information openly)
4. *empathy:* the ability to project one's own personality onto another person (this promotes understanding)
5. *caring*: the desire to help others on an individual and collective level[6]
6. *humor:* the ability to identify situations as ludicrous, comic, or happy[7]

All six tools require the integration of personal needs with goals and actions.

Communication Barriers

Communication can be blocked by internal or external forces. Internal forces, including both conscious and unconscious thoughts, may preclude listening, sharing, and caring so that the meaning of the exchange is confused and misinterpreted. Conscious behaviors that limit communication include facial expressions that are perceived as negative or inappropriate (e.g., smiling when reprimanding a subordinate), body postures that are perceived as rejecting or critical of the person (e.g., folding one's arms over one's chest although expressing a desire to share ideas), verbalizations that interrupt the flow of the exchange (e.g., saying "fabulous!" every time a speaker pauses), and interruption or disruption of the speaker's thoughts (e.g., changing topics abruptly, such as interrupting a request for assistance with a comment about football scores).

External forces also impede communication. Distractions, such as noise, motion, and confusion, compromise the quality of an exchange. The context for a communication adds to or subtracts from the interaction. For example, a crowded room with flashing lights and loud music is designed for sensory stimulation, not verbal communication. In this environment, intimate conversations are taxed and labored; communication is limited to nonverbal cueing.

Speaking to Groups

Much of a department manager's verbal communication, surely an overwhelming majority for most first-line managers, involves one-on-one, face-to-face interchanges with individuals or with collectives of perhaps two or three people at most. There are, however, regularly occurring needs for the manager to address larger groups such as an entire department or perhaps the organization's management group. Speaking before groups is unavoidable, yet some managers who do very well in face-to-face situations experience considerable problems with addressing groups. This is unfortunate because public-speaking ability is extremely important to the career-minded manager who wishes to advance in an organization.

The following story suggests the value of a manager's capacity for public speaking. To afford all managers with some development opportunity, the administrator of a small community hospital established the practice of rotating the chairmanship of the monthly meeting of the facility's 24 or 25 managers. Given a broad outline, each manager would develop a specific agenda and chair the meeting, making the month's announcements and calling on other participants as needed. It was felt that experience with speaking and with leading meetings could be acquired as painlessly as possible in this friendly, familiar setting in which everyone knew each other.

On the day when the supervisor of the hospital's small business office medical records was to chair the meeting, she called in sick. Having missed her turn, she was assigned the next month's meeting; that time she scheduled a day off for personal business. When spoken with privately by the administrator she admitted her intense fear of public speaking. When asked how she conducted department meetings, she pointed out that with just two employees other than herself a department meeting was more like three friends getting together. She declared she could not possibly address a group as large as the management team. Over the following few weeks she resisted all of the administrator's efforts to get her some assistance in overcoming her fear. She claimed that the mere thought of speaking to a group made her physically ill.

Shortly thereafter, the hospital's board of directors voted in favor of a merger with another, slightly larger, community hospital. Most department managers from the two facilities were put in the position of having to compete for the resulting single position for each combined department. The process involved having each pair of managers prepare proposals describing how they would administer the combined department, this proposal to be presented orally before the administrators and senior managers of both facilities, a group of five or six in total.

As one might expect at this point in the story, the supervisor who feared speaking was not chosen to head the combined department. She did everything possible to duck the appearance, and, when essentially trapped into it, delivered a brief, stammering start before excusing herself, pleading illness.

The person who was chosen as the department head was actually her equal in education and qualifications and had more experience. Yet she accepted a staff position in the combined department in the knowledge that she would probably never return to management.

At the very least, every group supervisor and department manager will have to conduct meetings of his or her own staff. In most organizations, it is also likely that from time to time one will also have to present a proposal or deliver an oral report to a management team or perhaps even to an administrative group or board of directors. And one who dodges assignments that involve speaking had best appreciate that doing so is decidedly a career-limiting practice.

It should not be news for many readers to learn that fear of public speaking is both common and widespread; it is one of the most frequently encountered fears in the population at large. However, it may not be news to most to learn that the majority of individuals who regularly, capably, and comfortably speak before groups of people once struggled with this same fear. Sure, there are some natural speakers to be encountered now and then, those who never had reservations about addressing many people at one time. But these natural speakers are a minority. Most people who regularly speak in public had to overcome a certain amount of apprehension about doing so.

To offer an all-encompassing shortcut to a subject that rates an entire book by itself, the keys to success in public speaking are *preparation, practice,* and *repetition.* Preparation should always go without saying; there are not a great many speakers who can go in cold and simply "wing it," especially on an important topic. Preparation—knowing what one will say and how it will be said—helps moderate the uneasiness felt by the new speaker. Practice simply makes sense, at least for the inexperienced speaker; this also helps quell the new speaker's apprehensions. The most significant key, however, is repetition. Take it as a given that for most people *the more public speaking you do the better you become at it, and the more speaking you do the less fearful you become about speaking.* Getting started requires preparation and practice, and getting better and becoming less fearful and more confident requires preparation and repetition.

The Meeting

Meetings, particularly those of smaller groups, are where most managers acquire their early experience in both speaking to groups and leading discussions. For convenience we can consider the department manager's meetings as being of two kinds: staff meetings and general meetings (all others). Staff meetings are those the manager convenes with his or her own employees; general meetings include problem-solving meetings or meetings held for various other purposes with people from a variety of departments or activities.

The Staff Meeting

The manager has considerable flexibility in determining how and when staff meetings are scheduled, how they are conducted, and what is covered at them. Some managers find it advisable to bring the staff together on a weekly basis; some do so monthly and occasionally even less frequently. Staff meetings may take different forms: sometimes it is necessary for the manager to carry most of the meeting for providing information and updates; sometimes it is appropriate to have each staff member report on his or her recent activities; sometimes one or two staff members will provide most of the meeting's substance. Regardless of frequency or form, however, some fundamentals should be observed:

- Employees should expect staff meetings to occur on some regular, planned frequency (except for the occasional emergency meeting).
- Staff meetings should happen; there should be only a few special circumstances under which a meeting is skipped or cancelled. (For activities in certain professional areas, regular meetings—and minutes thereof—are a requirement of regulatory and accreditation bodies.)
- Staff should be advised that meetings will start on time, that starting will not be delayed for the sake of latecomers and that information will not be repeated for latecomers.
- Meeting length should be limited, holding to specific starting and quitting times. Ending early is fine if all pertinent business has been transacted, but ending late should occur only under exceptional circumstances and then as seldom as possible.
- The meeting leader—assuming that this is the department manager—should not dominate but rather make every effort to secure employee participation.
- If decisions are made or specific subsequent actions are required, these should be committed to writing.

The General Meeting

Every manager should expect to become involved in specially scheduled meetings held for a variety of purposes—information sharing, exploratory discussion, problem solving, and so on—as both meeting convener and participant. Specific guidelines for calling and holding such meetings are as follows:

- Define the issue or problem and determine whether a meeting is truly required. Depending on the number of people who must be involved, the required timing, and other means of communication available, it might be possible to avoid a meeting. The most efficient meeting is the meeting that never takes place.
- Determine a goal for the meeting, deciding what it is that must be accomplished. It is necessary to be able to identify what one desires from the meeting—the solution to a problem, a group decision, the group's acceptance of an idea, or whatever.
- Select the participants, taking care to include the people who have the necessary knowledge of the topic and those who have the authority to commit to a solution, if this is necessary.
- Give participants sufficient advance notice—no last-minute surprises that create conflicts—and distribute needed materials, if any, along with the initial notice (it is highly inefficient to wait until meeting time to provide handout material pertinent to the meeting).
- Make certain a proper meeting area is secured well in advance of the meeting; it can be highly frustrating to have a bunch of people ready to meet with no place to gather.
- Prepare an agenda. It need not be elaborate; a brief list of points to cover will usually suffice.
- Start the meeting on time and reiterate its purpose. Describe up front what you wish to accomplish and by what time you expect to end the meeting.
- As meeting leader, do not lecture or otherwise dominate. Encourage participation by all; stimulate discussion.
- Do not let any particular participants monopolize or dominate; likewise, if possible do not allow anyone to remain silent the entire time.
- End with a decision, a plan, a schedule of subsequent activity, or whatever concrete results come of the meeting.
- Arrange for the production of meeting minutes, if necessary, or otherwise ensure that significant results are documented.

- If a follow-up meeting is necessary, if at all possible get it scheduled before the participants leave. If it cannot be scheduled then, schedule it as soon as practical.

WRITTEN COMMUNICATION

The Importance of Written Communication

Written communications are essential to the conduct of business in any organization. Some ways of doing business require that letters and memoranda pass between individuals and organizations, and in spite of advances in electronic record storage there remain many needs for filed hard copy. Also, written copy of various kinds must be produced and maintained for purposes of satisfying legal, regulatory, and accreditation requirements.

Many who work in the delivery of health care can attest to the volume of writing required of them. Complaints about "paperwork" are common and widespread, and there is undoubtedly much more paper generated than is truly needed. Nevertheless, much of the written material that is produced is inescapable; hard-copy documents of various kinds will remain with us for the foreseeable future.

As many professionals and managers resist speaking in public, so do many frequently resist writing. Thus many professionals and managers who resist writing chores do not write especially well. It could perhaps be argued forever whether some dislike writing because they are not especially good at it or they are not especially adept at writing because they dislike it. Add to the often widespread dislike of writing the fact that writing seems to consume more time than many wish to devote to it. The resulting resistance to writing is that any number of professionals and managers will write a letter or memo only when absolutely necessary and even then will react to the pressures of time and write something once through and send it on its way.

The biggest problem concerning writing in business is not that it takes too much time but rather that it is allowed to consume too little time. Writing well requires more time and effort than simply dashing something off to get it sent and out of the way. Writing well requires editing and rewriting, admittedly time-consuming activities but activities that will usually pay for themselves in improved understanding and fewer problems of misinterpretation. Any who regularly communicate in writing should heed the words of Blaise Pascal: "I have made this letter rather long because I have not had time to make it shorter."

E-mail: Helpful but Source of Many Problems

It is likely that no modern business technology is more misused and abused than e-mail. E-mail is even more problematic than the next most misused and abused business technology, the photocopier. Many photocopiers, as all know but frequently choose to ignore, handle a significant volume of non-business copying. E-mail not only carries a high volume of non-business material; unlike the photocopier, it also carries business information communicated in slapdash, generally careless fashion that frequently does more to raise questions than convey information.

When it is necessary to spend a third to half of one's e-mail time sorting through unimportant communications and personal information before getting into pertinent messages, many of which must then be interpreted or questioned before passing along or acting upon, e-mail is out of control. Appropriate use of e-mail requires attention to the handling of both that which is received and that which is sent.

In addressing incoming e-mail:

- First be attentive to deleting rather than reading. In most instances a quick look at the subject line along with one's knowledge of the sender will indicate whether a message should be read in full or discarded at once.
- Become familiar with frequent senders and what they are likely to be sending. There has never been and there will never be a beneficial technology that does not have a downside, and the downside of the personal computer is its appeal to some users as more of a toy than a tool. Learn where many of the important messages come from and who is likely to be sending junk.
- Similar to the age-old advice about handling each incoming piece of paper only once, try dealing with each e-mail message once and only once. Upon reading a message, reply to it, forward it, delete it, or store it in an electronic folder. Messages should not be allowed to accumulate; they fill up the inbox and increase the chances of importance messages getting lost in the clutter.

In sending an e-mail message:

- Use a clear, understandable subject line that tells the addressee in a few words what to expect of the communication.
- Write, edit, and rewrite each message as though it were an important letter or memo (more on this to follow).
- Inform employees of the proper business use of e-mail and train them in proper handling of incoming mail. Consider reminding employees that e-mail is not as private as they might believe; messages are regularly misdirected accidentally, and it is easy for some computer users to tap into oth-

ers' e-mail. It helps to imagine that any particular message could conceivably become as public as a bulletin-board notice.

Concerning the seemingly prevalent "casual" (or, less euphemistically, "sloppy") use of e-mail, it often seems that e-mail brings out the worst in many writers of business communications. E-mail is such a readily available and easily usable means of interpersonal communication that it is easy to overlook its relatively severe shortcomings. Speaking with someone face-to-face, in addition to words one also has the benefit of facial expression, vocal tone, and immediacy of feedback. Even in a telephone conversation there is vocal tone and immediacy of feedback. However, an e-mail message is like a letter or memo in that all that is available to carry the message are words someone must read.

Misunderstandings abound because so many users simply "dash off" messages minus the care they might apply to letters or memos. Some who would never allow a letter to go out containing obvious errors think nothing of e-mailing unedited ramblings devoid of capitalization and normal punctuation and overflowing with misspellings and incorrect terms.

Editing a letter takes time, and although this task is often ignored it is not ignored nearly as often as editing an e-mail message. What's different about an e-mail message that causes its writer to forget the need to edit and clarify? Perhaps it's the seeming immediacy of e-mail, the feeling it provides of talking directly to someone via the computer screen. But it is easy to forget that the key element present in dealing with someone face-to-face—immediacy of feedback—is missing in e-mail. Feedback is delayed, and all too often it becomes necessary to trade messages back and forth to achieve the appropriate transfer of meaning. Far better to edit and rewrite—and certainly spell-check—before sending each message. Clarity of content is most likely to accompany clarity of presentation.

E-mail is perhaps best thought of as one of a subset of tools in that versatile toolkit known as the personal computer. Like any good tool, to retain its usefulness it must be kept in good order and used for its intended purposes only.

Memos and Letters *

Letters and memoranda are essential—and unavoidable—in the operation of any business or other organization. To many people who work in various health care

---

*Portions of the section "Memos and Letters" were adapted from: Charles R. McConnell, *The Effective Health Care Supervisor, 6th ed.* (Chapter 19, "Communication: Not by Spoken Words Alone") (Sudbury, MA: Jones and Bartlett Publishers, 2007), pp. 302–317.

settings it often seems that more than enough paperwork is already required without adding more by creating documents in addition to necessary charting, covering the organization legally, and responding to external requirements. However, even though the paper volume seems almost overwhelming at times, much of this paper is nevertheless necessary. Many organizations function quite well in spite of hefty amounts of paperwork, but just try to run an organization completely without paper.

Any written communication serves one or more of several important functions. Specifically, a given written communication may be used to advise (or inform), explain, request, convince, or provide a permanent record. Letters and memos may be used for any one or a combination of these purposes.

No matter how well it is written, any letter or memo possesses a serious drawback: it is essentially a one-way communication, providing no opportunity for immediate feedback. The individual who writes a letter or memo is unable to amend, correct, clarify, or defend what is being written based on the reactions of the audience.

Because of the one-way nature of a letter or memo, the need for clarity in writing becomes critical. However, clarity is an attribute frequently lacking in written communications in the organizational setting.

This section offers some guidelines for communicating more clearly via letter or memorandum. However, although these guidelines will help improve the clarity of one's writing, no few pages of advice in a work such as this will make one a "good" writer. To become a writer of effective business communications two things are needed: (1) the desire to write better letters and memos and (2) the help provided by practically oriented teachers of business writing and good references on writing.

Numerous books on writing techniques are available, but the writer who wishes to use one single straightforward reference should turn to *The Elements of Style* by William Strunk Jr. and E. B. White. This short volume contains more solid, usable advice per page than any other writing book available.

For better letters and memos, conscientious use of the following guidelines will improve your writing in a minimum amount of time.

Write for a Specific Audience

A particular letter or memo may be going to one person, or it may be intended for several people. Before writing, the writer must decide to whom, specifically, the missive is to be directed. The person who will receive the communication, that person for whom the message is primarily intended, is the primary audience. However, there may also be a sizeable secondary audience—others who will receive, read, and perhaps make use of the communication.

Many managers write as though they believe that anyone picking up a particular document will completely understand its contents. This is a difficult task at best, however, and it becomes nearly impossible in the presence of a sizeable secondary audience including people of widely varying backgrounds and different degrees of familiarity with the subject.

Write specifically for the primary audience. You cannot successfully write for everyone. If there is difficulty identifying the primary audience, you need to sift through the likely recipients of the message with one question in mind: Who of all these people needs this information for decision-making purposes? Often the primary audience will be a single person, but it could just as well be two, three, or more people. For example, a nursing supervisor writing about the need for a specific change in departmental policy would likely be making all of nursing management aware of the issue, but it would be the supervisor's immediate superior, the director of nursing service, who would be the primary audience because this is the person who wields the decision-making authority concerning departmental policy. In contrast, if the director of nursing service is releasing a new policy with which all supervisors are expected to comply, then the memo announcing the policy will have all supervisors as its primary audience.

Use what is known about the primary audience in deciding how to structure a message. Can it be on a friendly, first-name basis? Must it be a formal letter, or will a brief, casual note suffice? Does this person prefer detail, or would a concise overview be enough? Let knowledge of the primary audience suggest how to communicate.

Avoid Unneeded Words

Understanding and exercising one simple concept, that of the "zero word," will go a long way in removing excess words from one's writing. Every word in a given piece of writing can be placed in one of three categories: necessary, optional, or zero.

A necessary word is essential to getting the basic message across. An optional word, as the name suggests, can be used at one's option to qualify or modify a necessary word or phrase. A zero word contributes nothing and should be removed.

Consider the following sentence:

Mary is certainly an exceptionally intelligent woman.

This sentence contains only three necessary words: *Mary is intelligent.* Note, however, that even with all zero words and optional words removed, what remains is still a sentence.

The word *exceptionally* is the only optional word in the sentence. It may well make a difference in what you are trying to communicate to say that "Mary is exceptionally intelligent" rather than simply, "Mary is intelligent." While this is perfectly acceptable, it is necessary to watch out for the excess use of such modifiers and qualifiers; after a while they not only become tiresome but they also lose much of their impact.

The sentence includes three zero words: *certainly, an,* and *woman.* At least they are zero under normal circumstances, assuming that Mary is a woman. The word *an* is there for structural reasons, and *certainly* is certainly unnecessary, since in terms of what we are trying to convey, Mary either is or is not intelligent and *certainly* does not make it any more binding. Zero words abound in most business writing. However, they are relatively easy to get rid of with conscientious editing.

Almost any sample of business writing will yield at least a few zero words. If in doubt about a word, try the sentence without it. If the sentence remains a sentence and continues to convey the intended message, the word is probably a zero word. One can usually find a surprising number of zero words, among which are often many uses of *the, that, of,* and other simple words.

Unnecessary words are often used in several-word phrases to do the work that could be done by one or two words. This is especially common in business correspondence in which some phrases have reached cliché proportions. Consider these examples:

- the use of "due to the fact that" when one can simply say "because"
- saying "be in a position to" when all that is needed is "can"
- saying "in the state of California" when "in California" says the same
- using the stuffy "with reference to" when the job can be done by "about"

Such phrases are to be avoided; they simply add bulk without adding clarity. In fact, such words not only fail to add clarity but also can actually harm your message by surrounding and obscuring the real meaning.

Use Simple Words

Almost every technical and professional field has its own jargon, with jargon defined as "the technical terminology or characteristic idiom of a special activity or group." However, this is the *second* definition of jargon appearing in several dictionaries—the first is "confused unintelligible language."

It is one thing for a laboratory technologist writing to an audience of other laboratory technologists; in this instance one can get away with the free use of the language of the field. However, the employees of the health care organization usually include highly educated, specialized professionals, unskilled and semi-skilled workers, and numerous levels between. Also, an organization's staff includes people in many different but medically related fields, all of which have their own "languages."

Medical and technical professionals are among the worst offenders when it comes to sprinkling correspondence with jargon. The excuse that writing is "in the language" of a field, however, should not allow one to cut across departmental lines to any considerable extent. As already suggested, technologist-to-technologist may be a safe channel for the use of jargon. However, technologist-to-finance director is a channel calling for a completely different approach. Again, consider the primary audience in preparing to write.

Edit and Rewrite

During editing and rewriting, zero words, roundabout phrases, and other verbal stuffing should come out of the intended correspondence. Few pieces of writing cannot be improved by careful editing or rewriting. Most people—and this statement includes professional writers—cannot go from thought to a completely effective finished message in a single pass. In fact, professional writers do much more editing and rewriting than do most writers of day-to-day business correspondence. This reveals the problem: much of what is wrong with our writing is wrong simply because not enough time is put into it. As the Pascal quotation used earlier suggests, it usually takes more time to write a shorter letter than it does to write a longer one.

Anyone who might think that better writing is too time consuming should think also of the cost of misunderstanding. Many a manager has had to spend valuable time and effort smoothing out some problem that developed because a written message was misunderstood. Many memos can be edited in the time it takes to solve a couple of knotty problems arising from missed communication.

Changing Old Habits

In our day-to-day writing many people are unconsciously still trying to please English teachers of years gone by. Throughout several decades of the 20th century, students were taught to write letters that sounded as though they were lifted from a Victorian secretarial handbook.

Most of what has been said up to this point is "legal" in terms of long-standing English usage. However, many practices that are acceptable (and even improve) business writing today would previously have been guaranteed to get users into trouble with the teacher.

Be Friendly and Personal   Feel free to use personal pronouns in letters and memos. People use *I, you,* and *we* when we are speaking to each other, so why not use them when writing? Many people were taught to avoid personal pronouns, and this warning sticks with them. Students were once taught never to say *I.* But for clarity and directness, *I* is far preferable to archaic affectations such as *the undersigned* or *the author.*

Most letters and memos should strive for a conversational tone; once this is achieved, correspondence will be direct, friendly, and personal.

Use Direct, Active Language   Ask direct questions when the situation warrants it. Some may have been taught to go out of the way to avoid questions and thus say things like, "Let me know whether or not you will attend." It is much more direct to ask, "Will you attend?"

Statements should be kept in the active voice, avoiding the likes of, "The contract was signed by your representative." How much cleaner it is to say, "Your representative signed the contract."

Use Contractions   It is preferable to use contractions such as *don't, wouldn't, can't, shouldn't,* etc., even though this usage in business was long discouraged. Contractions contribute to the natural, conversational tone one should be working to achieve. Even so, many writers of business correspondence squeeze the contractions out of their writing without realizing what they are doing. The result is a formalistic style, stilted and stuffy, that serves only to create more distance between writer and reader.

Write Short Sentences   Although it is difficult to set firm guidelines for sentence length, consider that any sentence much longer than 20 words is edging into questionable territory. Some teachers of business writing have suggested 20 words as maximum sentence length; others suggest that 14 or 15 words be considered maximum. Regardless, it is safe to say that the longer the sentence, the more opportunities there are for misunderstanding.

Forget Old Taboos about Prepositions and Conjunctions   It is likely that most people were repeatedly and sternly warned against committing two terrible transgressions: ending a sentence with a preposition and starting a sentence with a conjunction.

A story is told about Winston Churchill and the rule concerning prepositions. When reminded it was improper to end a sentence with a preposition, Churchill replied (paraphrased but retaining the point), "This is something up with which I shall not put." An extreme example, for sure, but it cleanly illustrates how far out of the way the writer may be led in search of so-called structure. Go ahead and say, "This is something I won't put up with."

A surefire way to lose points with many teachers is to begin sentences with conjunctions, especially *and* and *but*. Fortunately this archaic prohibition has been successfully shattered by professional writers. Of course, if every other sentence in a letter begins with *and*, the writer has created a different kind of monster. However, the freedom to open a sentence in this manner can help avoid long sentences and needless repetition.

Say It and Stop   Avoid starting a letter by repeating what was said in the letter being answered. Also, avoid opening with standard stuffing such as "In response to yours of the . . ."

Simply state the message. If the point of the letter is to tell a potential supplier that the bid was rejected, do not spend two paragraphs describing the evaluation process and building the rationale for the "no" to deliver in paragraph three. Deliver the answer in the opening paragraph, preferably in the first sentence. Then go on to explain why, if necessary.

Having delivered the message and explained it as necessary, do not spend another paragraph or two winding down by repeating what has already said. Simply say it—and stop. Also, watch out for standard closing lines that mean little or nothing. It may be quite all right to say something like, "Call me if you need more information"; this is thoughtful and it shows interest. But avoid phrases such as, "We trust this arrangement meets with your complete satisfaction." If the reader is not completely satisfied the writer is likely to hear about it.

Consider also the use of the collective *we* in the foregoing example. Few words are more likely to make a letter more impersonal to a reader than one who is made to feel that the communication is coming from a crowd. The *we* has its place, for instance, when writing to someone outside the organization and speaking for the organization. However, rather than being organization-to-person or organization-to-organization, most of one's writing will be person-to-person. As long as the thoughts are your own and yours is the only hand pushing the pen or tapping the keys, say *I*.

Sample Letter: Wrong and Right

Following is the text of a letter sent to a number of hospital chief executives by the director of a regional office of a state health department:

Dear Administrator:

I would like to call your attention to Section 702.4 (c) of the State Hospital Code which requires nosocomial infections in hospitals be reported immediately to the Regional Health Director.

We have recently experienced several hospital outbreaks in this region which have not been reported to this office by the hospital. It is recommended that you review Section 702.4, *Infection Control and Reporting,* of the State Hospital Code so that you understand what your responsibilities are regarding increased incidence of hospital infections or disease due to chemical or radioactive agents or their toxic products in patients or persons working in the hospital.

In counties where there is an organized county or city health department or a Commissioner of Health, it is also required that a report of communicable be made immediately to the County or City Health Commissioner. In the unorganized counties or districts, a report must be made to the District Health Officer immediately. This is no way eliminates or excuses the hospital from reporting immediately to the Regional Health Director.

Please note that failure to report nosocomial infections is a violation of Section 702.4(c) of the State Hospital Code. Violations of the Code are subject to penalty. In the future, such violations will leave us no alternative but to recommend that appropriate sanctions be taken against a hospital for violation of this section of the State Hospital Code.

Very truly yours,
Regional Health Director

It is certainly possible to correctly extract the true message from the foregoing letter, although a telephone call or two might be necessary before a recipient would feel comfortable about its meaning. Also, there is no denying the scolding tone and the threat contained in the letter (with threats of sanctions or punishment of some kind seemingly incorporated in a great many communications from government agencies). However, consider how the text of the letter could read if more thoughtfully written:

The State Hospital Code calls for the reporting of nosocomial infections to the Regional Health Director as soon as they are discovered. However, several recent outbreaks in this region have not been reported.

Please review Section 702.4 of the Code (Infection Control and Reporting) concerning your role in helping to control infection or disease resulting from the exposure of patients, staff, or others to chemical or radioactive agents or their toxic products.

If you community has a Department of Health, your timely report should go to the local Commissioner. If you have no local health department, your report should go directly to the District Health Office.

Please assist us in ensuring that Section 702.4 of the Code is observed as intended. Your cooperation will be appreciated.

Why should the author have bothered to edit and rewrite? One good reason for doing so is for clarity; in its rewritten form the letter is far less likely to be misunderstood. Also, the scolding and threatening have been removed; there is always the opportunity to communicate more sternly later with recipients who might remain noncompliant. And consider this as well: the text of the original letter contains 232 words; the rewritten version contains 127 words. This amounts to a reduction in length of 45 percent. Not only is the rewritten letter clearer, there is less to read. Is this at all important? It has been estimated that most business documentation contains anywhere from 25 percent to 100 percent more words than are actually needed. This suggests that the two-inch-thick stack of documentation in the manager's inbox need be only one to 1.6 inches thick if properly written.

Time spent editing and rewriting is time well spent in making a message more readily understood while greatly reducing the chances of misunderstanding.

Formal Writing and Reporting

Letters and memos constitute a significant percentage of most managers' writing chores. However, it may occasionally be necessary or desirable to tackle larger writing tasks such as informational or analytical reports, educational presentations, speeches, or perhaps even journal articles.

Many elements of the personal, direct style preferred for correspondence are applicable to other writing. For instance, some speeches or educational presentations can, and should, be handled with the same personal touch. However, some additional rules apply in writing more structured material such as formal reports, and still more rules apply when writing for publication in trade magazines or professional journals.

A thorough treatment of the topic of report writing is well beyond the scope of this book. If you need to author a formal report, obtain a manual or handbook on the subject and do some studying, with particular attention to outlining schemes if the report in question is likely to be lengthy. Also, be aware of the advisability of using one of the commonly recommended report formats, one that calls for a tight summary of objectives, conclusions, and recommendations early in the report.

Whether you are writing a letter, memorandum, or formal report, never lose sight of the fact that the initial step in preparing to write anything is to get a clear image of the intended audience, both primary and secondary.

COMMUNICATION IN ORGANIZATIONS

Considering that communication between two people may be difficult at times, and small-group communication may frequently be taxing, the task of communicating with a large group may at first seem overwhelming. As bureaucracies began to emerge at the dawn of the 20th century, when industrialization promoted the growth of large organizations, the need to develop complex communication patterns became more pressing as organizations added more and more members. Communication had to keep pace with production. The resulting strategies to increase organizational communication can be divided into two categories: formal and informal.

Formal Communication

Verbal

An organization is a stratified social system with a hierarchy of roles. The roles are arranged according to the degree of power and status assigned to each, and the assignment is based on the goal-oriented needs of the organization. Formal communication is sanctioned by the organization and is shared along communication channels established by the hierarchy of roles. The arrangement of roles determines the direction of the communication.

Formal communication is directional. The four traditional channels of communication are upward, downward, diagonal, and lateral (Table 14–2).

Table 14–2 Example of Directionality

Four Channels	Examples
1. Upward	Staff person communicating with supervisor
2. Downward	Staff therapist giving orders to an aide
3. Diagonal	Department head of social work conferring with patient registrar in Admissions
4. Lateral	Nurse sharing night orders with another nurse

Formal verbal communication in organizations takes place through orderly channels. The exchanges are directional and promote organizational goals, such as a verbal exchange of orders or instructions. Department meetings can also be formal. An aide who wants to register a complaint must go through a series of formal channels; the aide cannot walk into the president's office and discuss the grievance.

Because the size of organizations precludes face-to-face interaction among the majority of group members, they must rely on less personal means of communication (for example, written and transmitted communication). Common examples include goal statements, policy and procedure manuals, directives, direct mailings to employees, inserts in pay envelopes, mass e-mail communications, organizational bulletins, newsletters, magazines, bulletin boards, posters, and handbooks.

Nonverbal Elements

The use of space is a form of nonverbal communication. The goals of the organization determine the location and quality of space assigned to group members (who may resist adjustments and reassignments). The way that furniture is arranged, the selection of ornaments, and the care given to the space all reflect the values of the group. If an organization has an elaborate waiting room and sloppy offices, it can be inferred that the company is more interested in its public face.

The arrangement of furniture can stimulate or stifle communication. Managers rely on spatial relationships to strengthen their communication. For example, asking for a raise while the manager looks over a desk is more difficult than asking while both parties are seated next to each other.

Informal Communication

Because informal communication is not sanctioned by the social system, it may or may not promote the goals of the organization. Informal communication is not directional; it may—and frequently does—circumvent formal channels. Informal communication is frequently anonymous, and more often than not sources cannot be verified.

Informal communication, such as small talk and gossip, may not be accurate. Even so, the use of informal communication should not be neglected. Managers can use this type of communication to determine the success of formal communication patterns. Rumor and gossip, although inaccurate, may gauge the feelings of group members. Perceptions about events can also be examined. Informal communication is a barometer of the organization, because information can travel at a fast rate. Future events may be foreshadowed by listening to information communicated informally.

Informal communication within the organization may be accurately described by a single familiar term: the grapevine. This may perhaps be more accurately described as *the communications network of the informal organization.* Every organization has a formal structure of relationships governing relationships within the workplace. In addition, every person in the organization has a number of informal channels of communication, relationships with friends, acquaintances, and others with whom one might speak. Further, many of the relationships partially define the informal organization, which implied structure based on numerous interactions between and among people.

The informal organization is at work, for example, when two or three employees happen to stand out from the group, perhaps even speaking for others, although they have no official standing. This effect is also evident when a single manager is regarded as senior by the work group over a number of others at the same level because of longevity or perhaps because of strength of personality or some particular trait or combination of traits. In brief, interpersonal relationships and people's regard for one another describe the informal organization, at best a phantom structure that is always shifting and realigning.

People will talk. The grapevine is not required by management, and it is certainly not controlled by management. It runs merrily back and forth across departmental lines and rapidly changes its course. The grapevine is dynamic but unreliable. It carries a great deal of misinformation, but it is in the organization to stay.

It is best to remain acutely aware of the grapevine. Tune in, listen to what it is carrying, and learn from it. A manager is likely to be isolated from some of the bits and pieces the grapevine carries, or at least miss a few things until they have been around awhile. How much one hears is frequently dependent on how well one relates with employees, peers, and others.

When tuned in to the grapevine, a manager is going to hear some things that he or she knows are simply not correct. One who hears something that is disturbing or inappropriate should check it out if possible. Each manager is responsible for setting the facts of the story right whenever the opportunity to do so presents itself. You must be sure, however, to have the story straight—do not heap more speculation onto a growing rumor.

The grapevine sometimes possesses the distinct advantages of speed and depth of penetration. Some bits of news can travel through the organization at an astonishing rate and often reach people who would never think to read a bulletin board or look at an employee newsletter. The grapevine can carry the good as well as the bad, and since it will always be around it is best to feed it some real facts whenever possible so it will have something useful to carry.

Tools for Improving Communication

A number of formal and informal tools can be used to promote communication within the organization. Assessment instruments require analysis of the conscious and unconscious goals of group members. Some can be used to assess individual interaction styles, members' perceptions of each other, perceptions of leadership, roles that members play with each other in the work group, and members' feelings about the organization. Group members complete questionnaires, and the results are compared and discussed. The goals of the members are compared with the goals of the leaders. The results are discussed in nonthreatening ways. Strategies for promoting change can be generated in the group.

Sometimes, group communication becomes so difficult that outside experts, called facilitators, are brought in to resolve the issues. Facilitators are trained in a number of disciplines, including business, psychology, education, and sociology.

Barriers to Communication in Organizations

A number of obstacles can block communication or distort the goals of organizational exchanges:

1. *Language.* There may be a lack of common understanding of certain important terms. The use of slang, jargon, or technical language can create problems.
2. *Unconscious Motives.* Inner thoughts, ideas, and emotions not readily available for examination may cloud a group's ability to perceive or interpret events. A group may share a collective mentality that may not be based on real events. The collective thought has been shaped by emotions.
3. *Psychological Factors.* Past experience and ideas impinge on the communication process. Feelings such as mistrust, fear, anger, hostility, or indifference may shape group perceptions.
4. *Status.* Real or perceived differences in rank, socioeconomic status, or prestige may detract from the communication process. People develop preconceived notions about others and act on their preconceptions instead of reality.

5. *Organizational Size.* The larger the social system, the greater the number of communication layers. Each layer provides an opportunity for additional distortion.

6. *Logistical Factors.* Groups may lack the time, place, or space to communicate clearly. Feedback may be neglected because it is difficult to collect.

7. *Overstimulation.* Members may be bombarded with so many events that they are unable to process any more information. People who are stressed must be managed carefully so they are not additionally burdened.

8. *Cultural Clashes.* One group may misinterpret another's ideas because of a difference in cultural factors, such as age, socioeconomic status, the region of birth, and education level.

9. *Organizational Structure.* Communication may be blocked by the structure of the communication channels. One person's role may serve as a bottleneck for open communication. In another instance, roles may overlap, and some groups may not receive the information that they need.

10. *Phase in Life Cycle of Organization.* Communication may be taxed during the organization's developmental stage. In later stages, the old channels may not have been adapted to new situations. Sometimes, organizations rely on one type of communication and ignore other methods.

Special Consideration: Directional Flow Barriers

Communication within a work organization moves downward with far greater ease than it moves upward. The downward channels of communication are largely controlled by management and tend to be exercised at management's option. Letters and memoranda to employees, general e-mailings to employees, employee meetings and staff meetings, informational stuffers in paycheck envelopes, bulletin boards (except for occasional boards placed solely for employee use), policy and procedure manuals, most newsletters and employee newspapers, and public address systems all represent downward channels of communication controlled by management. Perhaps the most potent downward channels reside in the vested authority that each level of management has over its subordinates; in any vertical relationship in the chain of command, the person higher in authority is seen as exerting the greater measure of control in the communication that occurs within the relationship.

When a bit of information is set in motion in any of the downward channels, barring occasional breakdowns in flow, it moves as does anything moving from higher to lower—as though readily assisted by gravity. Moving a message up the chain of command, however, is often like attempting to make a physical object rise in spite of gravity. One can of course make an object rise in spite of gravity, but doing so requires the effort of lifting it plus whatever extra effort is required to over-come gravity. It is the same with communication; it usually requires a bit of extra effort to make a message travel upward against the normal downward-flowing ten-dency of organizational communication.

To obtain communication from employees the manager can and indeed should, through techniques such as proper delegation, build in requirements for all rea-sonable forms of employee feedback. If an employee clearly understands that he or she is to report to the manager on a given matter at a given time, then reporting usually takes place. It is likely that a large part of the effective group manager's time is consumed in the basic management function of controlling—ensuring, through regular follow-up and correction, that work is getting done as intended. This func-tion requires employee feedback.

Despite such efforts, the manager can never secure a considerable amount of valuable information by mandating feedback. Information that frequently remains hidden from the manager can include personal as well as work-related employee problems. It can also include difficulties employees experience with management and coworkers, problems understanding or adhering to certain policies and prac-tices, ideas for improvement that employees may not know how to structure or transmit, complaints about treatment from the organization, and numerous other indications of unmet needs. These kinds of information may be essential, or at least helpful, to the manager in running the department. Yet the manager may obtain such information not through mandate but rather by being visible and available to the employees and by earning the trust and confidence of the employees to the extent that they will volunteer such information.

Thus the manager may ordinarily communicate downward at will because of position in the hierarchy; however, employees can communicate upward effectively only if the manager makes it possible for them to do so.

CASE: THE LONG, LOUD SILENCE

Background

As the director of health information services recently hired from another organ-ization, it did not take you long to discover that morale in the department had been at a low ebb for quite some time. As you undertook to become acquainted with each of your employees, you quickly became inundated with complaints and other ev-idences of discontent. Most of the complaints concerned problems with adminis-tration, the financial division, and the records-related practices of physicians, but there were also a few complaints by staff about other members of the department and a couple of thinly veiled charges concerning health information services personnel who "carry tales to administration."

In listening to the problems it occurred to you that there were a number of common threads running through them, and that a great deal of misunderstanding could be cleared up if the gripes were aired in open fashion with the entire group. You then planned a staff meeting for that purpose and asked all employees to be prepared to air their complaints—except those involving specific department staff—at the meeting. Most of the employees seemed to think such a staff meeting was a good idea, and several assured you they would be ready to speak up.

Your first staff meeting, however, turned out to be brief. When offered the opportunity to air their gripes, nobody spoke.

This result—silence—was the same at your next staff meeting four weeks later, although in the intervening period you were steadily bombarded with complaints from individuals. This experience left you frustrated because you regarded many of the complaints as problems of the group rather than problems of individuals.

Instructions

1. Describe in detail what you believe you can do to get the group off dead center and to open up about what is bothering them.
2. Describe how you might approach the specific problem of one or more of your employees carrying complaints outside of the department—that is, "carrying tales to administration."
3. Describe several means of organizational communication at your disposal that you believe might be applied in helping to address this department's problems.

CASE: YOUR WORD AGAINST HIS

Background

You and six other department managers are at a meeting chaired by your immediate superior, the vice president for patient services. The subject of the meeting is the manner in which members of this group, as well as other supervisors and managers, are to conduct themselves during the present union organizing campaign.

The vice president makes a statement concerning one way in which all managers should conduct themselves. You are surprised at what he said because earlier that day you read a legal opinion describing this particular action as probably illegal.

You interrupt the vice president with, "Pardon me, but I don't believe it can be done quite that way. I'm certain it would leave us open to an unfair labor practice charge."

Obviously annoyed at being interrupted, the vice president says sharply, "This isn't open for discussion. You're wrong."

You open your mouth to speak again, but you are cut short by an angry glance.

You are absolutely certain that the vice president is wrong. He had inadvertently turned around a couple of words and described a "cannot do" as a "can do." Unfortunately, you are in a conference room full of people, and the document that could prove your point is in your office.

INSTRUCTIONS

Describe in detail any options you believe you can pursue in an effort to set the matter straight for all parties who received the wrong information as well as with the vice president, while incurring the minimum possible public disfavor by the vice president.

NOTES

1. Evelyn W. Mayerson, *Putting the Ill at Ease* (Hagerstown, MD: Harper & Row, 1976), 1–36.
2. Sigmund Freud, *A General Introduction to Psychoanalysis*, trans. Joan Riviere (New York: Washington Square Press, 1964), 40.
3. Joseph Luft, *Group Process* (Palo Alto, CA: National Press Books, 1963).
4. E. T. Hall, *The Hidden Dimension* (Garden City, N.Y.: Anchor Books, 1966), 113.
5. A. C. Mosey, *Three Frames of References for Mental Health* (Thorofare, N.J.: Charles B. Slack, 1970), 52. Taken from J. Mazer, G. Fidler, L. Kovalenko, and K. Overly, *Exploring How a Think Feels* (New York: American Occupational Therapy Association, 1969).
6. Naomi I. Brill, *Working with People* (Philadelphia: J. B. Lippincott, 1973), 31–46.
7. V. M. Robinson, *Humor & the Health Professions* (Thorofare, N.J.: Charles B. Slack, 1977).

15

Day-to-Day Management for the Health Professional-as-Manager

CHAPTER OBJECTIVES

- Examine the dual role of the health professional working as a manager.
- Explore some potential problems and barriers often encountered by health professionals who enter management.
- Confirm the legitimacy of management, necessarily a second career for many health professionals, as a profession in its own right.
- Identify the nonmanagerial professional employee as a sometimes-scarce resource, suggesting a necessary focus on employee retention.
- Introduce the high-skill professional and review the special management problems of directing such personnel.
- Discuss several aspects of day-to-day management in which the manager must put more into the relationship with each employee because the employee is a professional.
- Establish the manager's critical role as the essential link between the employees' profession and the remainder of the organization.

TWO HATS: SPECIALIST AND MANAGER

The professional who is asked to assume a management position is being asked to take on a second occupation and perhaps even pursue a second career. Management positions turn over as other positions do, and vacant management positions are often filled from within the ranks of the work group. There are both advantages and disadvantages to having a particular member of a work group step up to the position of group manager. On occasion, however, the new manager of a group will come from outside of the organization.

Although familiarity with the specific organizational setting may be helpful to the new manager, such familiarity is certainly not a requirement of a group's new manager. There is one firm requirement of the individual who is to assume command of any work group: the individual must be intimately knowledgeable of the kinds of work the group performs. Because many work groups within the health care institution include professional employees and because the manager's technical qualifications must essentially be equivalent to the qualifications found in the department, the career ladder of a professional may logically be extended to include the management of that specialty.

The professional who enters management must exist ever after in a two-hat situation. This person must wear the hat of the professional—that is, the technical specialist—and render judgments on countless technical matters concerning the profession, but this person must also wear the hat of the manager and effect the application of generic techniques—processes that apply horizontally across the organization regardless of one's individual specialty. The professional in a management role must be both specialist and generalist. As a professional, the person is trained as a specialist in a particular field. As a manager, however, it remains largely up to the individual to recognize the need to become a generalist and to independently seek out sources of education and assistance.

The average employee who progresses from the ranks into management is usually well grounded in a working specialty. In this sense all employees, professionals and nonprofessionals alike, are functional specialists. For instance, the individual who works for several years in the housekeeping department and has performed a variety of housekeeping tasks and has become a specialist in the work of that department brings all this experience into supervision when promoted. At the least, the nonprofessional is a specialist by virtue of experience.

While the professional employee is usually also a specialist by virtue of experience, that is only a part of the professional's qualifications as a specialist; the remaining criteria defining the professional as a specialist are education and accreditation. The professional entering management brings both credentials and experience to the job. In this regard the person is usually eminently qualified to wear the manager's technical hat but may not be nearly as well qualified to wear the managerial hat.

The professional who enters management is usually extremely well trained in the specialty but trained minimally or not at all in matters of management. Health care professionals become professionals by seeking out appropriate programs, gaining entry, and working toward the necessary qualifications, but these same people become managers by virtue of organizational edict; that is, they are simply appointed. Precisely at this stage some employees and organizations commit a classic error—assuming that because people have been promoted and given appropriate titles, they are suddenly managers in the true sense of the word. Unfortunately, organizational edict does not automatically make a manager out of someone who is not adequately trained or appropriately oriented to management any more than the mere conferral of the title could turn an untrained person into a nurse, an accountant, a biomedical engineer, or any other professional.

The professional entering management, then, is usually well trained at wearing the hat of the specialist and trained little or not at all in wearing the hat of the manager. Although each side of the role is equally important, and even though one side or the other may dominate at times, many such persons exhibit a long-run tendency that is fully understandable under the circumstances. This is the tendency to favor the wearing of the hat that fits best, leaning toward the one of the two roles in which they find themselves more comfortable.

By listening carefully to some of the common complaints of certain managers, it is possible to identify the aspects of the management job that lie at the heart of the complaints. Such complaints will then identify the individuals on whom the management hat does not fit especially comfortably. Common areas of complaint that indicate the presence of ill-fitting management hats include the following:

- *Budgeting.* As one manager complained, "Budgeting is an annual chore that seems to come around every two or three months." If the management hat does not fit well, budgeting is likely to be a dreaded chore filled with frustration and only partly understood.
- *Performance appraisals.* Appraisals are also a common annual responsibility that seems to come around sooner than it ought to. When the management hat does not fit well, appraisals are likewise dreaded, tend to run late or perhaps not get done at all, and may make the manager feel uncomfortable and perhaps inadequate.

- *Employee problems.* The essence of the management role is getting things done through people, and this requires maintenance of the manager's most valuable resource—the employees. When the management hat does not fit well the manager may exhibit a tendency to shy away from people problems and resent them as intrusions that keep one away from the "real work."
- *Identification with the work group.* "Listen, gang, I know I'm the manager of this group but don't forget that my background is the same as yours and I'm a lot more like you than those people in top management." The tendency to identify with the group and join with them in condemnation of the infamous "they"—as in "It's not my fault, *they* made me do it"—is another sure sign of the ill-fitting management hat.
- *Disciplinary issues.* Rarely is any manager completely comfortable with exercising the disciplinary process, and indeed, he or she should never become completely comfortable with something of this importance. Often, however, out of discomfort the manager wearing the ill-fitting management hat will ignore disciplinary issues altogether or take action that is too little or too late.
- *Personnel policies.* The wearer of the ill-fitting management hat may have little familiarity with pertinent personnel policies and thus may simply tell employees to "call human resources" rather than help them answer policy questions.
- *Work priorities.* One sure sign of the ill-fitting management hat is the apparent inability to plan one's work and establish priorities. The manager so afflicted will often seem to be spending each day reacting to crises or continually responding to the demands of the moment regardless of their relative importance.
- *Delegation failure.* The manager who is constantly juggling an overload because of inability to delegate, or whose behavior seems to be saying, "If you want something done right, you'd better do it yourself," is wearing the ill-fitting management hat. This manager is failing to use staff to the full extent of their capabilities and is overlooking the important employee-development role of the manager.

The foregoing list could be made longer, but the point is made. When such symptoms appear the manager is feeling the pinch of the management hat, reacting out of frustration and insecurity, and taking refuge under the technical hat. Those processes that can be described as generic to management—because they apply across the organization regardless of the function managed, such as budgeting and performance appraisal—appear as mysterious, somewhat misunderstood activities. These come to be regarded as elements of interference rather than the vital elements of management. Disciplinary problems and other people problems are likewise seen as annoyances rather than as legitimate obstacles to overcome in the process of getting things done through people. What is seen as "real" work is the basic work of the technical specialty. Overlooked is the reality that the true task of the manager is largely to serve as a facilitator in the process of getting the real work done by the employees.

The signs of the ill-fitting management hat are numerous, and many managers continually take refuge under the hat of the technical specialist. This is understandable considering the professional employee's degree of familiarity with the occupation and unfamiliarity and discomfort with some of the processes of management. Yet simply being aware of the likely imbalance between the two halves of the role should be sufficient to inspire some managers to improve their capability and performance in the management sphere. Both sides of the manager's role are extremely important. A working knowledge of the technical specialty remains important at most levels in the health care hierarchy. Particularly in the lower levels of management, the generalist side of the role—that is, the management side—is neither more nor less important than the specialist side; it is simply different.

Although most managers in the health care organization's hierarchy have a need to be both technical specialist and management generalist, as there is a place in the working ranks for the pure technical specialist there is also a place in the management hierarchy for the pure management generalist. In general, however, the few management generalists in the organization are found in the upper reaches of the hierarchy in positions of multidepartmental responsibility.

In the health care organization, administration is the province of the pure management generalist. Administrators of health institutions come from a variety of backgrounds, with many of them arising out of the management of certain specialties and having perhaps broadened their scope through studies in administration. It matters little whether the institution's chief executive officer may have originally trained as an accountant, a registered nurse, an attorney, or a physician as long as that person made the necessary transition from specialist to generalist while rising toward the top. Still, it is rare to encounter, for example, a director of nursing service who is not a registered nurse, a health information services manager who was not first a health information practitioner, a director of finance who was not an accountant, or a manager of physical therapy who was not a physical therapist.

A CONSTANT BALANCING ACT

Some professionals who take on the management of departments never completely adapt to the dual role of professional and manager and never develop an appropriate balance between the two sides of the role. Their behavior often sums up their attitude; once a specialist, always a specialist. Such persons tend to give the technical side of the role the majority of their interest and attention, their priority treatment, and certainly their favor. Never having become sufficiently comfortable with the management role to enjoy what they are doing, they take refuge in their strengths and minimize the importance of their weaknesses.

The dedicated professional often has far more difficulty than the nonprofessional in balancing the roles of professional and manager. The professional has devoted far more time, effort, and commitment to becoming a specialist and has probably done so at least partly because of an attraction to or an aptitude for that kind of work. Some may indeed like their work so well that, although they do not necessarily refuse promotion to management, they show an inclination to subordinate the management side of the role so that it does not intrude too far into their favored territory.

Just as the liking for their specialty is important to success in their basic fields, so too is a liking for management essential for success in management. Usually a liking for a given activity is strongly influenced by one's degree of familiarity or level of comfort with the elements of that activity. Quite simply, the more a person knows about a given activity, the more the person is inclined to like that activity. Conversely, one may be more readily inclined to dislike an activity that seems bewildering, strange, or discomforting.

It has been suggested that the professional who enters management is faced with becoming grounded in management and getting up to speed. Once in management, the individual discovers that to remain effective as a technical professional and as a manager it is necessary to try to remain current in two career fields.

Staying current with the latest developments in a technical specialty is a sizable task in itself; getting fully up to speed and remaining current with the elements of one's management role is an unending task, considering the scope and breadth of management. Often, both sides of the role suffer to some extent; however, the technical side is more likely to receive most of the conscientious attention. The professional employed as a manager has all the problems of any other manager and also has most of the problems that confront the working professional who is not a manager.

THE EGO BARRIERS

Probably few if any health professionals do not believe that their professions are of considerable importance to their organizations. This is to be expected; to find any significant measure of fulfillment in work, health care professionals must regard their occupations as being of significant value to the organization and its patients. The potential for problems exists when an individual professional behaves as though his or her particular working specialty is more important than other occupations in the organization. If a professional who carries an inflated regard for the importance of a given profession happens to be the manager of a department, the seeds of interdepartmental conflict are present.

Managers without a particular background or origin—neither technical specialist nor management generalist—are not immune to inappropriate organizational behavior. Both generalist managers and technical-specialist managers can display self-serving tendencies at times. Some managers, however, frequently differ in how they pursue their objectives of service according to whether they see themselves as generalists or technical specialists. The generalist who is on a self-serving track often tends toward empire-building, working to acquire every function or responsibility that can in any way be connected under a common head. This manager is working toward elevation of self by acquiring far-reaching control throughout the organization much as some nations extend their authority by acquiring colonies throughout the world.

The self-serving technical specialist manager, however, is often limited by the inability to absorb functions that are not technically related to the profession of the manager. Rather than building an empire, much like the feudal baron who remained in his castle but devoted most of his time and energies to making it the grandest and strongest castle in the country, the manager strives to build an elegant structure that will surely dwarf its neighbors. Thus the "most important" specialty eventually has the most elegant quarters, the most generous budget, the most favorable staffing relative to the amount of work to be done, and the strongest voice in influencing institution policy. The results convey the belief that one's own profession is somehow better than the other professions in the organization.

Another ego problem to which the technical-specialist manager may fall victim, one of perhaps significantly more impact than the preceding effect, is found in the tendency to place management in an inferior role relative to the profession. This may also appear as a tendency to consider the profession itself as so necessary to management that one could not possibly be an accomplished manager of anything without knowledge of this particular profession.

The behavioral message sent by some technical-specialist managers is: knowledge of my technical specialty is critically important in health care management. Therefore, it is implied that you must originally be a social worker, psychologist, registered nurse, physical therapist, registered health information administrator, or whatever to become fully effective as a manager in health care.

In fact, to become a well-rounded and effective health care manager one need not be a social worker, speech pathologist, laboratory technologist, registered nurse, or any other health care specialist. It is automatically conceded that in all but the most general of support activities the manager must be some kind of specialist as well as a manager; however, no one specialty has a monopoly or even a modest edge regarding management expertise. The fundamental task of management—getting things done through people—is reflected in practices such as proper delegation, clear and open two-way communication, budgeting and cost control, scheduling, handling employee problems, and applying disciplinary action. All true management practices are transportable across departmental lines, and to believe otherwise is to fall into the ego trap of the technical specialist.

The professional employee who enters management is literally adopting a second career. If a potential manager thinks of management as a profession, and to many people management is indeed a profession of considerable breadth and depth, then he or she must recognize the necessity to enter management with as much preparation as possible. In their academic training most professionals receive a few credit hours in management courses. On this basis some then claim expertise as management generalists. But consider the reverse situation; assume that a student of general business managed to take a couple of social work courses (perhaps as electives) and after graduation claimed to be a social worker as well as a management generalist. The individual's claim to social work expertise would of course be automatically rejected. Yet time and again the technical specialist who has had a management course or two lays claim to equivalent expertise in management.

To summarize, the ego barrier to managerial effectiveness can surface in two important dimensions:

1. an inflated view of the importance of one's profession relative to the importance of management;
2. the failure to recognize management, devoid of all implications of any other particular occupation, as a specialty in its own right.

The obstacles presented by ego are overcome with great difficulty. In many instances they are never overcome. This is unfortunate because the most significant effects of the ego barrier are the tendency to place organizational interests second to departmental interests, and the proliferation and perpetuation of middle-management mediocrity.

THE PROFESSIONAL MANAGING THE PROFESSIONAL

The Professional as a Scarce Resource

From time to time some health care specialties experience conditions of oversupply. On the other hand, on numerous occasions many parts of the country experience shortages of certain skills, and organizations are forced to compete for the services of available workers. Once a department's personnel needs have been met, however, the focus of the manager—and certainly much of the focus of the organization's human resource department—should turn from recruitment to the important matter of retention. In short, when certain human resources are scarce, it is necessary to concentrate on keeping the people who are in the organization.

Consider, for example, professional nurses. The management of professional nurses, especially in the hospital setting, has become increasingly complex over the years. Financial restrictions, technological innovations, professional labor unions, and the changing attitudes of nurses have had a considerable impact on the practice of nursing. In some parts of the country the recruitment of professional nurses has become highly competitive and is likely to remain that way for some time.

The retention of professional employees is emerging as one of the more challenging tasks ever faced by health administrators. Where once it was possible to accept relatively high turnover among some professionals—again nurses, for example, many of whom were seen as entering or leaving the work force essentially at will—organizations have been finding supplies of help drying up and have had to turn their attention to reducing turnover. Thus, attention naturally shifts to factors and conditions that have a bearing on job satisfaction, such as better pay scales, more generous benefits, more attractive schedules, additional compensation for less popular assignments, a more clearly defined role for the professional, and a stronger voice in matters of patient care.

Generally, the health care organization should be interested in retaining employees who are functioning satisfactorily, but the organization may not be inclined to do any more about retention than has already been done as long as replacement employees are available. When a particular specialty is in short supply, however, an organization should do what it can to retain those skilled employees—but always within limits, because to take steps that seem to favor one class or group of employees over others is to invite trouble; what is done for one group is often done for others, as well.

There are costs associated with active retention efforts because factors like improved benefits and generous staffing patterns certainly cost money. For specialties in short supply, however, the cost of retaining employees is not nearly as high as the ongoing cost of continually recruiting, hiring, orienting, and training replacements. It is true that some professionals may be considered scarce resources because of their limited numbers; however, it behooves the manager to consider all steadily and satisfactorily performing employees, professional and otherwise, as equally worthy of the best efforts at retention.

The High-Skill Professional: Some Special Management Problems

The high-skill professional usually has extensive education, frequently possesses a master's degree or a doctorate (medical or otherwise), and is likely to work in a position that entails the exercise of a great deal of operating autonomy. High-skill professionals found in health care might include

- an employed physician or dentist
- a professional administrator engaged to operate a hospital or to run a major organizational unit
- a certified public accountant engaged to audit the organization or perhaps to oversee the organization's finance division
- a chemist, physicist, physician, or other scientist engaged in research or in day-to-day operations
- a management consultant engaged to solve a problem for the organization

Such persons have two obvious factors in common: they are extensively educated, and they are on their own much of the time in the performance of their work.

The high-skill professional often presents the manager with some special problems and unique challenges. Frequently these problems and challenges exist because of some of the same factors that contribute to the professional's ability to perform as desired.

The high-skill professional may generally be described by some or perhaps all of the following:

- As are many employees, the high-skill professional is accountable for results; however, this person is primarily responsible for getting things done and then later, if at all, reporting the results. There is only limited or occasional need for clearing actions or decisions in advance. In this regard the high-skill professional possesses a significant degree of operating autonomy.

- The high-skill professional may have a great deal of geographic mobility, ranging throughout an entire facility or, as in the case of a management consultant or an auditor, from organization to organization and even from city to city.
- Being a solitary operator much of the time, the high-skill professional must consistently exercise individual discretion and judgment.
- The successful high-skill professional generally exhibits a high degree of self-confidence and independence of thought and action.
- The successful high-skill professional appears as a self-starter who is also highly self-sufficient in work performance. He or she is able to function with minimal supervision or direction, sometimes for prolonged periods.

In general the high-skill professional is a highly educated specialist who largely operates independently, determining what needs to be done and doing it without direct management. Yet many characteristics that make for an effective high-skill professional also tend to make that employee difficult to manage at times. This is especially true of the characteristics related to independence, those factors that make an individual an effective lone operator. While it is certainly important to cultivate independence in those persons who are on their own much of the time, at times even the lone operator must be counted on to be a team player.

Some might say that one should also have a healthy ego to be able to presume to operate in a mode that can often be described as that of the visiting expert. The high-skill professional is indeed one who may often be viewed as needing to be in control of the situation. The healthy ego, so helpful to the professional while on assignment, can sometimes be troublesome to the manager. The successful manager of the high-skill professional must adhere to a number of guidelines:

- Be thorough and cautious in recruiting and selection, ensuring that educational requirements have been met and that all necessary credentials are possessed. For an experienced candidate, the manager should look for a demonstrated record of success and for sound reasons for wishing to make a change. For a newly graduated professional, the manager should look for self-confidence and a strong desire to do that particular kind of work.
- Try to learn what most strongly motivates the individual. Often the effective high-skill professional has a strong liking for the work and a strong desire for achievement and accomplishment. The best independently functioning

professionals like the work, are driven to do the work their own way, and have a great need to see the results of their efforts.

- Pay close attention to the orientation of every new employee. Even the well-experienced professional, new to the organization, needs to be thoroughly oriented to the organization, its policies, and its people before being turned loose.

- In addition to knowing the rules and policies of the organization, make certain that the new hire knows the results expected on each assignment. The manager should take care to thoroughly define the boundaries for independent action, such that the individual is able to develop a sense for how much may be done independently and when it is necessary to call for management assistance.

- Once the boundaries for independent action are established, give the professional employee complete freedom to operate within those boundaries. Strive to develop trust in the individual and, by reflecting this trust, endeavor to instill in this person the belief that management has confidence in his or her ability. Do not violate the boundaries by trying to dictate from afar; besides generally not working, absentee management serves only to frustrate the employee.

- Finally, introduce changes—whether changes in policies, practices, operating guidelines, or whatever—with plenty of advance notice. If at all possible, allow and even encourage the employee to take part in determining the scope and direction of each change.

A number of characteristics that make a high-skill professional an effective employee may also make the person difficult to manage at times. On one hand, independence and self-confidence must be encouraged; on the other hand, the same characteristics must be controlled. The manager is most likely to succeed with the high-skill professional by applying an open, participative approach to management.

Credibility of the Professional's Superior

When there are professionals in a work group, there is always the potential for differences in professional opinion, and there is always the likelihood of varying degrees of unwillingness of professionals to accept direction from the manager.

Whether or not such credibility problems exist in a given work group depends on the background and qualifications of the employees. Problems arise from the presence of a certain amount of ego, from the belief that one's profession is at least a bit more important than other occupations. Some problems arise from a sense of territorialism exhibited by some professionals, the belief that no one should hold sway over any aspect of professional performance without being perceived as at least equal in professional status and capability to the perceiver.

Management credibility problems may exist when the manager is not of the same profession as the individual employee. For example, the director of nursing service who is a registered nurse may be viewed or responded to differently by an employee who is also a registered nurse than by a certified nurse anesthetist. Similarly, an employed physician may question the credibility of an administrative superior who is a professional administrator or who perhaps stepped into administration from dentistry. Likewise, a professional trained as a chemist may have problems relating to an immediate superior whose background is that of a medical technologist. In all such cases there may be tendencies to differ on professional judgments, as in, "He's only a medical technologist, so who is he to tell me what I should be doing as a chemist?" and there may be feelings of territorialism: "Chemistry is my area, and only a chemist can legitimately make judgments that involve chemistry."

Credibility problems are also likely to arise when the manager is thought to be on a lower professional level than the employee. Thus, the clinical psychologist with a doctoral degree may be less than completely willing to accept the leadership of a manager whose education stopped at the master's degree level, and the certified public accountant may balk at the direction of a managing accountant who is not similarly certified. It again becomes a matter of one person, the "higher" professional, being unwilling to accept the judgment of another person, who happens to be "lower" on the professional scale. In such situations there are also more hints of territorialism; there appear to be more exclusive territories within broader territories that are mentally reserved for those of greater status.

Problems of management credibility are highly likely in situations in which employees see their managers as nonprofessionals. To fully understand such credibility problems, one must appreciate that many individual professionals do not regard management as a profession in its own right. Occasionally a nonmanagerial professional must report directly to a nonprofessional. In one organization, for example, a registered health information administrator (RHIA) and a utilization review coordinator who was a registered nurse reported to a director of health information services who was a management generalist and held no professional credentials. These two professionals were inevitably in some degree of conflict with their manager and frequently questioned the manager's direction. A direct reporting relationship between a nonmanagerial technical specialist and a generalist manager is often marked by many disputes concerning managerial judgments and may also be marked by a strong territorialism on the part of the professional.

Automatic management credibility is likely to be greatest when the manager is a professional of obviously higher standing than the employee. At the other extreme, management credibility is most strained when the manager's standing is rejected by the professional as being nonprofessional.

LEADERSHIP AND THE PROFESSIONAL

Leadership style may be simply described as that pattern of behavior projected by the leader in working with group members. Leadership styles run the gamut from completely closed to thoroughly open. At the closed end of the scale are the autocratic leaders, those who rule by order and edict. The harshest style is that of the exploitative autocrat, a leader who literally exploits the followers primarily in the service of self-interest. One major move along the scale takes one to the style of the benevolent autocrat. The benevolent autocrat also rules by order and edict, but it is a paternalistic rule imposed supposedly for the good of all.

Approaching the middle of the scale of leadership styles one encounters the bureaucratic style. In many ways fully as onerous as the autocratic styles, the bureaucratic style ordinarily subordinates human considerations to the service of the "system" or the "book."

Toward the open end of the scale one encounters the consultative style of leadership. Under this approach the employees are often given the opportunity to provide their thoughts, ideas, and suggestions, but the ground rules are such that the leader recognizes no obligation to utilize anything the employees provide. In this style the guiding philosophy of management is "the buck stops here," and management reserves the right to make all decisions at all times regardless of employee input.

Consultative leadership often exists when management claims to practice true participative leadership, the most open style on the leadership scale. With participative leadership, all members are included in all decision-making processes so that all members own a piece of all decisions. The greatest flaw of participative leadership is the ease with which managers, most of whom grew into their positions under authoritarian role models, can unconsciously hinder participative processes such that they become consultative and perhaps even manipulative at times.

The higher the professional level of a work group, the more the manager will find it necessary to move toward the open end of the scale of leadership types to accomplish the work of the department. Given the nature of professional work and the advanced state of most professionals' education, the average professional does not willingly suffer authoritarian management. It falls to the manager to examine basic assumptions about human behavior, to get beyond mere verbal tribute to modern management, and to take some of the risks inherent in open leadership styles.

SOME ASSUMPTIONS ABOUT PEOPLE

Douglas McGregor, in his landmark work *The Human Side of Enterprise,* wrote of two opposing approaches to management: Theory X and Theory Y.[1] Theory X in its pure state is autocratic leadership. Pure Theory Y is participative leadership. Each of these management theories is based on a number of assumptions. The first, relating to management in general, is common to both and states that management remains responsible for organizing the elements of all productive activity—that is, bringing together the money, people, equipment, and supplies needed to accomplish the organization's goals. Beyond this assumption, however, the theories diverge. Theory X assumes the following:

- People must be actively managed. They must be directed and motivated, and their actions must be controlled and their behavior modified to fit the needs of the organization. Without this active intervention by management, people would be passive and even resistant to organizational needs. Therefore, people must be persuaded, controlled, rewarded, or punished as necessary to accomplish the aims of the organization.
- The average person is by nature indolent, working as little as possible. The average person lacks ambition, shuns responsibility, and in general prefers to be led.
- The average person is inherently self-centered, resistant to change, and indifferent to the needs of the organization.

Theory Y, on the other hand, includes the following assumptions:

- People are not naturally passive or resistant to organizational needs. If they appear to have become so, this condition is a response to their experience in organizations.
- Motivation, development potential, willingness to assume responsibility, and readiness to work toward organizational goals are present in most people. It is management's responsibility to enable people to recognize and develop these characteristics for themselves.

- The essential task of management is to arrange organizational conditions and methods of operation so people can best achieve their own goals by directing their efforts toward the goals of the organization.

STYLE AND CIRCUMSTANCES

Professional or not, not every employee responds to the same leadership style; however, the average professional is generally more receptive to open styles—to Theory Y approaches. Thus it is in the manager's best interest to begin a manager-employee relationship with reliance on an open style. Management style may depend largely on the individual circumstances, but in starting the relationship with an employee the manager should initially extend every benefit of the doubt regarding the employee's motives.

The autocratic leader simply operates under Theory X assumptions, choosing to make all the decisions and hand them down as orders or instructions. The participative leader generally ascribes to Theory Y assumptions and encourages employees to participate in joint processes.

The manager has a choice of leadership styles ranging from extremely closed to extremely open. The trick is to know which style to apply and when to apply it. There may be some Theory X–style people in the department; these are the few who actually prefer to be led and have their thinking done for them. There may also be a number of Theory Y–style people who are self-motivated and capable of significant self-direction. This should be especially true in departments employing large numbers of professionals. Although the same personnel policies apply uniformly to all employees, the manager deals differently with individuals in other ways. Some the manager consults with and invites their participation; others the manager simply directs.

Theories aside, a manager must avoid making assumptions about people. Rather, it is necessary to know the employees and to try to understand each one as both a person and a producer. By working with people over a period of time, and especially by working at the business of getting to know them, one can learn a great deal about individual likes, dislikes, and capabilities. Learn about the people as individuals and lead accordingly. If a certain employee genuinely prefers orders and instructions, and this attitude is not inconsistent with job requirements, then use orders and instructions. Although many health care workers seem to prefer participative leadership, not everyone desires this same consideration. Sufficient flexibility must be maintained to accommodate the employee who wants or requires authoritarian supervision. It is fully as unfair to expect people to become what they do not want to be as it is to allow a rigid structure to stifle those other employees who feel they have something to contribute.

No single style of leadership is appropriate for all people and situations at all times. Today there are more reasons than ever to believe that consultative and participative leadership is most appropriate to modern health care organizations and today's educated workers.

Much can be said about what leadership is and what it is not, but in the end, only a single factor characterizes or defines a leader. That factor is acceptance of the followers. For this critical factor to be present in the manager-employee relationship, the professional employee must:

- respect the manager's technical knowledge
- accept the manager's organizational authority and respect the manager's skill in utilizing that authority
- respect the manager's ability to blend the technical and managerial sides of the management role fairly and justly

The manager accrues little if any acceptance by virtue of organizational authority. Most of what the manager acquires in the way of willing acceptance must be earned. It can thus be suggested that to lead the professional employee successfully, the manager must provide a broad framework for employee action. This means that it is necessary to provide the employee with every opportunity to be self-led and to impose specific direction only after all else has failed and the employee has demonstrated the need to be taken by the hand.

THE PROFESSIONAL AND CHANGE

No single group or classification of employee has a monopoly on resistance to change. Rigidity and inflexibility are found at all levels of the organization. This being stated, the professional employee is expected to be on the average more amenable to change because of the professional's advanced education and broader perspective. But as many managers have discovered, the professional employee may be fully as resistant to change as any other employee. It depends entirely on how the employee is approached and how the particular change is presented.

The Basis for Resistance

As far as the majority of people are concerned, change is threatening. Change threatens one's security by altering the environment; it disturbs the equilibrium, the state of balance that most people automatically seek to maintain with their surroundings.

As set forth in Chapter 2, most people tend to seek a state of equilibrium with their surroundings and they continually make adjustments intended to preserve their equilibrium. Unwanted or unheralded change threatens to disturb this equilibrium and thus becomes a threat to a person's sense of security. People often react to change in completely human fashion by countering the threat with resistance.

It is primarily the unknown that fosters resistance or intensifies what otherwise might be nominal resistance. In short, almost any change can generate resistance even if approached with full knowledge and plenty of warning, but if it comes on the employee by surprise, then intense resistance is almost certain. When a change is not a surprise, when it is approached in the full knowledge of everyone involved, much of the unknown becomes known and the chances of success are greatly increased.

The Manager's Approach

Chapter 2 suggests that in approaching the employees with a change the manager can: tell them what to do; convince them of what must be done; or try to involve them in assessing the need for the change and in determining the form and substance of the change. Yet the manager, who after all is but another employee and susceptible to the same fears and insecurities as the rank-and-file, may also automatically tend toward resistance.

The manager, however, must strive to overcome the tendency toward resistance that likely afflicts the majority of employees. It is an important part of the managerial role to be a driver of change and at times even an originator of change. Therefore, there is no room in the effective manager's approach to the job for automatic or unfounded resistance. Rather, the truly effective manager recognizes his or her responsibilities as an agent of change.

To enjoy the greatest chance of successfully functioning as a change agent the manager should:

- inform employees, as early as possible, of what is likely to happen
- plan thoroughly
- communicate fully
- convince employees as necessary
- involve employees whenever circumstances permit
- monitor implementation and ensure that decisions are adjusted and plans are fine-tuned as necessary

Employee knowledge and involvement are the keys to success in managing change. The employee who knows what is happening and is involved in making it happen is less likely to resist.

METHODS IMPROVEMENT

Every worker has a potentially valuable role in methods improvement. As noted, nobody knows the inner workings of a job nearly as well as the people who do it every day. This detailed knowledge is essential in methods improvement activities. Precisely how a task is performed is the necessary starting point in working to improve the performance of that task. The professional, whether employee or manager, is especially important in methods improvement because the professional's depth of knowledge in the field, both theoretical and practical, is a source of a variety of work-improvement options. In addition, the creative nature of much professional work suggests that the professional knows not just what to do but also how to determine what to do.

The professional employee is often a key person in a methods improvement undertaking, such as in chairing a quality circle or leading a work simplification team. In all probability the professional knows the work far better than the manager does. The manager, even though a professional as well, has necessarily been moving away from the technical work in some respects while growing as a manager. To succeed in improving the methods by which the work is accomplished, the manager must regard the department's professionals as the most potentially valuable source of improvement knowledge.

EMPLOYEE PROBLEMS

Occasionally managers tend to treat their professional employees much like parents often treat the older children in the family: "You're more advanced, so we can expect more of you." The you-should-know-better attitude is fine as long as it is expressed properly and is not carried to extremes, as far as the technical work of the profession is concerned; however, this attitude is not generally appropriate regarding adherence to the policies and work rules of the organization.

Rules and policies must be applied consistently among all employees. The professional employee should not be held to more rigid standards of behavior simply because of being professional. On the other hand, neither should the professional be allowed to get away with more simply because of professional status. Rather, policies and work rules must apply equally to all employees regardless of qualifications or classification, and the manager must take pains to ensure that all receive equal treatment.

The professional is as fully human and unpredictable as any other employee when it comes to the likelihood of personal problems, variations in personality, and behavior that might give rise to employee problems. The manager's long-run experience shows that professional employees are fully as great a source of discipline and behavior problems as nonprofessional employees. When the kinds of problems presented by employees are considered, one often finds that the problems presented by professionals are more complex and more difficult to deal with than the problems presented by others. Especially troublesome is the occasional professional who takes advantage of professional status to demand professional treatment without extending the appropriate behavior in return.

COMMUNICATION AND THE LANGUAGE OF THE PROFESSIONAL

For the professional who manages professionals it would be pertinent to repeat the preceding chapter as well as pass along all of the additional advice that can be offered for communication as it applies to the manager of any employees, professional or otherwise. This discussion, however, is limited to a few aspects of organizational communication in which professional status or professionalism may make a difference.

Each function within the modern health care organization includes a certain amount of what can be called inside language. Those who work in rehabilitation services, for example, have special terms that they use regularly. A few of these terms may be unfamiliar to persons who work in other areas and completely foreign to persons not involved in health care. Likewise, health information practitioners, respiratory therapists, computer specialists, microbiologists, and numerous others have inside languages that have evolved within their respective disciplines.

Inside languages are an inevitable outgrowth of the development of any area of concentrated specialized activity. The more concentrated the specialty and, in the case of health professions, the higher on the professional scale an occupation resides, the more extensive this inside language is and the more incomprehensible it is to outsiders. Inside languages develop for perfectly logical reasons. As advances are made in any aspect of life or any area of business activity, needs arise for describing concepts, conditions, problems, and even physical objects in a way that clearly identifies these within the context of the growing specialty as different from anything else in the world.

The needed words come from two sources: existing words that are given new meanings for specific purposes, and new words coined to represent new concepts. As a simple example, consider a small part of the effect caused in the English language in the 20th century by the advent of the internal combustion engine and specifically by the automobile. The automobile gave us terms such as *overdrive, carburetor, spark plug, headlight,* and *crankshaft* that may not have previously existed or that resulted from the combination of existing words in a new context. The automobile also gave new meaning to old words in the language such as bumper, starter, distributor, clutch, and differential. Every bit of advancing technology has thus expanded the language, and every profession that has emerged and evolved has built its special language along the way.

Clearly, our language must be dynamic, must be able to shift and expand as knowledge increases. It is thus fully understandable that an inside language should develop within any activity. It serves a clear purpose in describing, in terms as specific as possible, what goes on within that activity. Some may also say, however, in perhaps less-than-kindly fashion, that the purpose of the inside language is to elevate the specialty and define it as a closed club of sorts. Though probably not a purpose of an inside language, this is undoubtedly an effect of such a language. An inside language certainly heightens the mystique surrounding any given occupation and in addition helps to define the territory about that occupation. Relative to territory, the presence of the inside language is a qualification, admittedly superficial but certainly highly visible, for entry into another's territory.

Nurses have a language of their own, and human resource practitioners have a language of their own. Laboratory employees, radiology employees, physical therapists, psychologists, social workers, occupational therapists, physicians, and many others have their own inside languages. Fortunately many of these inside languages have some terms in common so they are not entirely different from each other. For example, some of the nurse's inside language is the same as part of the physician's inside language, and it is largely these areas of overlap that provide the interprofessional points of contact through which much communication flows. Occasionally, however, there emerges an inside language that has few if any points of overlap with other inside languages.

A glaring example of a highly restrictive inside language is found in computer science. This specialty area is filled with terms and abbreviations and acronyms that are used freely in normal interchange, often without explanation. One hears about *RAM, ROM,* and *CPU* often without being told that these mean *random-access memory, read-only memory,* and *central processing unit,* respectively. Old, otherwise familiar words are used in new combinations and with entirely new meaning, such as *mainframe, terminal, disk, peripheral, online,* and *real time.* Beyond the limited number of terms that many of us mange to absorb as computer users, "computerese" stands as very nearly a language in its own right.

One of the major problems commonly encountered in communication involving professionals is the disregard for the need to structure any given communication to suit the needs and capabilities of the audience. In communicating, the professional

- may freely use inside language when communicating with others in the same specialty
- must use a lesser level of special terminology when relating to persons outside of the specific specialty but still within health care
- must use a third and general level of language when relating to persons outside of both the specialty and the industry

The manager has a key role to fill in professional communication. It is all too easy for the manager to perpetuate foggy communication by simply joining in with other professionals in the group and relying on restrictive inside language in all contacts. This is not unusual when the manager has risen from the ranks in the same profession. Rather, it should fall to the manager to serve constantly as a facilitator and a translator in communication between the professional group and others. This role should extend to instruction and guidance in how to structure reports, memoranda, and other documentation to the needs of a specific audience and how to do likewise for the audiences to the professionals' oral presentations.

While some professionals tend to use language to make themselves appear knowledgeable and important, to elevate the mystique of the profession, and to isolate and protect its territory, the primary purpose of language should be to communicate, that is, to transfer meaning. As a primary source of worker guidance and the department's major point of contact with the rest of the organization, the manager has a strong interest in ensuring that the department's contributions are presented so that they are completely understood by those who need to know.

AN OPEN-ENDED TASK

On any given day the professional employee can present the manager with a problem or challenge that can be brought by the nonprofessional—and then some. Any advice that may apply to the management of anyone can apply to the management of the professional. Additional requirements on the manager call for the constant awareness of the sometimes subtle and sometimes glaring differences presented by the professional employee. In addition to the normal requirements of managing any employee, in the day-to-day management of the health care professional, the manager has several key objectives:

- Help the professional employee identify and pursue objectives that are consistent with the objectives of the department and the objectives of the organization.

- Work to ensure consistency between the priorities of the employee's profession and the priorities of the department and the organization.
- Strive to establish and maintain management credibility in a clear leadership role relative to the individual professional employee.
- Establish and maintain a working communications link between the individual professional and all other employees.

CASE: PROFESSIONAL BEHAVIOR— THE BUMPING GAME

Background

Dr. Gable, chief of anesthesiology, said to vice president Arthur Phillips and human resource director Carl Miller, "There are no two ways about it. We're going to have to raise the pay of our nurse anesthetists by at least 10 percent. With Don Williams leaving us and going to Midstate Hospital for a lot more money, we're going to have to pay more than we're now paying to fill that spot. Of the nine hospitals in this city our nurse anesthetists are by far the lowest paid."

Carl Miller said, "Since we spoke of this a week ago I personally surveyed every hospital compensation manager in town. We're not the lowest paying of the nine. In fact, we're the third highest paying."

Dr. Gable shook his head. "That doesn't wash," he said. "Some of our people moonlight at other hospitals and they've told me the hourly rates they're getting for part-time work. They said they'd bring in pay stubs to prove it."

Arthur said, "A week ago you said you were going to bring in some of those pay stubs from other places. Did you get them?"

"No. They forgot."

Carl said, "Moonlighting rates aren't relevant. Most of these places pay their part-time or casual nurse anesthetists a rate that amounts to more than their full-time employees get. That's because these casuals work only when called and they don't receive vacation, sick time, or other benefits, and they don't get retirement credit."

Arthur asked, "How about Midstate? I understand they have more than one scale for nurse anesthetists, with a second scale that might not readily be shared with other places."

Carl nodded and said, "That's right. Midstate is the highest paying hospital in the area, based on this sort of hidden scale that it applies to some of its people. It pays up to 15 percent more for this one small group, all of whom have agreed to an extra-long work week and a certain amount of weekend call. But it's not really comparable to our situation."

Arthur said, "In all the years I've been here, it seems I can depend on this same exercise coming up every time one of our nurse anesthetists leaves. I've also come to count on it happening with the pathologists and radiologists every few years— they go to work at one hospital to get their compensation increased, then they use this new pay leader as a wedge to get the other hospitals to pay more."

Carl said, "I'm sure that all of the nurse anesthetists in town know what the others earn. All it takes is a few people in one hospital to get a strong advocate to go to bat for them, and the pressure to bump pay rates is felt throughout the region."

Dr. Gable said, "I take it that you're seeing me in that strong advocate role." Miller did not respond.

Arthur said, "Anyway, Dr. Gable, you obviously see the nurse anesthetist pay rates as a problem and we're willing to listen to any potential solutions that you may have to offer. However, the budget year is barely one-third over and there is no more money to play with until the first of next year. As a first pass at the problem, we'll be happy to take a close look at any creative solutions you can come up with that lie within the limits of this year's budget."

Questions

1. What does this case say about the supply of the particular skill in the area? And what might come of Dr. Gable's arguments if the realities of supply were different?

2. Do you believe that the interorganizational "bumping" of pay rates, if indeed a fact, constitutes professional behavior? Why or why not?

3. Because it might be reasonably suggested that the nurse anesthetists in the area are acting together, at least in a loosely organized way, one might be tempted to suggest that the area's nine hospitals get together and establish fair and consistent pay rates for this occupation. What hazards are inherent in this approach, and in what sense has one of the case's participants already ventured into hazardous territory?

4. How would you suggest that Arthur and Carl proceed in their consideration of Dr. Gable's request?

CASE: DELEGATION DIFFICULTIES— THE INEFFECTIVE SUBORDINATE

Background

Nursing supervisor Kate Dyer was finally forced to admit, at least to herself, that she was going nowhere in her attempt to get nurse manager Susan Foster to behave as a manager ought to behave. Summarizing the recent occasions on which

Susan and her performance had come to Kate's attention, Kate had assembled the following:

- Whenever Kate went through Susan's unit she found Susan's desk in disarray and invariably found Susan herself behind in her work.
- Susan seemed to experience a great deal of difficulty in making important meetings; she had missed three of the last four nursing management meetings, and at the one she did attend she did not show up until it was half over.
- Kate's specific suggestions as to tasks that Susan might consider delegating to some of her subordinates have apparently been ignored.
- Some weeks earlier Kate had asked Susan for a detailed written list showing how the various nursing duties on her floor might be divided among the unit's staff members. Susan did not comply with the request.

In general, Susan seemed to have but two answers for many of the questions put to her by peers and supervisors alike. To questions that were general and non-threatening, such as "How is everything going?" she would simply answer, "Just fine." However, if a question seemed intended to determine why something had not been done, Susan could be counted on to answer, with a pained expression on her face, "I simply haven't been able to get to it."

Questions

1. Although Susan's performance is obviously lacking in a number of ways, Kate might best begin by examining some elements of her own performance and her own leadership style. What are the elements of the case that may have prompted this statement, and what are the implications of those elements regarding Kate's style and performance?
2. What appear to be the weakest elements in Kate's style? Why are they weak?
3. Assuming that Kate is able to successfully address the deficiencies in her own approach to management, where should she begin in trying to determine if Susan has the potential to become a truly effective nurse manager?

NOTE

1. Douglas M. McGregor, "The Human Side of Enterprise," *Management Review* 46, no. 11 (November 1957): 22–28, 88–92.

INDEX

A

Absoluteness of authority principle, 175
Accommodation, patterns of, 349
Actuating. *See* Directing
Adaptation
  organizational, 17–18
  to organizational life, 346
Age Discrimination in Employment Act
    (ADEA), 95, 456
Agency, regulatory, features of, 2
Agenda, preparation of, 327
American Health Information Management
    Association (AHIMA), 11, 16, 39,
    40–41, 79
American National Standards Institute
    (ANSI), 11
Americans with Disabilities Act (ADA), 95,
    472
Appeal procedure, 447–448
Appreciative inquiry, 354–356
  defined, 354–355
  motivational aspects of, 355–356
  process of, 355
Argyris, Chris, 57
Audit, general, 303–304
Authority, 173–176, 170, 181
  charismatic, 421
  of committee, 31–322
  consent theory of, 419–420

consolidation of, 316
counterbalancing of, 316–317
of the facts, 423
functional, 423
holders, characteristics of, 424
manager's use of sources of, 424–425
principle of absoluteness of, 175
rational-legal, 421–422
restrictions on use of, 425–426
  See also Organizational authority

B

Barnard, Chester, 152–153
Barth, Carl. G. L., 56
Benchmarking, 251–253
  defined, 251
  sources of measures for, 251
  studies, sample, 252, 253, 254
Benefits, administration of, 460
Body language, 484
Budget(ing), 275–304
  approaches to, 281–281
  basis of procedures for, 276
  capital expenses in, 287, 289
  cost centers in, 281
  cost comparison in, 299–300, 301
  cuts to, 299
  expenses, direct and indirect in, 298, 298
  general audit in, 303–304